Chronic Fatigue Syndrome

INFECTIOUS DISEASE AND THERAPY

Series Editors

Brian E. Scully, M.B., B.Ch.
Harold C. Neu, M.D.

College of Physicians & Surgeons
Columbia University
New York, New York

Additional Volumes in Production

Chronic Fatigue Syndrome

edited by

Stephen E. Straus

*National Institute of Allergy
and Infectious Diseases
National Institutes of Health
Bethesda, Maryland*

Marcel Dekker, Inc.   New York • Basel • Hong Kong

Library of Congress Cataloging-in-Publication Data

Chronic fatigue syndrome / edited by Stephen E. Straus.
    p. cm. — (Infectious disease and therapy; v. 14)
    Includes bibliographical references and index.
    ISBN 0-8247-9187-8
    1. Chronic fatigue syndrome. I. Straus, Stephen E. II. Series.
RB150.F37C473   1994
616'.047—dc 20   94-14914
                                    CIP

The publisher offers discounts on this book when ordered in bulk quantities. For more information, write to Special Sales/Professional Marketing at the address below.

This book is printed on acid-free paper.

Marcel Dekker, Inc.
270 Madison Avenue, New York, New York 10016

Current printing (last digit):
10 9 8 7 6 5 4 3 2 1

PRINTED IN THE UNITED STATES OF AMERICA

To Marc, for whom
medicine is art,
art is poetry, and
poetry is medicine.

Series Introduction

Marcel Dekker, Inc., has for many years specialized in the publication of high-quality monographs in tightly focused areas in a variety of medical disciplines. These have been of great value to both the practicing physician and the research scientist as sources of detailed and up-to-date information presented in an attractive format. During the last decade, there has been a veritable explosion in knowledge in the various fields related to infectious diseases and clinical microbiology. Antimicrobial resistance, antibacterial and antiviral agents, AIDS, Lyme disease, infections in immunocompromised patients, and parasitic diseases are but a few of the areas in which an enormous amount of significant work has been published. The Infectious Disease and Therapy series covers carefully chosen topics that should be of interest and value to the practicing physician, the clinical microbiologist, and the research scientist.

Brian E. Scully, M.B., B.Ch.
Harold C. Neu, M.D.

Foreword

This series has addressed a number of infectious diseases that are clearly established and have symptoms that are understandable in terms of pathophysiology and their infecting bacteria or viruses. Chronic fatigue syndrome, however, has rather nonspecific symptomatology, and its pathophysiology and pathogenesis are poorly understood. Also, chronic fatigue syndrome has no physiological markers. Therefore, epidemiologists are forced to use patient-reported symptoms, ocasionally unrelated physical signs, and unusual criteria to rule out other possible causes of fatigue.

Certainly the findings vary and most cases are sporadic. Person-to-person transmission does not occur, and, except in a few outbreaks that have never been substantiated, family members rarely suffer from the same syndrome. It is clear that there is fatigue following hepatitis A, B, or C, infectious mononucleosis, and influenza A, but this tends to go away with time. It is also of note that in Austrialia individuals tend to recover from chronic fatigue syndrome, and there are localized problems with chronic fatigue. Most of the individuals with chronic fatigue syndrome have been women under the age of 50 and, in recent years, in their late teens. Whether chronic fatigue syndrome should be called epidemic neuromyasthenia is unclear.

Basically this monograph addresses the problem of chronic fatigue syndrome, which has gained prominence over the past decade in the United States and is a significant cause of work absenteeism. Insights are provided into detailed epidemiological information regarding the virology and other studies in which therapy was directed at various viruses, for example, the Epstein-Barr virus and herpes type 6.

Although it is clear that this monograph cannot provide the answer to this disease at this time, it should be a useful reference for scientists, epidemiologists, and physicians who see patients with this frustrating illness.

Harold C. Neu, M.D.

Preface

In the theater of human misery fatigue may be only a minor player, but in the context of a healthful and largely unchallenged society such as ours, it has gained center stage. Chronic fatigue now occupies a degree of acceptance, both within and outside the domain of established medicine, as a veritable and corrosive malady unto itself.

Fatigue has perplexed generations of physicians, as it has frustrated and disabled their patients. Our literature is replete with countless attempts to categorize the fatigue, to discern its essence and origins, and to find the reasons for its persistence in some instances. Recent years have witnessed an energetic engagement with the problem through the application of powerful scientific tools and the formulation of imaginative new hypotheses by individuals of remarkably diverse training and interests.

In recognition of this evolving synthesis of perspectives on chronic fatigue I became motivated to capture our current knowledge of it within the bounds of a multidisciplinary book. In so doing, I aimed to assemble a volume that fairly represents a spectrum of creditable and authoritative positions from virtually all established disciplines engaged in the study of chronic fatigue and the subset of individuals who could be said to suffer chronic fatigue syndrome.

This is by no means a comprehensive compendium, for the field has always been, and remains still, open to extravagant claims. I view that my role as editor is to assure that each vantage point is presented as clearly as possible. The reader will discern inconsistencies in some arguments and even frank disagreements among them. This is inevitable in an area as unsettled as this one.

The chapters are organized to present to the clinician or highly informed lay reader a statement of the problem and its deep historical and multidisciplinary perspectives. There is a series of refined analyses of putative causes for the syndrome and of body systems affected by it or affecting it in turn. The volume closes with a discussion of well-considered contemporary approaches to management.

Consensus has not been achieved on many of these issues, and the flow through the book is not entirely seamless, as would be more likely were it penned by one hand. But then it would be devoid of the exhilarating tension that arises from rational discourse and collegial debate and might fail to offer as broad a conceptual palette as it does.

Stephen E. Straus, M.D.

Contents

Part II: Infection and Immunity

Part III: Neurological, Psychological, and Psychiatric Issues

Part IV: Relation to Other Disorders

Part V: An International Perspective

Contents

Part VI: Approaches to Treatment

Contributors

Susan E. Abbey, M.D., F.R.C.P.(C) Director, Program in Medicine and Psychiatry, The Toronto Hospital and Assistant Professor, Department of Psychiatry, University of Toronto, Toronto, Ontario, Canada

Dedra Buchwald, M.D. Associate Professor, Department of Medicine, University of Washington and Harborview Medical Center, Seattle, Washington

John E. Clague, M.D., M.R.C.P. Englert Lecturer in Neuromuscular Disease, Department of Medicine, University of Liverpool, Liverpool, England

Michael R. Clark, M.D., M.P.H. Assistant Professor of Psychiatry, Director, Consultation/Liaison Psychiatry, Department of Psychiatry and Behavioral Sciences, Johns Hopkins University, Baltimore, Maryland

Mark A. Demitrack, M.D. Assistant Professor, Department of Psychiatry, University of Michigan Medical Center, Ann Arbor, Michigan

Richard H. T. Edwards, Ph.D., F.R.C.P. Professor, Department of Medicine, University of Liverpool, Liverpool, England

Robert Fekety, M.D. Professor of Internal Medicine and Chief, Division of

Infectious Diseases, Department of Internal Medicine, University of Michigan Medical Center, Ann Arbor, Michigan

Thomas M. Folks, Ph.D. Chief, Retrovirus Diseases Branch, Division of Viral and Rickettsial Diseases, National Center for Infectious Diseases, Centers for Disease Control and Prevention, Atlanta, Georgia

Henry Gibson, Ph.D. Clinical Physiologist, University of Liverpool, Liverpool, England

Don L. Goldenberg, M.D. Chief of Rheumatology, Newton–Wellesley Hospital, Newton, Massachusetts, and Professor of Medicine, Tufts University School of Medicine, Boston, Massachusetts

Jordan Grafman, Ph.D. Chief, Cognitive Neuroscience Section, Medical Neurology Branch, National Institute of Neurological Disorders and Stroke, National Institutes of Health, Bethesda, Maryland

Charles E. Halstenson, Pharm.D. Co-director, Drug Evaluation Unit, Minneapolis Medical Research Foundation, Hennepin County Medical Center, and Professor, University of Minnesota College of Pharmacy, Minneapolis, Minnesota

John Hay, Ph.D. Grant T. Fisher Professor and Chairman, Department of Microbiology, School of Medicine, State University of New York at Buffalo, Buffalo, New York

Timothy R. Helliwell, M.A., M.D., M.R.C.Path. Senior Lecturer in Pathology, Department of Pathology, University of Liverpool, Liverpool, England

Walid Heneine, Ph.D. Visiting Scientist, Retrovirus Diseases Branch, National Center for Infectious Diseases, Centers for Disease Control and Prevention, Atlanta, Georgia

Ian Hickie, M.D., F.R.A.N.Z.C.P. Associate Professor, Mood Disorders Unit, Department of Psychiatry, The Prince Henry Hospital, Little Bay, New South Wales, Australia

Cheryl A. I. Hirata-Dulas, Pharm.D. Clinical Scientist, Drug Evaluation Unit, Minneapolis Medical Research Foundation, Hennepin County Medical Center, and Assistant Professor, University of Minnesota College of Pharmacy, Minneapolis, Minnesota

Frank J. Jenkins, Ph.D. Associate Professor, Department of Microbiology and Immunology and the Neuroscience Program, Uniformed Services University of the Health Sciences, Bethesda, Maryland

Wayne Katon, M.D. Professor and Chief, Consultation/Liaison Psychiatry, Department of Psychiatry and Behavioral Sciences, University of Washington Medical School, Seattle, Washington

Anthony L. Komaroff, M.D. Professor of Medicine, Department of Medicine, Harvard Medical School, and Director, Division of General Medicine, Brigham and Women's Hospital, Boston, Massachusetts

Andrew Lloyd, M.D., F.R.A.C.P. Staff Specialist in Infectious Diseases, Infectious Diseases Department, The Prince Henry Hospital, Little Bay, New South Wales, Australia

Phillip K. Peterson, M.D. Director, Division of Infectious Diseases, Hennepin County Medical Center, and Professor, Department of Medicine, University of Minnesota Medical School, Minneapolis, Minnesota

Michael Sharpe, M.A., M.R.C.P., M.R.C.Psych. Tutor in Psychiatry, Department of Psychiatry, University of Oxford, and Warneford Hospital, Oxford, England

Warren Strober, M.D. Head, Mucosal Immunity Section, and Deputy Director of Intramural Research, Laboratory of Clinical Investigation, National Institute of Allergy and Infectious Diseases, National Institutes of Health, Bethesda, Maryland

Denis Wakefield, M.D., F.R.A.C.P., F.R.C.P.A. Associate Professor and Chairman, Immunopathology Department, The Prince Henry Hospital, Little Bay, New South Wales, Australia

Norma C. Ware, Ph.D. Assistant Professor of Medical Anthropology, Department of Social Medicine, Harvard Medical School, Boston, Massachusetts

Simon Wessely, M.A., M.Sc., M.R.C.P., M.R.C.Psych. Senior Lecturer, Department of Psychological Medicine, King's College Hospital and the Institute of Psychiatry, Camberwell, London, England

I

THE ILLNESS

1

The History of Chronic Fatigue Syndrome

Simon Wessely
*King's College Hospital and the Institute of Psychiatry,
Camberwell, London, England*

The history of diseases can take two forms. One, the easiest, is a straightforward account of the attempts of scientists to solve a problem—the classic medical detective story. This is the approach frequently adopted by the media coverage of chronic fatigue syndrome (CFS), allied to that other stereotype, the small-town doctor confronting the skeptical medical establishment. For example, two doctors who have played major roles in the current resurgence of interest in chronic fatigue syndromes in the United States are described as "medical sleuths" and "dogged small-town doctors," involved in a "quest" until they inevitably "crack the case" [1]. The history of CFS is replete with claims of major advances, significant progress, and medical breakthroughs, all of which conform to an optimistic view of medicine as a continually improving scientific discipline.

Yet despite all the breakthroughs, CFS remains an enigma. This chapter will argue that little real progress has been made and, in many respects, we are little better informed than our Victorian counterparts. The simple story of progress and discovery is, as in many other aspects of medical history, more often fiction than fact, reflecting wishful thinking, since medicine rarely moves in a smooth path from ignorance to knowledge, but frequently in a more circular fashion. This was reflected in the perhaps unintentional choice by Melvyn Ramsay [2], whose single-minded efforts are agreed to have played a major role in bringing one variant of CFS, myalgic encephalomyelitis (ME), to wider public attention in the United Kingdom, of the title *The Saga of Royal Free Disease* for his account of the history of the condition. A saga, with its echoes of myth, is indeed an appropriate word to describe the history of this elusive condition.

I chose to begin the story of chronic fatigue syndrome with the illness known as neurasthenia. There are many reasons for this. At a simple level it is because the symptoms of neurasthenia and those of CFS are so similar, but the resonances between the two go beyond clinical descriptions. Neurasthenia is an appropriate historical starting point, and continues to have many lessons for understanding our contemporary concern, chronic fatigue syndrome.

NEURASTHENIA: THE FIRST CHRONIC FATIGUE SYNDROME

Many writers have assumed that neurasthenia was first described by New York neurologist George Beard in a brief paper in 1869 [3]. However, a psychiatrist, Van Deusen, has an equal claim to the authorship of neurasthenia, as he introduced the term in the *American Journal of Insanity* in the same year [4]. The rival claims of Van Deusen, an alienist treating farmers in unfashionable Kalamazoo, and Beard, an East Coast neurologist with clients drawn from the Social Register, mirrored the wider confrontation between neurology and psychiatry at that time [5]. As with the larger professional conflict, it was Beard who triumphed, and although the *American Journal of Insanity* would later resurrect Van Deusen's claim, it was the neurologist who became most credited with the "discovery" of neurasthenia.

The concept of nervous exhaustion was not new, and a few contemporaries took pains to elaborate the history of the disease before Beard, tracing its origins to nervosisme, neurospasm, spinal irritability, and so on [e.g., 6,7], whereas later historians have pointed out the debt Beard owed hypochondria, spinal irritation, and asthenia [8,9].

Beard's views were not fully articulated until his two books written toward the end of his life [10,11]. In them he drew on several contemporary scientific sources, including Marshall Hall's discovery of the spinal reflex arc, Edison's electricity, Du Bois Reymond's electrical nervous impulse, and others [12]. His skill lay in mixing scientific advances with social theory and moral exhortation, and constructing out of these sources a single disease entity, designed to appeal to many of the concerns of the age, but couched in what seemed to many (but not all) acceptable scientific terminology.

Whatever the provenance of neurasthenia, its rapid spread and popularity owed much to Beard, especially in France and Germany. By the turn of the century a French physician wrote that "everything could be explained by neurasthenia, suicide, decadent art, dress and adultery" [13]—"since the works of George Beard . . . the name of neurasthenia was on everybody's lips, the fashionable disease" [14], the "maladie a la mode" [13]. When Levillain published his important text he subtitled it *La Maladie du Beard* [15]. Many of Charcot's pupils wrote texts on the illness, although the most popular was probably that by Adrien Proust, ironically the father of the most famous neurasthenic of the age, Marcel. It was as successful in Germany—Bumke later wrote that there was probably no instance in the history of medicine of a label having the impact of neurasthenia [16].

What Was Neurasthenia?

Perhaps the most succinct description was provided toward the end of the neurasthenia period: "Neurasthenia is a condition of nervous exhaustion, characterised by undue fatigue on slightest exertion, both physical and mental, with which are associated symptoms of abnormal functioning, mainly referable to disorders of the vegetative nervous system. The chief symptoms are headache, gastrointestinal disturbances, and subjective sensations of all kinds" [17]. This definition outlines the core concepts of neurasthenia—that it was the disease of excessive fatigability, and that fatigability could affect physical and mental (which meant the processes of thought, speech, and memory) functioning equally. There was a consensus that although the symptoms of neurasthenia could vary, essential to the diagnosis was that the patient be "incapacitated for all forms of mental and physical exertion" [18].

Beyond that core concept, neurasthenia was an exceptionally broad church: "all things to all men" [19]. Several strands can be discerned [20]. First, neurasthenia was simply chronic fatigue—the fatigue neurosis [21,22]. In neurasthenia, chronic fatigue was always the primary or essential symptom [23], it was "an enfeeblement or fatigue neurosis, its cardinal characteristics being an inordinate sense of physical or mental fatigue" [24]—remember that neurosis did not have its modern meaning. The most common manifestation of fatigue was a "neuromuscular weakness—by all writers this is accounted for as the most frequently observed objective sign of disease" [25], although for others the "unusually rapid exhaustion mainly affects the mental activities; the power of attention becomes quickly exhausted and the capacity for perception is paralysed" [26]. Whether mental or physical, fatigue had certain characteristics: "it comes early, is extreme, and lasts long" [27], and is "the first, and most important symptom" [28]—hence, neurasthenics had abnormally quick fatigability and slow recuperation [29], their fatigue not being relieved by rest. Jewell noted that neurasthenics, with "every appearance of normal values of power, are speedily exhausted in the process of moderate exercise," and that "prolonged or severe mental effort" was equally impaired [30].

Second, neurasthenia was depression. Cowles listed depression as a first-rank symptom of neurasthenia [31], and Clouston viewed it as a minor form of melancholia [32]. This could mean depression of cortical activity [e.g., 33] or latterly depression in a more psychological sense. Déjerine and Gauckler felt that melancholia and neurasthenia could be distinguished only on the basis of history, previous episodes of depression, or mania, favoring the former diagnosis [34]. Many authors equated neurasthenia with a mild melancholia [e.g., 25], although the differences remained as instructive as the similarities; thus, Friedman stated that although both neurasthenics and depressed patients required treatment away from the family, only the latter should be admitted to an asylum [35].

Third, neurasthenia was male hysteria: "neurasthenia is to men what hysteria is to women" [36]. Freud felt that the "male nervous system has as preponderant a disposition to neurasthenia as the female to hysteria" [37]. Again, as with neurosis, it is important to remember that hysteria did not have its modern meaning of nonorganic—indeed, almost the opposite was true.

Fourth, Beard himself viewed neurasthenia as the prototype of many diseases, both physical and mental. In particular, it occupied the "broad borderland between mental health and outspoken mental disease (insanity)" [38]. These intermediate stages are "the various anomalies usually combined under the common name of neurasthenia" [39].

Regardless of the classification of neurasthenia adopted, most noted the discrepancy between physical disability and physical examination. Despite all the symptoms, neurasthenia was "destitute of the objective signs which experimental medicine of our times more particularly affects" [40]. Sufferers looked normal, and were typically well nourished, muscularly well developed [41], despite often profound functional disability, which could reach states of complete motor helplessness, in which case authors coined terms such as atremia and akinesia algera [see 42]. Despite this, it had no significant mortality (indeed, Beard and others claimed the opposite [10]).

The Etiologies of Neurasthenia

Peripheral

During the early years of interest in neurasthenia the prevailing neurological paradigm remained the reflex hypothesis. Excessive irritation or stimulation of the nervous system led to exhaustion of the peripheral nerves, which could spread to any tissue [see 9,20]. However, the remarkable flourishing of neurophysiology soon discredited the reflex hypothesis, while the related belief that female genital reflexes were the cause of nervous disease in women was also under pressure by 1870 [20]. In ridiculing the reflex theory, Allbutt explained that neither muscles nor reflex arc were in a state of exhaustion, nor were the neurasthenic cells too excitable: "to be excitable is their business" [43]. All these authorities espoused the new central paradigm of nervous disease, which soon replaced reflex theories.

Central

As views of the nervous system changed, especially under the influence of the new laws of thermodynamics and conservation of energy [9,12,44], so did the nature of neurasthenia. Physicians were beginning to discuss not only the body, but also the mind in terms of heat and energy before the arrival of neurasthenia, so it was only a short step to see neurasthenia as an exhaustion of that supply of energy within the central nervous system. The consequence was cortical weakness [45] or cortical irritability [46]. Irritable weakness of the brain permitted some remnants of reflex theory to survive, but many other causes of cerebral exhaustion were identified: a failure of cerebral blood flow, a deficiency in energy sources, or, alternatively, excessive demands made by the body. These could result from overwork or the demands made by toxic or metabolic insults. Chief among these insults were infections and fevers which, given their modern importance, will be discussed in greater detail later. Thus, the late Victorian physician was in little doubt that in neurasthenia fatigue was of central origin [47], or that "neurasthenia is a neurosis essentially located in the brain" [40]. This central, organic paradigm was perhaps the dominant mode of medical thinking during the Golden Age of this, the first chronic fatigue syndrome.

Social

The doctrine of overwork and nervous exhaustion linked neurasthenia with a variety of contemporary changes in society. Medical authorities viewed over-work, the agent by which the nervous system became exhausted (which could be purely physical, mental, or a mixture of both), as the inevitable consequence of a host of new social ills. Even before the introduction of neurasthenia, a variety of medical authorities were writing about the dangers of overwork [48–50]. Once again, it was Beard, with his facility for similes, who joined together a number of discontents into an explanatory model for his disease. For example, Beard, and many others, ascribed neurasthenia to the new, acquisitive nature of society, singling out wireless telegraphy, science, steam power, newspapers, and the education of women, summed up as modern civilization [11]. Much of this was conveyed by metaphors drawn from business or new technologies: the exhausted businessman overdrawn on his nervous capital, overspent nervous resources, flat batteries, and others [see 19,51,52].

Beard succeeded because he articulated his ideas to a receptive audience. For example, a series of investigations during the 1880s had revealed the poor health of many French youths. One favored explanation blamed this on the alleged excessive mental demands (*surménage*) made by the new education system [52], an idea that was echoed in Beard's writings. It was popular because it allowed medical thinking to move away from the old, outdated doctrines of sentiments and passions no longer suitable for a society preoccupied with "La Vie Moderne" [53]. Neurasthenia, like CFS now, was thus up to date, both in its scientific and social context, and was expressly seen as a disease of modern life [see 52,54].

Neurasthenia was new, increasing, and alarming. It was held to be both a consequence and the cause of numerous social problems. It was the price to be paid for industrialization, the rise of capitalism, and the consequent strains to which the business and professional classes were exposed [55]. Neurasthenia was labeled the *the disease of the century* [56–58]. Contemporaries often referred to the time as the Age of Nerves, but also the Age of Fatigue [52].

Psychogenic

Unfortunately for the organic view of neurasthenia, the central paradigm could not be sustained either. Fatigue could not be measured objectively [29,59], nor could any discrete neuropathological lesion be located. Adolf Meyer later wrote that the "remarkable changes in the nerve cells" which others had found, which were "highly fashionable and a matter of pride to both patient and diagnostician . . . could not be replicated. Fatigue exhaustion is no longer tenable" [60]. The consequence was a loss of faith in simple neurological explanations. Donley, in the first issue of the prestigious *Journal of Abnormal Psychology*, criticized the previous "mechanical symbolism" of descriptions of neurasthenia for the false belief that "for every pathological manifestation there must be an underlying, definite 'disease process'," and noted the "futility of the purely anatomical concept" expressing itself in "apologetic reproductions of nerve cells in a state of fatigue" [61].

Social etiologies were also changing. It was doubted if neurasthenia really was a disease of modern life except that "we had become more tender in our ills" [14]. It was hinted that neurasthenics suffered from under-, rather than overwork [62], reflected in the changing nature of rest cure. Other etiologies, considerably less attractive to the potential neurasthenic, were now suggested, such as bad housing [63], and poor dental hygiene due to the "fashion of eating ice cream . . . prevalent among the children of the lower classes" [64].

These last quotes suggest a further change, that of class. Neurasthenia had been sustained by the belief that it was a condition of the most successful people in society. "It is a disease of bright intellects, its victims are leaders and masters of men, each one a captain of industry" [65], a view shared by many, including Freud and Kraepelin. Many noted the large number of doctors afflicted. The male doctor who, like Beard, Dowse, and Mitchell, willingly admitted he had suffered the illness, played an important role in establishing the legitimacy of neurasthenia [66,67], and will reappear later in the story.

However, the preponderance of the male professional classes among sufferers began to alter. Charcot was among the first to point this out in 1889 and, by 1906, a series of papers were produced describing the illness in the working class [63,64,68–70]. The records of the Vanderbilt Clinic in New York [71] show that neurasthenia was now mainly a disease of the lower social classes and, as most of these comprised Jewish immigrants, it could no longer even be called the "American disease." In 1906 Stedman pleaded in his presidential address to the American Neurological Association for more attention to the need for facilities for the neurasthenic poor [72], and the illness had become the most common cause of absenteeism among the garment workers of New York [73]. Cobb noted sardonically that those who continued to believe the disease was restricted to the upper social echelons were those whose commitment was entirely to private practice [17]. Even the excess of male medical sufferers began to alter: it was the female doctor who was particularly vulnerable, because "only the strong can survive" [74].

The failure of the organic paradigm, and the change in social class and etiologies, prepared the way for the psychological model. This took two stages. First, neurasthenia was retained, but viewed as a psychological rather than a physical illness. The pendulum shifted—rather than psychological symptoms being a consequence of neurasthenia, they first became linked in a vicious circle, with neither having supremacy [e.g., 75], and, finally, were seen as causing the condition. Thus, Déjerine writes that "many manifestations [of neurasthenia] are by nature purely phobic in origin" [34]. Second, the category itself was dismembered and replaced by new psychiatric diagnoses. It is well known that by 1894 Freud considered sexual exhaustion to be the sole cause of neurasthenia, either directly or indirectly. The following year [76] saw his famous removal of anxiety neurosis from neurasthenia (although he later acknowledged that earlier Hecker had anticipated his work in the previous year in a paper distinguishing anxiety neurosis [*Angstneurose*] and neurasthenia). As important was the work of Pierre Janet. Influenced by both William James and Weir Mitchell, he also regarded fatigue as the key to psychological disorder [52]. Similar to his contemporaries, he blamed modern life for fatigue neurosis. However, he followed William James in deriding the conventional economic metaphor of the neurasthenic overdrawing on a limited capital of physical energy, but empha-sized, instead, the emotional demands on the psychic economy. Eventually, Janet detached obsessional and phobic neuroses from neurasthenia, through the agency of psychasthenia [see 77]. Freud, Bernheim, and others continued to believe in a physical neurasthenia, not amenable to psychotherapy, labeled by Freud an *actual neurosis*, in which sexual energy was lost by masturbation, but thought it was rare: Freud's biographer and disciple Ernest Jones later wrote that fewer than 1% of neurasthenics were correctly diagnosed [78].

The organicists countered such observations in two ways. First, the present methods of investigation were simply too crude to detect the organic changes that must be present [e.g., 26]. Second, psychological symptoms, if present, were part of the physical neurasthenic state [79,80], or were an understandable reaction to the illness. In a speech to the American Neurological Association, Weir Mitchell referred to his own early neurasthenia and pointed out how depression could not be an explanation for his condition, since he had "no depression that was abnormal or unreasonable" [28]. He used his own example and that of "an eminent president of the college" to reaffirm that it was impossible that neurasthenia could be "a malady of the mind alone."

Nevertheless, these became increasingly minority views. The neurologist Charles Dana read an influential paper to the Boston Society of Psychiatry and Neurology urging adoption of the new psychiatric classifications [81]. Only 2 years later, the new president of the Neurological Association described an eminent patient as suffering from "neurasthenia or mild melancholia" [72]—the *or* being unlikely a decade earlier. When the London Medical Society debated neurasthenia in 1913, Kinnier-Wilson wrote that "it was clear . . . from the discussion that Beard's original description of 'American Nervousness' as a physical and not a mental state was evidently not accepted by several of the speakers" [82]. The successive editions of several textbooks show how neurasthenia moved from the neuroses (meaning a disease of the nerves, an organic neurological diagnosis) to the psychoneuroses [83]. Neurologists at the Massachusetts General Hospital had already done the same [84], while in France, both Dutil and Déjerine, pupils of Charcot, wrote that "Beard's illness" must now be seen as of mental origin, a psychoneurosis. In our own time, the word neurasthenia is discussed almost exclusively in psychological terms (at least in the West), but one must emphasize that this represents only one aspect of its complex heritage.

Treatment

The replacement of organic by psychological models of etiology was mirrored in changes in treatment. The first category of treatments was pharmacological, drugs used either to stimulate a fatigued system, or to sedate an overexcitable one. These all proved unsatisfactory, since they rarely worked, and the patients were exquisitely sensitive to side effects [41]. The concept of a deficiency in energy also led to the flourishing of electrical treatments for neurasthenia, since, in the age of electricity, the notion that the deficiency of nerve energy could be made up by electrical stimulation was a seductive one [44]. However, authorities gradually conceded that electrical treatments were effective more for psychological reasons, rather than any organic modifications of the nerve centers [56]. This shift from organic to psychological explanations of treatment efficacy was most visible in the progression of ideas concerning the rest cure.

It seemed logical that if neurasthenia was due to overwork, then the solution was rest. Rest conserved energy, the quantity that neurasthenics lacked. This was given the necessary scientific respectability by reference to the new laws of thermodynamics, and institutionalized in the rest cure. Rest cure consisted of five elements: rest, seclusion, massage, electricity, and diet. Weir Mitchell, the doyen of American neurology, first described the cure in 1875, and then popularized it in a series of best sellers (although not initially concerned with neurasthenia), summed up in the contemporary catch phrase "Doctor Diet and Doctor Quiet" [see 85]. By 1881 the "cure" was being used in England, largely owing to society obstetrician William Playfair, who proclaimed it "the greatest advance of which practical medicine can boast in the last quarter of the century" [86].

It was in Germany and the United States that the rest cure found its most ready acceptance. Playfair's book was available in German in 1883, only a year after its publication in English, and a German edition of Weir Mitchell was available by 1886, reviewed by Freud in the following year. Large numbers of "retreats," private clinics, and rest homes appeared in these countries between 1880 and 1900 [55,66,87], although business was also good in the United Kingdom. It was financially vital to the neurologist, since, as one wrote in 1894, the neurologist should not *undertake a thoroughgoing course of this sort of treatment unless in a private institution*" [88]. Fortunately, the author continued, "We have in Germany an abundance of good private institutions." The rest cure became the most used treatment for nervous disorder across Central Europe and America. It "provided the raison d'etre for the clinic, since isolation could not by definition be procured at home, nor could the expensive apparatus of electrotherapy." Mitchell himself may have earned 70,000 dollars in private practice per year [66]. As Shorter points out, "physicians in these competitive, profitmaking clinics were happy to comply with the patients' desire for face saving [organic] diagnoses, and made great use of such expressions as . . . chronic fatigue and neurasthenia" [87].

The rest cure has attracted many criticisms over the years. The writings of several patients treated by the cure, such as Virginia Woolf and Charlotte Perkins Gilman, have been important in highlighting how male stereotypes of women, especially their moral and physical weaknesses, intruded into treatment [see 89,90]. Contemporaries, however, noted other failings. Principal among these was failure of the somatic model. If there was no cellular basis to exhaustion, then what was the purpose of rest? The growing awareness that all the business of the cure, the diet, massage, electricity, and so on, were just props for the physician to exhort and encourage the patient meant that they could be dispensed with [see 91–93]. It became increasingly difficult to deny the role of suggestion, of the doctor–patient relationship, upon which "everything depends" [34], and ultimately of the newer psychotherapies [see 5]. If rest cure worked, it was more to do with Mitchell's charisma, which was considerable [93,94]. Furthermore, even if effective, few could afford it [25].

Others felt that it was not even effective for psychological reasons, but might actually make the patient worse. Few changes were so dramatic as that of Dutil. In his contribution to an 1894 textbook he espouses a standard Weir Mitchell approach [95], but by 1903 he wrote that the inevitable consequence of Mitchell's regimen was "the patient, condemned to complete inactivity, lying on her chaise-longue for days and nights . . . constantly alert to the most minute sensations, surrounded by those excessively concerned for her health" [91].

The consequence was rest cure was first modified, and then abandoned. By 1892, in the same volume as Playfair's strict Mitchell approach, Arndt was advocating "for some patients exercise is needed, for others rest is beneficial" [96]. Absolute rest was soon to be followed by a restoration of activity [80,97]. Everywhere activity or exercise, allied to psychotherapy, began to replace the rest cure [14] and, instead of sanatoria, came the first occupational therapy programs [98]. "Frequently these patients have indulged in rest for months, or even years, without beneficial results. This has been so much recognised by many of the sanatoria that facilities for exercise and occupation have to a large extent replaced those of rest and seclusion with gratifying results" [93]. Rest cure did survive for a while—in 1907 it was still followed at the Edinburgh Royal Hospital, but the physicians attributed its efficacy solely to suggestion [99]; however, eventually, it was only practiced at Mitchell's old hospital [100]. Elsewhere, rest cure vanished and, with the new, albeit short-lived, era of psychiatric optimism, Karl Menninger was able to look on the whole episode with disdain [101].

The Reaction Against Neurasthenia

What were the consequences of the failures of the simple organic models of both etiology and treatment, and the rise of the psychological models? Physicians could either abandon the concept, or concede that the patients were best cared for by the psychiatric profession. Many neurologists were soon persuaded that neurasthenia should be abandoned. Browning wrote that neurasthenics were rare in his neurological service (although not, he admitted, in his private practice), because "Many of our best neurologists do not now recognise such as disease" [102]. Particularly in the United Kingdom, neurology was establishing itself as a scientific speciality, and many soon turned their backs on this now discredited diagnosis. This happened with alacrity in the United Kingdom and, albeit with less speed, in the United States. Diller noted that between 1894 and 1916 the proportion of neurasthenics and hysterics in his case load had halved [103], an even more precipitous decline occurring at the New York Neurological Institute. This should be contrasted to the preponderance of the diagnosis at the Vanderbilt Clinic in the previous decade, but, although pleas were made for the same process in the United States [e.g., 81], the concept was more deeply entrenched there and in France. As late as 1927, one-third of patients seen by American neurologists were still either neurasthenic or psychasthenic [104]. Many physicians retained the diagnosis (and, therefore, the patients), but began gradually to incorporate the new psychological insights into their treatments—the rational psychotherapy of Paul Dubois [14] being particularly influential, perhaps because it so clearly repudiated notions of the unconscious that were often unpalatable to many neurologists.

The rapid abandonment of neurasthenia by British neurologists was because the illness had never found a fertile soil there anyway. Beard himself had a dismal reception when he visited this country in 1880 and 1881, committing one social gaffe after another [105,106]. Sir Andrew Clark, an eminent physician at the London Hospital, launched a blistering attack in the *Lancet* [107] and, although Playfair made a spirited defense [108], he was forced to concede that he had been unable to persuade the Collective Investigation Committee of the BMA to take an interest. Neurasthenia was never accepted by the neurological establishment. The giants of the profession, such as Gowers, Gordon Holmes, Ferrier, Buzzard, and Kinnier-Wilson based at the National Hospital for Nervous Diseases, declared themselves in various ways against an organic view of neurasthenia and in favor of psychological interpretations. Gower devoted only one page of his 1888 two-volume text to the subject [109], writing "the use of the word [neurasthenia] has brought with it a tendency to regard the condition as a definite disease. Books have even been written about it. . . ." The next edition, in 1899, was even briefer: neurasthenia "occurs especially in those of a neurotic disposition" [110]. This should be contrasted with the extensive coverage given in Oppenheim's equally monumental German neurology text [26]. Unlike the United States, France, and Germany, in the United Kingdom the neurasthenic flag was flown by only a few, the most prominent being Clifford Allbutt in Cambridge. Despite such efforts a reviewer in 1907 conceded that neurasthenia had "not taken deep root in Britain" [111], and by 1913, its "serviceableness as coin of the realm" [112] was doubtful.

Issues of class and gender were intimately related to those of etiology and treatment. The more "organic" the account, the more likely was the author to insist on the preponderance of upper social classes, the distinction from hysteria (the archetypal disease of women [see 19]), and the overrepresentation of men and "civilized" races. Physicians, then and now, were more likely to view sympathetically those whose illnesses had been acquired by praiseworthy, rather than contemptible, means—neurasthenia, the disease of overwork, came into the former, hysteria the latter [113]. Groups not subject to such overwork, such as women, lower classes, degenerates, American blacks, and all uncivilized races, thus were spared neurasthenia [see 11,74,114,115]. Playfair, writing in Tuke's dictionary, stated that the difference between neurasthenics and hysterics was that the former "give all they possess to be well, and heartily long for good health, if only they knew how to obtain it" [116]. Neurasthenics cooperated with the doctor, unlike hysterics [117]. The bluntest was Ernest Reynolds, Professor of Medicine in Manchester, who wrote that, whereas hysteria was "purely a mental condition, whose basis is a morbid craving for sympathy and notoriety," neurasthenia was "entirely different," a "functional disorder of chronic overuse of neurones" due to "gross overwork and worry" [118], although the symptoms seemed much the same.

Even within the sexes, such moral judgments were frequent; thus, Sir Frederick Mott wrote that "neurasthenia . . . was more likely to be acquired in *officers of a sound mental constitution than men of the ranks*, because in the former the prolonged stress of responsibility which, in the officer worn out by the prolonged stress of war and want of sleep, causes anxiety less he should fail in his critical duties" [119].

The consequence was the decline of the diagnosis. This was partially intended, as physicians dismantled the now overstretched concept, that "mob of incoherent symptoms borrowed from the most diverse disorders" [107]. However, as the hostile reception accorded Beard in the journals showed, academic disdain was not new. It now vanished for more practical reasons. Neurasthenia had survived academic dissatisfaction because it was "useful to the doctor" [112] as a code for nonpsychotic illnesses for which the only effective treatments were psychologically based. The diagnosis was made "for the comfort of the relatives and peace of mind of the patient" [120], since it avoided the stigma of psychiatric illness and the necessity to seek treatment in an asylum, where the neurasthenic would "soon be subject to the usual stigma attached to the abode of mental patients . . . only in a general hospital could the psychic problem be solved under the happiest auspices" [121]. Others commented that even if the symptoms were "purely mental," it was better to talk about nervous diseases and neurasthenia since "the patients and the patients friends usually have a horror of mental disease" [38]. Several anecdotes attest to the consequences of not keeping to these codes, one of which represents a situation still familiar to readers of this volume. Drummond [92], a physician in Newcastle upon Tyne, describes a scene he witnessed when a "kindly physician," actually Sir Andrew Clark, during a consultation with a neurasthenic patient, let slip the word "melancholia." "The outcome of that visit was disastrous, involving serious trouble all round, in which even Sir Andrew himself shared, for he was pestered for weeks with letters to know whether in using the term 'melancholia' he had the idea of insanity in his mind."

As more doctors publicly accepted the new psychological models, it became harder to maintain the code. Statements such as "functional illness means pooh poohed illness" [122] and "neurotic, neurasthenic, hysterical and hypochondriacal are, on the lips of the majority of clinical teachers, terms of opprobrium" [92] show that the codes were being broken, and the demise of the category was a matter of time. In 1868 patients were only too willing to confess to "weakness of the nerves" [123], but 30 years later the *Spectator* observed that neurasthenia was "no longer interesting," it was "discredited and disgraceful . . . shameful to confess" [124]. The changes in social class and the rise of the psychogenic school meant that etiologies had also changed. Infection remained, but in place of overwork came laziness, fecklessness, degeneration, and poor hygiene. Neurasthenia, once almost a badge of honor, was now considerably less praiseworthy. In place of the hard-pressed businessman came the stereotype of the work-shy laborer or the pampered hypochondriacal upper-class female invalid [125].

From its dominant position in the Surgeon General's Index neurasthenia began to disappear. The space devoted to it in the classic neurological texts dwindled, and finally disappeared, or received a brief psychiatric coverage. In the first edition of Cecil's prestigious textbook of medicine neurasthenia has its own chapter [104]. By the third edition in 1934 it is listed under "The Neuroses or Psychoneuroses" and is reduced to a single sentence in the 1947 seventh edition. One edition later it disappears from the index.

Neurasthenia was replaced mainly by the new psychiatric diagnoses. The symptoms were now listed as psychological—painful fatigue became anhedonia [126], whereas a 1937 textbook of anxiety could include the symptom "fatigue on slightest exertion [127]. For a period psychasthenia contained much of obsessional and phobic neuroses [128], but this soon gave way to the current classifications. The greatest beneficiary was the new concept of depression. Even De Fleury acknowledged the change. In 1901 his first book was called *Les Grands Symptômes Neurasthéniques*, but by 1924 the title had changed to *Les États Dépressifs et la Neurasthénie*. With the support of such figures as Jaspers and Bleuler, the latter commenting that "What usually produces the so-called neurasthenia are affective disturbances" [129], the view became widespread that "all neurasthenic states are in reality depression, . . . perhaps minor, attenuated, atypical, masked, but always forms of anxious melancholia" [130]. In current neurological practice, neurasthenia, when mentioned at all, is seen as synonymous with depression [131].

In conclusion, there were several reasons for the decline in neurasthenia. First, the neuropathological basis of the illness was discredited. Second, rest cure was seen either to be unsuccessful, or to be efficacious principally for psychological reasons. Third, the social class distribution of the illness altered. Finally, the interest and optimism shown by the neurologists was transferred to the new profession of psychiatry.

The Disease That Did Not Disappear

The consequences of the psychogenic explanations of neurasthenia were not entirely as intended. In 1930, Buzzard had warned that although the advances in both neurology and psychiatry had illuminated the plight of the neurasthenic, the same could not be said of the exclusively psychogenic theories, which would lead to a polarization among doctors [132]. "On the contrary, Freudian doctrines have produced a reaction in the minds of medical men which has taken the form of a desire to ascribe all mental disorders, including neurasthenia, to some physical or chemical agent the result of disturbed glandular secretions, of septic tonsils or teeth, of intestinal stasis or infection, or of a blood pressure which is too high or too low."

Buzzard was right. Before the acceptance of the psychogenic paradigm neurasthenia served a purpose: "At a time when physicians felt comfortable only with clearly organic disorders, a diagnosis of neurasthenia permitted some to address themselves to tangible clinical issues and to provide an essentially psychological therapy under a somatic label" [66]. With the rise of the psychogenic school, this ability, acquired by physicians with difficulty, was lost. For a time the good physician now "wanted to study all sides of the question" [60], which meant attention to emotional issues, but "without overlooking the possibilities of infective and organic factors." Conversely, the informed psychiatrist also accepted the possible role of organic factors; hence, Tredgold in 1911 doubts the existence of a structural basis to neurasthenia, but accepts the probable role of a cerebral "bio-chemical" abnormality" [133].

However, the introduction of psychoanalysis to the United States, with its exclusive emphasis on mental origins, ended this appropriately labeled holistic approach [134]. Narrow somaticism had failed, but in its place came belligerent Freudianism, as illustrated by statements such as "there is only one certain cure for neurasthenia—viz psychoanalysis" [83]. Ironically, this treatment attracted criticisms reminiscent of those of the rest cure, namely questionable efficacy, but unquestionable expense [5,112,132]. Others disliked the new approach because it appeared to encourage introspection, the quality that the neurasthenic apparently already possessed to excess [e.g., 104].

Paradoxically, it was the solely psychological explanations in the new "official" consensus on neurasthenia that ensured the survival of a contradictory view familiar to Beard and Mitchell. One reason was financial. Beard had made a virtue out of the preponderance of upper classes among his patients, claiming that "the miseries of the rich, the comfortable and intelligent have been unstudied and unrelieved" [11]: 40 years later A. J. Cronin was still making a decent living in fashionable London by treating society ladies for the illness [135]. American physicians and neurologists were particularly reluctant to abandon it—as late as 1927, Adolf Meyer was writing to Abraham Flexner complaining that neurologists continued to see neurasthenics in their clinics, although it was psychiatrists who had the necessary training [136].

As important as the financial rewards was the rejection by sympathetic physicians of what they perceived as the implications of the now ascendant psychological views. Such physicians usually endorsed a division between organic and psychological, usually synonymous with a division between real and unreal, illnesses. The argument revolved around the status to be accorded neurasthenia. Those continuing to diagnose the condition would thus energetically refute "the idea, now strongly held that neurasthenia is basically psychiatric, almost imaginary in nature" [80]. Only by continuing to affirm the organicity of neurasthenia could many doctors continue in their dealings with chronically fatigued patients. It was the survival of such attitudes that prolonged the survival of neurasthenia, and prepared the way for its modern reemergence.

The result was that, despite the obituaries and the consignment of the condition to the garbage can [117], rubbish heap [137], or waste basket [82], neurasthenia survived. Writing in 1933, Dicks observed that "Everywhere we meet with the statements that it is rare . . . yet no name is more often on the lips of both our profession and the laity" [138]. Buzzard noted, with regret, that although he felt that most of the patients referred to him were depressed, nearly all came with a label of neurasthenia [138]. Brill commented "in spite of all that was said and done about the inadequacy of the name, as well as the concept itself, neurasthenia is still very popular with the medical profession" [117].

Modern Neurasthenia

Nevertheless, neurasthenia did gradually disappear, with only two exceptions. The term does survive in some parts of the world, and is retained in the International Classification of Diseases (ICD-9 and ICD-10). It is a common neurotic diagnosis in the Netherlands, Eastern Europe, and the old Soviet Union, and flourishes in parts of Asia, especially China, where it is seen as a physical illness, without stigma, describing what Western observers label as depression [139]. The second exception is the line of illnesses known as the effort syndromes (Da Costa's syndrome, Soldier's heart), in which one synonym, neurocirculatory asthenia, continues to attract professional and academic attention. Nevertheless, even here the same shift from organic to psychological formulations is visible [140]. A variety of organic explanations initially dominated the literature, including infective etiologies [e.g., 141], but these gradually altered. For example, no figure was more associated with these diagnoses than the influential cardiologist Paul Wood, but by the end of his career he saw them as synonymous with anxiety disorder [142]. Recent authors have claimed that effort syndromes and CFS are synonymous, seeing them both as essentially psychophysiological conditions [143].

Other inheritors of part of the neurasthenia heritage, and another historical pathway between neurasthenia and CFS, are illnesses such as candidiasis, hypoglycemia, brucellosis, food allergy, and total allergy syndrome. These illnesses, none of which attract much professional support, instead flourish in what Kleinman has called the *folk sector*, the nonprofessional healing specialists who lie between professional medicine and lay explanations of illness, incorporating elements of each to produce a popularly appealing, but technically based system [see 144].

There is no shortage of those who claim links between these conditions and CFS. Both Straus [145] and Stewart [146] have shown the clinical overlap between each of the foregoing conditions and CFS. Stewart [147] went on to describe how each of the conditions overlap in the illness careers of individual patients, with CFS-like diagnoses appearing in recent years. Many self-help books effortlessly link candida, allergy, hypoglycemia, chemical sensitivity, and food intolerance, to which list has now been added CFS. William Crook, the author of the phenomenally successful (except with the medical profession) *Yeast Connection* has recently published *Chronic Fatigue Syndrome and the Yeast Connection* [148]. The advocates of all these conditions are keen to point out the similarities between all of them, and are indeed correct to do so. The symptoms overlap, but so do the social characteristics. The gender and class distribution, the existence of support groups, media campaigns, dissatisfaction with traditional medicine, the necessity to reorganize lifestyles, and the hostility to psychiatric illness, coupled with high rates of psychological distress, all find parallels with some aspects of ME/CFS [see 147,149,150]. However, it is important to emphasize that these diseases are only part of the heritage of CFS, and may apply to only a small group of patients, albeit highly visible.

THE BEGINNINGS OF POSTINFECTIVE FATIGUE

Conditions such as candidiasis, hypoglycemia, total allergy, and so on, have never become an established part of medical practice. Their lack of empirical support and their cultural aspects, prevent substantial professional affirmation and, hence, the links between these conditions and CFS are only rarely considered in the modern medical literature. Professional support for CFS emerged from a different source, the postinfective fatigue syndromes [54].

Even the first descriptions of neurasthenia included a link with febrile illness. Van Deusen highlighted malaria, since he worked in an area in which the disease was endemic [4], whereas Beard drew attention to wasting fevers [3]. The latter's descriptions of neurasthenia continue the infective theme: key symptoms included "general and local chills and flashes of heat." The link with infection persisted in the earliest accounts in France [6], and one of the first cases to be treated in this country by the Weir Mitchell regimen was a woman with a 14-year history of neurasthenia, permanently confined to bed in a darkened room, whose illness had begun with a persistent cold [151].

By 1914 the observation that neurasthenia frequently followed an infection was widely acknowledged. For many, including Osler, Ely, Oppenheim, Cobb,

Horder, Ladova, Clarke, Kraepelin, Althaus, Arndt, and others, influenza was a prominent, and sometimes the principal, cause of neurasthenia, but claims were also made for many others, especially typhoid and, more recently, the effects of vaccination [152]. As the microbiological revolution spread, each organism was linked with neurasthenia. The clinical evidence of neurasthenic conditions after infection was, however, a two-edged sword. Everybody had a favorite culprit, until it was conceded that any infective agent could produce the state of chronic exhaustion [14,26,138], especially in combination with depression [153], worry [58], or emotional disturbance [24]. Furthermore, most individuals with infections, even influenza or typhoid, did not develop neurasthenia [24]. To a generation schooled on Virchow and Koch, these were major hurdles. As clinical research became less inclined to accept uncomfirmed clinical observation, skepticism increased [154]. Streckler's caution is worth quoting in full, as it remains relevant. "There can be no valid objection to the bacteriologic method of approach, providing that each study is rigorously controlled and that conclusions do not exceed the premises" [154].

Such efforts did not cease after the decline of neurasthenia, since, starting with Reiter's disease [155], attempts to link infective organisms with previously mysterious clinical conditions had reaped dividends, and the list of bona fide postinfective conditions was growing, especially in the neurological field. Specific postinfective syndromes identical with neurasthenia continued to be described as each new infection was discovered, although such descriptions, for example, of the fatigue states arising after hepatitis [156] and schistosomiasis [157], continue to be noticeable for their psychological flavor.

One of these conditions, chronic brucellosis, exemplifies in microcosm many of the issues surrounding neurasthenia and CFS. By 1930, the diagnosis of acute brucellosis was well established. There was less certainty about the condition of chronic brucellosis, but it had many adherents. One of them, the public health specialist Alice Evans, noted the similarities between neurasthenia and chronic brucellosis, but only to highlight the plight of the large numbers of those afflicted who suffered the indignity of receiving the erroneous, and "dishonorable," diagnosis of neurasthenia [158]. Thirteen years later she was still championing the disease, which remained "extremely difficult to diagnose . . . however, an unrecognised mild form of brucellosis is a common ailment in this country" [159].

The end of the syndrome encapsulates on a smaller scale the eclipse of neurasthenia. Spinks studied a series of patients with acute brucella infection, and noted that a proportion failed to recover—the chronic brucellosis group [160]. However, neither he, nor anyone else, found objective evidence of disease, and instead noted high rates of psychological disorder. Researchers from Johns Hopkins Hospital, in the first of a series of papers on the relation between infection and psychological vulnerability, studied subjects with the label of chronic brucellosis in greater detail. They found no evidence of chronic infection [161], but high levels of psychiatric morbidity, coupled with reluctance to discuss psychological issues and a strong attachment to the "organic" diagnosis [162]. Once this evidence became widely disseminated, chronic brucellosis disappeared, reappearing only in an editorial on the social construction of mental illness [163]. Table 1 summarizes some links between fatigue syndromes and infection.

THE BEGINNINGS OF MYALGIC ENCEPHALOMYELITIS: FROM LOS ANGELES TO THE ROYAL FREE

In the United Kingdom, the first mention of the term myalgic encephalomyelitis (ME) was in a leading article in 1956 [164]. It was proposed as an explanation for a series of outbreaks of a contagious condition, causing symptoms referable to the central nervous system, that had occurred in various parts of the world in the preceding three decades. Some of these had been named by their place of origin (hence, Iceland disease), others by the neuromuscular weakness that was

Table 1 Infectious Agents and Fatigue Syndromes

Organism or disease implicated	Year
Malaria	1869
Influenza	1892
Typhoid	1892
Alimentary bacteria	1911
Streptococci	1922
All vaccination	1922
Encephalitis lethargica	1931
Brucellosis	1934
Yellow fever vaccine	1946
Schistosomiasis	1946
St. Louis encephalitis	1970
Epstein–Barr virus	1982
Varicella	1984
Coxsackie B virus	1985
HHV-6	1988
Rubella immunization	1988
Tick-borne encephalitis	1989
Lyme disease	1990
Hepatitis B vaccine	1991
HTLV-2	1991
Spumavirus	1991
Rubella vaccine	1992
Rickettsiae	1992

a frequent feature (hence, neuromyasthenia), and others by the presumed relation to poliomyelitis (hence, atypical poliomyelitis). An exhaustive, if uncritical, bibliography of these outbreaks is provided by Parish [165] and Hyde [166].

Two episodes have attracted most attention. These took place at the Los Angeles County Hospital (LAC) in 1934, and the Royal Free Hospital (RFH) in London in 1955. Both concerned the nursing and medical staff of these hospitals, and not patients. The symptoms of these epidemics remain unclear, but at the core were mixtures of unusual motor and sensory symptoms, accompanied by myalgia and signs of emotional distress and lability. On the whole, the laboratory tests available to the clinicians of the day were unhelpful.

Some of the contemporary professional concerns about many of these epidemics centered around possible links to poliomyelitis, a theme that remains relevant today. Aronowitz elegantly demonstrates how these links began [167]. He shows before the LAC epidemic in 1934 the incidence of polio in California had been declining for several years, and that, by the prevailing opinion of the time, this heralded a new severe episode. The cases were thus viewed with polio very much in mind, and described as atypical poliomyelitis. McEvedy and Beard make similar points about the Middlesex hospital outbreak in 1952 and, although physicians at the Royal Free Hospital 3 years later were less taken with the similarity to polio, this was not the case among the nonmedical personnel [168].

Despite the label, the nature of the outbreaks was unlike polio. Most of the cases in the LAC epidemic had unusually mild symptoms, and physicians experienced considerable diagnostic difficulties. The fatality rate was remarkably low, the cerebrospinal fluid (CSF) normal, paralysis was nearly absent, and muscular atrophy rare [169]. The public health report was unable to contain a calculation of the ratio of paralytic to nonparalytic cases, a conventional statistic of polio epidemics, because of the scarcity of paralytic cases. Instead, what was often recorded as paralytic polio was, in fact, minor neurological impairment detected by overvigorous testing [167]. Overall, the head of the infectious diseases unit reported that "it was the scarcity of the usual and the large volume of the unusual which gave the epidemic its bizarre aspects" [170]. Similar arguments soon convinced the Royal Free physicians that the illness was not poliomyelitis.

Having raised the possibility of infection, many of the original observers were reluctant to abandon it. Despite the lack of objective evidence of infection, and the observation that emotional disturbance was an integral part of nearly all of these outbreaks, the initial authors were keen to reinforce the organic etiology of the syndromes, and in introducing names such as neuromyasthenia or myalgic encephalomyelitis, effectively ruled out any alternative explanation. For some years this position remained publicly unchallenged (although this might be because many professionals remained either unaware of, or indifferent to, neuromyasthenia, ME, and so on during this period).

The most influential critique of the organic position came from McEvedy and Beard [171, 172]. They suggested that certain epidemics, such as the Royal Free, were due to transmitted emotional distress ("mass hysteria"), whereas others were not epidemics at all, but clustering of small numbers of cases of heterogeneous illnesses combined with altered medical perception. This was not the first time such a suggestion had been made: similar accounts had been in circulation during the Royal Free outbreak itself [173], and two epidemiologists had made the same suggestion in print [174]. Paul, the historian of polio, came to a similar conclusion [175]. However, McEvedy and Beard's was the most public statement. Their evidence against an infective origin was strong: the disease affected almost invariably female staff, and never patients. It was a similar observation, of an illness that affected patients, and never staff, that led to Goldberger's classic work refuting the alleged infectious origins of pellagra.

The evidence for an emotional origin to symptoms was less compelling, although there was little doubt that emotional factors were responsible for a proportion of the cases in the best-documented outbreaks. One case in Los Angeles developed "physic blindness," as well as psychosis [170], yet was still included as an epidemic case of atypical poliomyelitis. Observers constantly used terms such as *bizarre* or *remarkable* to describe the nature of the symptoms and signs, involving "frank hysterical manifestations" [176]. Many suggested that the illness represented the "functional end of a disorder with an organic beginning" [164]. Ramsay himself noted that the Royal Free disease resembled both polio and hysteria [177], and others felt the illnesses displayed features remarkably akin to hysteria [178]. McEvedy and Beard's second proposition, that of altered medical perception, also received support from later inquiries [179].

What did happen? We will never know. An infective agent, albeit not polio, cannot be dismissed, and has been cogently argued by Acheson [169] and, subsequently, Jenkins [180]. It is possible that cases were admitted of an infective disease that resembled, but was not, polio, but what is known about the epidemiology of the episodes is, in general, unlikely to be explained on a solely microbiological basis. On the other hand, there are also several arguments in favor of an emotional nature to the contagion [171,172]. Perhaps the initial infective cases served as a focus for natural anxiety and, in turn, triggered others whose illnesses cannot be explained by an infective agent, but it is only in a very few, isolated, cases that the diagnosis of factitious illness can be sustained [181,182]. The social pressures common to both hospitals and the subsequent history of the condition must be at least one factor in the sad tale of the future fate of those afflicted. In conclusion, it seems probable that the outbreaks grouped together under the label of ME/neuromyasthenia, and so on, are more heterogeneous than implied by a single label [183].

As with neurasthenia, the arrival of the psychogenic hypothesis was a very mixed blessing. Just as Buzzard had observed following the rise of Freudian theories, the mass hysteria hypothesis led to a retrenchment of the organic school of thought, and a polarized, bitter, and acrimonious debate that continues to this day. As with neurasthenia, many of the most active advocates of the organic camp remain afflicted physicians, especially since health service professionals continue to be dramatically overrepresented among sufferers [2,184]. Again, as the available evidence failed to determine the etiology of the outbreaks, prejudice was called on to affirm their organic nature. Poskanzer suggested that rather than ME being a psychoneurosis, all cases of psychoneurosis were sporadic ME [185]. In so doing he acknowledged that both conditions lay claim to the same clinical territory; hence, nonclinical factors were needed to assert the organic etiology. ME and more recently CFS are thus claimed to affect professionals of impeccable moral stature: level headed [186], extravert types of stable personality [187], and so on, all were used as evidence against a psychiatric origin.

FROM CHRONIC EPSTEIN–BARR VIRUS TO THE CHRONIC FATIGUE SYNDROME

Between the demise of neurasthenia and the last 10 years, fatigue syndromes were not a major issue for physicians or professional or lay journals. Certainly fatigued patients did not disappear. After the demise of neurasthenia, general physicians continued to encounter the patient with chronic fatigue, often arising after a variety of insults, including infection. Perhaps mindful of the neurasthenia experience, rather than develop specific nosological entities, physicians generally resorted to descriptive labels, such as chronic nervous exhaustion [188], tired, weak, and toxic [189], fatigue and weakness [190], or fatigue and nervousness [191]. The main emphasis was on psychological mechanisms.

Some patients did receive diagnoses of new fatigue syndromes. As already discussed, syndromes such as chronic brucellosis enjoyed some popularity in the United States. Myalgic encephalomyelitis, or ME, was a term in circulation from 1957, but had little public or professional prominence. None of these labels made much impact. Norma Ware has appropriately noted that throughout this period "chronic fatigue had become invisible," with "no name, no known etiology, no case illustrations or clinical accounts in the medical textbook, no ongoing research activity—nothing to relate it to current medical knowledge" [192].

The reconstruction of chronic fatigue began in the mid-1980s, with the emergence of chronic Epstein–Barr virus (EBV) syndrome. It appeared first with the publication of two papers from reputable researchers appearing in prestigious American journals [193,194], although one of the earliest appearances of the new condition was a paper from researchers in Israel [195]. These papers sought to link evidence of infection by the Epstein–Barr virus to chronic fatigue. The high point of this endeavor was a consensus conference organized in 1985 by the National Institute of Allergic and Infectious Diseases [196]. The technical aspects of the papers, and of chronic mononucleosis, have been discussed elsewhere [197]. It is now clear that the role of persistent EBV in the new condition was exaggerated (although very recent work from Peter White in London shows a clear role for EBV in postinfectious fatigue). The same authors who had presented the original data themselves concluded that chronic mononucleosis was a misnomer and should be abandoned.

This did not happen. The original proposers of chronic mononucleosis later declared themselves unprepared for the public and media attention that followed: "Physicians throughout the United States were inundated with requests to evaluate chronic fatigue" [198]. This was not just a response to the chronic mononucleosis papers, but also followed the publicity given to an epidemic of a mysterious disease that began in the Lake Tahoe region of Nevada. The confluence of these two events made an extraordinary impact, described by one medical journalist as a "proliferation of support groups, research foundations dominated by patients with the syndrome, and fund raising and lobbying groups" [199]. By 1990 a hotline at the Centers for Disease Control was attracting over 2000 calls a month [200], a figure now nearer 4000. Only the acquired immunodeficiency syndrome (AIDS) attracts more calls to the National Institute of Health [201].

Chronic mononucleosis had captured the public imagination. The professional disillusionment with the role of EBV in the syndrome did nothing to diminish or delegitimize this; the new syndrome appeared to be here to stay. The medical reaction, therefore, was to change the label. During a meeting of infectious disease physicians in 1987 it was proposed that a new term, chronic fatigue syndrome, be applied to the syndrome. Operational criteria, universally known as the CDC criteria, were published [202; also see Chapter 2]. Researchers in Australia had independently reached the same conclusion and made the same suggestions [203]. Two years later the United Kingdom followed suit [204].

It is the task of the social historian to determine why CFS became so popular during the mid-1980s. Patients with chronic fatigue were nothing new. The ill-defined epidemic at Lake Tahoe is often cited as the start of the emergence of CFS, but there have been other publicized epidemics before. Media coverage was extensive, but as Aronowitz has shown, so was coverage of the Los Angeles 1934 epidemic [167]. What is new is the scale of the response. In the United Kingdom a broadcast in 1980 on "Woman's Hour" led to 1000 letters [205], but many credit the article by Sue Finlay in the *Observer* of June 1, 1986 ("An illness doctors don't recognise"), relating her own experiences as a sufferer, as playing a pivotal role in the surge of interest in ME in this country and the founding of the ME Action Campaign [206]. The first medical advisor to the ME association noted how the dramatic rise in membership of the other patients' organization in the United Kingdom, the ME association, was also assisted by media coverage [207]. It was an article in the local newspaper in Portland, Oregon, that led to the founding of the first self-help group of CFS in the United States in 1985 [208]. A similar role is often given to a campaigning article by American sufferer Hiliary Johnson in *Rolling Stone* in 1987 [209]. Media coverage increased public awareness in both the United Kingdom and United States: increasing media coverage is an acknowledged task of the CFS organizations.

Did this coverage, itself labeled a media epidemic [200], actually create the demand? Stewart's finding of the overlap between CFS, environmental illness, and candida [147] may owe something to media publicity, but perhaps more the choice of label than the decision to be sick. Interest must have preceded the media attention—Sue Finlay's article provoked an immediate response: 14,000 fact sheets were requested in the following weeks [206], suggesting that the demand was already there and was not created by the article. Similar media coverage has been afforded other explanatory systems, such as allergy, candida, hypoglycemia, and so on. However, the size and speed of the response to CFS suggests that coverage was tapping an already present need, and not creating the phenomenon, although it may well shape illness beliefs.

What about epidemic forms of CFS? There are many clear-cut, noncontroversial examples of how media coverage facilitates the spread of mass hysterical outbreaks. One of the simplest measures to combat outbreaks of mass hysteria is either to prohibit media coverage, or to ensure that it clearly indicates the emotional nature of the contagion [see 207]. How relevant is this to CFS?

The two best described epidemics remain those at the Los Angeles County Hospital and the Royal Free Hospital. In both, social pressures were apparent from the start, fueled by the fear of polio. At the Royal Free "the anxiety of the lay population on this score was not at first appreciated" [168]. In Los Angeles, the chief of the California Department of Public Health stated that "There is a well founded fear of this disease, and there is also an unfortunate terror that is wholly unnecessary" [quoted in 167]. Aronowitz details the alarmist media coverage, often at the instigation of the authorities to enforce hygiene regulations. The fear of disease was not restricted to nonprofessionals: staff at the LAC, running the risk of exposure, were not well supported by their colleagues. Aronowitz notes how the attending physicians preferred not to visit the contagion wards, instead carrying out consultations on the telephone [167]. Staff on the ward were required to have their temperature taken every day. The severe stress to which the professional staff was subjected was commented on in an early account of the outbreak [211].

The Lake Tahoe epidemic occupies a similar symbolic place in the modern history of CFS to those taken by the LAC and Royal Free episodes in the early history of ME. Here media attention was not guided by the authorities, as at Los Angeles, but may have increased the number of cases. The investigators sent by the Centers for Disease Control to investigate the outbreak at Lake Tahoe reported that media attention had led large numbers of subjects from outside the area to refer themselves to the interested doctors for testing [212], while other doctors in the area were not seeing anything unusual [213]. It seems unlikely that the media created cases of CFS, but could have influenced a distorted perception of a local increase in rates. In all epidemics both media and professional attention could also have led to a gradual relabeling of existing morbidity as a new disease.

Several factors may be responsible for the dramatic reemergence of CFS. One is the coincidence of scientific legitimization and media coverage of a mysterious epidemic at Lake Tahoe. Feiden notes the key events in the story of CFS in the United States as the Lake Tahoe epidemic [208], which coincided with "two path-breaking articles in the *Annals of Internal Medicine*" [see 193,194]. This may be set against a background of increasing dissatisfaction with orthodox medicine and a decline in medical authority [see 20]. As the knowledge and attention given to ME/CFS spread, media attention may precede increased numbers of sufferers presenting to doctors. This has been well described in the United States [198] and mirrors the experience of many infectious disease and neurological specialists in this country. The same process is observed in other countries, such as Spain [214], and no doubt many others.

MYALGIC ENCEPHALOMYELITIS: FROM EPIDEMIC TO SPORADIC

As epidemic ME gave way to sporadic CFS, the nature of the illness itself was changing. In 1976, a group of physicians, including both sufferers and those involved in the Royal Free outbreak, formed a study group [215] and were instrumental in organizing a symposium at the Royal Society of Medicine. The content of the meeting showed that epidemic ME was still the dominant concern, but few new outbreaks were appearing for further study. Attention shifted to the problem of sporadic cases. These had been considered before—some had been noted in the community surrounding the Royal Free Hospital, and others had also described sporadic cases elsewhere [216], but these were not the predominant concern until the early 1980s.

The balance shifted toward nonepidemic cases. The result, largely unnoticed, was a gradual, but profound, change in the character of the illness. In the index episodes neurological signs, of whatever etiology, were recorded in the majority, and were divided into cerebral, brain stem, and spinal [168] (just as in the first series of neurasthenic texts). An early report of two cases of sporadic ME had neurological signs (and both required assisted ventilation) [217]. On the other hand, persistent severe fatigability was either not mentioned, or given little prominence, in the reports of epidemics [168,181], but gradually increased in importance until it became the hallmark of the disease. Neurological signs disappeared [183]. Unfortunately, whereas most epidemic cases recovered [218], this was no longer true for sporadic CFS [219,220]. Contagion, the key feature of the index episodes, all but disappeared.

It must be emphasized that the link between these epidemics and modern CFS is largely historical. The two conditions were very different. Epidemic ME was contagious, acute, and accompanied by paralysis and neurological signs (albeit of disputed origin). Sporadic CFS or ME, as seen today, is noncontagious, chronic, fatiguing, and has no neurological signs—I doubt whether any of the contributors to this volume would consider a diagnosis of CFS in a patient requiring assisted ventilation, nor would many consider a diagnosis of hysteria in a patient with CFS. Few aficionados of CFS appreciate this difference, and continue to lay claim to either the Los Angeles or Royal Free episodes as the origin of the disease. Because the same name has been attached to the two processes, supporters of ME continue to affirm the organicity of the original episodes with a vehemence at variance with the quality of the evidence available.

The shift from epidemic to sporadic occurred in both the United Kingdom and United States, but transatlantic differences remained. Although there are no reliable methods of distinguishing between ME and CFS, and the professional literature treats them as largely synonymous, some cultural differences can be discerned. British texts on ME frequently assume a neuromuscular pathogenesis and emphasize neurological symptoms and signs. American writings on CFS are less concerned with muscle symptoms and pathology, but instead emphasize central (cognitive or neuropsychiatric) symptoms. Similar differences exist in etiological theories. In the United Kingdom, more attention is given to viral causes, with the principal culprit the enterovirus family. In the United States immunological theories have achieved greater prominence and, although viral etiologies are by no means absent, the chief culprit has been the Epstein–Barr virus.

In the United Kingdom the link between enterovirus and ME started with the controversial association between poliovirus and some outbreaks of epidemic ME. The next stage was when two eminent Glasgow virologists, Norman Grist and Eleanor Bell, who had already played a major role in linking coxsackievirus to the pathogenesis of several diseases, joined forces with Glasgow neuroimmunologist Peter Behan, who was interested in ME. Together they studied new outbreaks of what appeared to be acute epidemic ME in the west of Scotland, and reported finding an association with high neutralizing antibody titers to coxsackievirus, to be succeeded by similar findings in sporadic cases. They were also instrumental in reintroducing the term postviral fatigue to replace ME [221]. Although the serological tests used are no longer seen as reliable [222,223], it served as a spur to further work, and more discoveries were made as newer and more refined techniques were introduced [see 223].

Particularly important to the rapid rise of interest in CFS/ME in the United Kingdom was the work carried out at St. Mary's Hospital, London, on enteroviral involvement in CFS [224]. This was greeted with immense enthusiasm: "all ME sufferers must have been elated by the news in January 1988 that a specific blood test for ME had been perfected" [206], and a physician congratulated those responsible for "the magnificent work with the VP-1 estimations" [225]. The scientific findings appear not to have stood the test of time, but the significance of the early work on enteroviruses in the United Kingdom, coming as it did from eminent researchers in prestigious institutions, was to confer the same degree of professional legitimacy to CFS in the United Kingdom as did the papers from Denver and the National Institutes of Health in the United States.

I have emphasized the role of historical continuity throughout this essay. Of course, some modern work has no previous counterpart; for example, the recent introduction of a new paradigm—that of persistent viral infection [223,226]—to challenge the concept of a postinfective syndrome. However, even modern ideas of viral or immune origins to CFS do show some consistency. The concern with postviral fatigue is nothing new, although explanations of possible mechanisms have advanced [see Table 1]. One example of this was the recent talk among British scientists of developing a vaccine against postviral fatigue, based on the work implicating the enterovirus. Rabinbach described the enthusiasm for a fatigue vaccine that first appeared among researchers at the turn of the century, and was only abandoned before the outbreak of the World War I, with the realization that the work on which it was based was faulty [44].

CHRONIC FATIGUE SYNDROME, MYALGIC ENCEPHALOMYELITIS, AND NEURASTHENIA

CFS, ME, and postviral fatigue have all the characteristics of neurasthenia in its heyday. All the symptoms, in particular profound fatigue, exhaustion after minimal effort, mental confusion and depression, chills and fevers, are present. Many have now recognized these links [e.g., 145,227,228]. The resemblances are not purely symptomatic, but are also social and cultural [54,229–231]. Upper-social classes appear to be overrepresented among sufferers, and medical and paramedical professionals are particularly affected. These conditions are frequently labeled "yuppie flu" in the media, reflecting the stereotype of the overstressed, overachieving urban professional, a characterization more than familiar to the readers of Beard, Osler, and Kraepelin. Adherents of the conditions emphasize the impeccable moral stature of those afflicted, to prove that the illness is not psychological. Just as Mott's neurasthenic officers fell ill because of their adherence to their duty, and not because of lack of will power, so are CFS sufferers "the last types to stay away from work without good reasons" [232]. A common theme of the personal stories of CFS sufferers in the media and self-help literature is that they fell ill because of their refusal to cease work and recover from a viral infection [see Chapter 4].

The etiological theories advanced are strikingly similar to those of neurasthenia, with claims made for peripheral (neuromuscular), central (central nervous system), and psychological hypotheses [20]. In the United Kingdom (although not the United States) peripheral explanations of the extreme fatigability have been popular, linked with evidence of biochemical, metabolic, structural, and virological abnormalities of muscle. However, more recent research has cast doubt on simple neuromuscular explanations of abnormal fatigability [see Chapter 9], and the division of fatigue into peripheral and central components first made by George Poore [48] has been resurrected, with most authorities favoring a central origin to fatigue in CFS. Several attractive hypotheses of central nervous dysfunction are currently the subject of investigation [see Chapters 10 and 11].

Finally, no one will be surprised to learn that the third and final etiological theory for neurasthenia, the psychological paradigm, is also the subject of much speculation [see Chapter 13]. As with neurasthenia, writers unsympathetic to CFS have claimed the illness is either hysteria, effort syndrome, depression, or anxiety, whereas supporters either deny any psychological involvement, or claim that psychiatric disorder is simply the normal reaction to physical disease.

The resonances between CFS and neurasthenia extend beyond the professional texts. In the current popular literature, one does not have to search hard for metaphors well known to Beard and the Victorians: concepts such as limited energy resources, lack of nervous energy, flat batteries, and so on. One popular characterization of neurasthenia was of the body giving way under attack from outside, becoming, as Beard described it, "overloaded" [11]. Writers on the illness ascribed this overload to the deteriorating quality of life, to new organisms, new stresses, new ways of working, the decline of leisure, and the increasingly decadent and acquisitive nature of society. This concept of overload remains relevant in CFS; indeed, a popular book on the subject chooses the word as its title [233]. The new overload is from viruses, pollution, pesticides, the deteriorating quality of our food and air, stress, and so on [e.g., 234]. The extreme end of this spectrum is reached with the concept of "total allergy syndrome" or "20th century disease" (curiously, neurasthenia was frequently called "19th century disease"—"this bitter comment on 19th century life" [124]).

The exact nature of the overload varies according to culture: in France, it can be due to educational practices; in Scandinavia, leakage of dental amalgam is a very popular concept; whereas in Britain and the United States, viral agents remain very popular. In her fascinating comparison of different medical cultures Lynn Payer [235] observes the popular tendency of American physicians and patients alike to ascribe many ailments to viruses that would be given different explanations in other Western countries: "America has a virus mentality" [235]. The chapter on American medical culture is titled "The Virus in the Machine."

Explanations of viruses and overload derive their resonance and legitimacy from the scientific evidence concerning immune dysfunction. The technical evidence is reviewed elsewhere in this volume [see Chapters 8 and 15], but it will be seen that there exists an association between immune dysfunction, atopy, and CFS. However, the nature and meaning of that association remains unclear. Nevertheless, the doubts and uncertainties articulated by Lloyd and Strober are rarely reproduced in the popular literature, where ideas of immune dysfunction are frequently cited, and indeed appear in the title of the most active of the current patient organizations in the United States. Abbey and Garfinkel have written that "just as neurasthenia was a compilation of ideas which captivated the imagination of both public and medical professionals, so too is CFS built upon two of the most interesting themes in modern medicine, infectious disease and immunology" [230]. The popular characterization of CFS/ME can thus, like the ideas of Beard, be seen as both dependent on, and a parody of, the current scientific concerns and paradigms. These are succinctly expressed in one article, chosen from a considerable literature, in which the author explains how viruses alter the immune system making the body susceptible to the effects of bacteria, toxins, candida, chemicals, stress, and so on [236].

The most extreme expression of this comes in the frequent analogies drawn between CFS and AIDS [237]. It may be an "AIDS epiphenomenon" [238], and it was not surprising that when claims were made for a retroviral etiology [see Chapter 7], much of the subsequent publicity drew an explicit link between the two conditions, and also raised doubts about the noncontagious nature of sporadic CFS. Interestingly, analogies between CFS and AIDS are rarely encountered in the United Kingdom, where theories of a primary immune dysfunction and CFS are not widely supported, even among those sympathetic to the illness.

The gradual shift in the clinical picture from epidemic ME to sporadic CFS appears to have been accompanied by the introduction of social concerns into the popular etiologies of CFS. That this might happen was hinted in one of the very first articles specifically addressing sporadic neuromyasthenia [216], which began with the phrase A "New Disease" is spreading in the civilised world—a phrase that could have reproduced without alteration from a large number of neurasthenia texts. Similar to neurasthenia, enthusiasts for CFS sometimes allege it is restricted to developed societies [184,239]. Like neurasthenia, CFS seems not to be diagnosed among ethnic minorities. Edes wrote that he did not "recall hearing of a case among negroes" [125], whereas a distinguished contemporary physician "can count on the fingers of one hand the number of blacks I've seen with chronic fatigue" [Dubois, cited in 208].

By the late 1980s CFS, like neurasthenia, had become a vehicle for the expression of wider social concerns, such as the state of our environment, both physical and social. It is remarkable how often very different concerns can find expression through the agency of CFS. In perhaps the first major press article on CFS in France [240], which may yet have the same effect as those already described in the United Kingdom and United States a few years ago, one article resurrected, without realizing it, an idea that was frequently expressed in the old French neurasthenia literature, that CFS was in some way linked to excessive educational demands made upon French schoolchildren *(surménage)*. As the cultural historian Peter Gay observed about neurasthenia "the symptoms of contemporary culture they liked to adduce in proof were, though plausible villains, not easily demonstrated agents of nervousness" [67].

A HISTORICAL PERSPECTIVE ON THE TREATMENT OF CHRONIC FATIGUE SYNDROME

Turning to treatment, a Victorian physician visiting a contemporary hospital would fail to recognize, and even comprehend, many of the treatments offered. However, the physician might feel more at home in some CFS clinics, especially in private practice. The Victorian physician had a vast range of drugs at his disposal, intended to increase the body's supply of energy. Taking one of many examples, Julius Althaus, a London neurologist, used a tonic extracted from the brains of young animals to restore brain power [241]. This "cerebrine alpha" stimulated cerebral oxidation, influenced the emotional centers of the midbrain, and speeded the elimination of "leucomaines." Some modern physicians use a variety of drugs to increase cerebral energy supplies: one popular physician lists 13 drugs for "energy improvement treatment" in addition to 24 other substances used for other purposes [242]. The use of extracts continues. German physicians recently described use of extracts of thymus and spleen in the treatment of CFS [243]. These are justified as immune stimulants and, although the concept of immunotherapy or immune modulation was not specifically available to the Victorian physician, the ideas behind such treatments would have fitted well with Beard's concept of neurasthenia.

Electrical therapy was frequently practiced for neurasthenia: George Beard was as well known for his writings on the therapeutic uses of electricity as on neurasthenia. Even that has not entirely vanished—a New Zealand physician treats ME with electromagnetic therapy: "a small pad giving off a low electrical field on her back" [233]. A well-known English physician recently gained publicity for an electrical device that sufferers must wear to "replace their missing brain waves" and another uses "galvanic currents" in treatment [244]. Finally, colonic lavage was frequently prescribed for neurasthenia, since one popular (both with the public and the medical profession) etiological theory was that the illness was the result of autointoxication, the absorption of "toxic" products from the colon. This was revived by the ME Action Campaign, the most active of the patient organizations in the United Kingdom, who produced a broadsheet entitled the *ME Hypothesis*, which quoted from a classic paper on autointoxication and neurasthenia. In consequence, colonic lavage continues to be advocated as a treatment for ME.

Similar to views of etiology, the jargon of treatment of neurasthenia and chronic fatigue syndrome contains within it elements of an everchanging parody of contemporary scientific terminology, set against a more stable background in which it remains true that "The mass media advertising of cures for fatigue over the past century provides a remarkably consistent theme during the midst of social change. Tonics, potions, herbs, vitamins and an incredible array of other substances have been advised as cures for pseudoanergic symptoms" [245].

Nowhere are the resonances between neurasthenia and CFS more obvious than in the views concerning the role of rest in treatment. During the organic heyday of neurasthenia, the approach that dominated therapy was the Weir Mitchell rest cure. This has been resurrected for the treatment of CFS/ME. An American self-help book contains a chapter entitled *Rest, Rest and More Rest* [208], whereas a British equivalent introduces "aggressive rest therapy" as treatment for ME [206]. A factsheet produced by one patient organization in the United Kingdom stated in bold type "For the majority of M.E. sufferers, physical and mental exertion is to be avoided, and adequate rest essential." A popular self-help book tells sufferers that they must only do "seventy five percent of what you are capable of . . . unless you want to plummet down with another relapse soon, you really must follow the rule of doing less than you think you can" [234].

Just as the Victorians became disillusioned with the rest cure, so have many modern physicians. Unlike the popular literature, the professional literature on CFS is less enthusiastic about the virtues of rest, and many are reaching the same conclusions as did Dubois, Déjerine, and many others. There is now interest in the possible benefits of modern rehabilitative approaches, such as cognitive behavior therapy [see Chapter 17]. It is thus salutary to read articles such as that written by Waterman in 1909 [93] to realize that, although the jargon has changed, the principles of treatment are nothing new.

CONCLUSION

When writing about CFS, Eichner notes that the problem has "long been here. Each generation of physicians rediscovers it; each generation of adults confronts it" [246]. He might have added, "and argues about it." One of the characteristic features of neurasthenia then and CFS now is their capacity to cause dissent. Nonbelievers have consistently attacked the gullibility of those who willingly accepted neurasthenia (or latterly ME) in toto: the reviews that greeted Beard's books between 1880 and 1882 are remarkable for their combination of skepticism and ridicule [247]. In his monumental textbook Clifford Allbutt was forced to attack those "medical men who reject neurasthenia as in part a sham, and in part a figment of complacent physicians" [43]. Believers gave as good as they got: Weir Mitchell once reacted to a copy of Freud by saying "Throw that nonsense on the fire" [94]. The accounts of the Congrès des Médicin Aliénists et Neurologist de France [248] (in which such figures as Bernheim, Dubois, and

Déjerine argued against well-known organicists such as De Fleury and Hartenberg), the American Neurological Association on numerous occasions between 1880 and 1914, the American Medical Association in 1944 [249], and so on, follow a similar pattern, which will be familiar to those who have attended recent meetings on CFS/ME. Doctors have always disagreed about chronic fatigue and show little signs of ceasing to do so.

Controversy seems inseparable from CFS, and consensus rare. A journalist has written that "there is no middle ground when it comes to CFS" [250]. Paul Cheney stated that "we who believe that this is a real disease are almost in a death grip with those forces who would stifle debate, trivialize this problem, and banish patients who suffer from it beyond the edges of traditional medicine" [251]. Many will have had similar experiences to one medical journalist, who wrote that "at any dinner party you will find the friends of sufferers, who will either support or hotly dispute this view," usually with "ferocity" [252]. Chronic fatigue syndrome "falls into the category of illnesses that cannot be debated dispassionately" [253].

With dissent comes dismissal, as the personal scorn about which Beard and Mitchell so often complained became transferred to the patients themselves. In 1886 Sir Andrew Clark called neurasthenics "always ailing, seldom ill" [107], and the "wealthy neurasthenics will be a useless, frivolous, noxious element of society" [254]. Yellowlees talked about the frequent specialist who regarded "a neurasthenic patient as little short of a personal insult" [255], whereas Charles Beevor [256] joined Clifford Allbutt in reminding doctors that "on no account should the patient's symptoms be laughed at," but it was to little avail. At the Johns Hopkins Hospital "the neurasthenic patient is treated by physicians . . . with ridicule or a contemptuous summing up of his case in the phrase 'there is nothing the matter, he is only nervous'" [257], views echoed in the popular press: "The majority of sufferers have better reason to complain of the weakening of their moral fibres than of either their mental or physical ones" [124]. A modern observer will be aware that although most physicians are more circumspect about committing such views to print, prejudice and dislike of the CFS or ME patient remains frequent, and the modern self-help texts are replete with examples of discourtesy, rudeness, and disbelief shown to sufferers by health professionals. In a direct echo of Clifford Allbutt and Charles Beevor, Paul Cheney told a journalist that "there are doctors who leave the room after speaking to one of these [CFS] patients and can't stop laughing" [209].

Even those sympathetic to neurasthenics could not avoid a note of irritation and condescension. Patients were the terror of the busy physician [57], occupied by their symptoms beyond reason [40], going from physician to physician (even Beard called them "rounders") where they write down their sensations in long memoranda which they hasten to read and to explain [40].

This dissent largely revolves around differing interpretations of the physical and psychological. The most common dialectic in both neurasthenia and chronic fatigue syndrome is that these must be physical illnesses, not because of the evidence, which remains inconclusive, but because psychological illnesses are unreal, malingered, or imaginary. This tendency of those committed to an exclusively organic view of such illnesses to juxtapose psychiatric and imaginary was criticized by both Dutil [91] and Tinel [130] in France, both of whom also denied that neurasthenia was a *malade imaginaire*, and by Drummond [92] in England. The latter attacked with equal vigor those who viewed neurasthenia as a solely physical illness, and those who regarded it as a malingerers' charter. The same arbitrary divisions apply today, and influence not just diagnosis, but also treatment, as the following extract from a newsletter produced by a patients' organization demonstrates:

> I have been diagnosed as having M.E. and believe that antidepressant drugs have been largely responsible for major improvements in my condition. However I am convinced that this has nothing to do with the antidepressants effect of these drugs, and everything to do with their effect on neurotransmitters in the central nervous system [258].

Neurasthenia, and now CFS/ME, provides both a haven for those uncomfortable with the psychological aspects of illness, who either insist on its solely organic basis, or see it as a refuge for the mentally infirm. Such views seem contradictory, but are closely related, both being based on the premise that psychological illness is unreal, or at least not as worthy of attention as "real, organic" disease. The only dissension continues to be the status to be accorded CFS. These arguments create passions because what is at stake is the issue of legitimacy: what constitutes an acceptable disease, and what is legitimate suffering, deserving of support and sympathy? It is this question and the differing answers that lie at the heart of first neurasthenia, and now CFS, and fuel the fire of the disputes that accompany them.

ACKNOWLEDGMENTS

Many people have influenced my views on the history of chronic fatigue syndrome, but I am particularly grateful to Susan Abbey, Peter Behan, Anthony David, Ian Hickie, Andrew Lloyd, Anthony Pelosi, Michael Sharpe, Ned Shorter, and Stephen Straus, none of whom bear any blame for the final product.

REFERENCES

1. The Charlotte Observer, Sept 4, 1990; Readers Digest, Sept 1991; Newsweek, November 10, 1991.
2. Ramsay M. Postviral fatigue syndrome: the saga of Royal Free disease. London: Gower Medical, 1986.

3. Beard G. Neurasthenia or nervous exhaustion. Boston Med Surg J 1869; 3:217–20.
4. Van Deusen E. Observations on a form of nervous prostration (neurasthenia) culminating in insanity. Am J Insanity; Supplement to the Annual Report for 1867 and 1868; 1869; 25:445–61.
5. Hale H. Freud and the Americans: the beginnings of psychoanalysis in the United States, 1976–1917. New York: Oxford University Press, 1971.
6. Huchard H. Neurasthénie. In: Axenfeld A, Huchard H, eds. Traite des nevroses. Paris: Germer Baillière, 1883:873–907.
7. Arndt R. Neurasthenia. In: Tuke D, ed. Dictionary of psychological medicine. vol 2. London: J Churchill, 1892:840–50.
8. Fishcher-Homberger E. Hypochondire. Melancholie dis neurose: krankheiten und zustandbilder. Bern: Hans Huber, 1970.
9. Lopez Pinero J. Historical origins of the concept of neurosis. Cambridge: Cambridge University Press, 1983.
10. Beard G. A practical treatise on nervous exhaustion (neurasthenia). New York: William Wood, 1880.
11. Beard G. American nervousness. New York: GP Putnam's, 1881.
12. Rosenberg C. The place of George M Beard in nineteenth-century psychiatry. Bull Hist Med 1962; 36:245–59.
13. Certhoux J. De la neurasthénie aux neuroses: le traitement des neuroses dans le passe. Ann Med Psychol 1961; 119:913–30.
14. Dubois P. The psychic treatment of nervous disorders. 6th ed. (Jelliffe SE, White W, trans). New York: Funk & Wagnalls, 1909.
15. Levillain F. La neurasthenia, maladie de Beard. (methodes de Weir-Mitchell et Playfair, traitement de vigoroux). Paris: A Malvine, 1891.
16. Bumke O. Die revision der neurosenfrage. Munch Med Wochenschr 1925; 72:1815–9.
17. Cobb I. A manual of neurasthenia (nervous exhaustion). London: Balliere, Tindall & Cox, 1920.
18. Deale H, Adams S. Neurasthenia in young women. Am J Obstetr 1894; 29:190–5.
19. Oppenheim J. "Shattered nerves": doctors, patients and depression in Victorian England. London: Oxford University Press, 1991.
20. Shorter E. From paralysis to fatigue: a history of psychosomatic illness in the modern era. New York: Free Press, 1992.
21. Knapp P. The nature of neurasthenia. J Nerv Ment Dis 1896; 21:688–9.
22. Weiss E. A consideration of neurasthenia in its relation to pelvic symptoms in women. Am J Obstet 1908; 57:230–5.
23. Dercum F. Rest, suggestion and other therapeutic measures in nervous and mental diseases. Philadelphia: Blakiston's Son & Co, 1917.
24. Neu C. Treatment and management of the neurasthenic individual. Med Rec 1920; 97:341.
25. Berkley H. A treatise on the mental diseases. London: Henry Klimpton, 1901:445.
26. Oppenheim H. Text-book of nervous diseases for physicians and students. vol. 2, 5th ed. (Bruce A, trans). London: Foulis, 1908.
27. Mitchell S. Fat and blood. 3rd ed. Philadelphia: JB Lippincott, 1883.

28. Mitchell SW. The treatment by rest, seclusion etc, in relation to psychotherapy. JAMA 1908; 25:2033–7.

29. Jaspers K. General psychopathology. (Hoenig J, Hamilton M, trans). Manchester: Manchester University Press, 1963:441.

30. Jewell J. Nervous exhaustion or neurasthenia in its bodily and mental relations. J Nerv Ment Dis 1879; 6:45–55.

31. Cowles E. The mental symptoms of fatigue. NY Med J. 1893; Apr 1:345–52.

32. Clouston T. Clinical lectures on mental diseases. 3rd ed. London: Churchill, 1892.

33. Hartenberg P. La psychothérapie chez les neurasthéniques. Encephale 1907; 7:266–7.

34. Déjerine J, Gauckler E. Les maniféstations functionelles des psychonevroses; leur traitement par la psychothérapie. Paris: Masson, 1911.

35. Friedman M. Über neurasthenische melancholie. Monatsschr Psychiatr Neurol 1904; 15:301–18.

36. Gerhardt C (1893). Cited in Fishcher-Homberger E. Hypochondire. Melancholie dis neurose: krankheiten und zustandbilder. Bern: Hans Huber, 1970.

37. Freud S. Hysteria. In: Villaret A, ed. Handworterbuch der gesamtem medizin. vol 1. Stuggart, 1888:886–92. In: Strachey J, ed. Standard Edition. vol 3. 1966:39–57.

38. Barker L, Byrnes C. Neurasthenic and psychasthenic states, including the new phobias. In: Forchheimer F, ed. Therapeusis of internal diseases. New York: Appleton, 1913:516–81.

39. Durkheim E. Suicide: a study in sociology. (Spaulding J, Simpson G, trans). Glencoe, Ill: Free Press, 1951.

40. Blocq P. Neurasthenia. Brain 1894; 14:306–34.

41. Ferrier D. Neurasthenia and drugs. Practitioner 1911; 86:11–5.

42. Osler W. The principles and practice of medicine. New York: Appleton, 1913:1106–16.

43. Allbutt T. Neurasthenia. In: Allbutt T, ed. A system of medicine. vol 8. London: Macmillan, 1899:134–64.

44. Rabinbach A. The body without fatigue: a nineteenth century utopia. In: Drescher S, Sabean D, Sharlin A, eds. Political symbolism in modern Europe: essays in honour of George Mosse. London: Transaction Books, 1982:42–62.

45. Foster G. Common features in neurasthenia and insanity: their common basis and common treatment. Am J Insanity 1900; 56:395–418.

46. Pershing H. The treatment of neurasthenia. Med News 1904; 84:637–40.

47. Tanzi E. A textbook of mental diseases. (Ford Robertson W, Mackenzie TC, trans). London: Rebman, 1909.

48. Poore G. On fatigue. Lancet 1875; 2:163–4.

49. Johnson G. Lectures on some nervous diseases that result from overwork and anxiety. Lancet 1875; 2:85–7.

50. Savage G. Overwork as a cause of insanity. Lancet 1875; 2:127.

51. Lutz T. American nervousness; 1903. Ithaca: Cornell University Press, 1991.

52. Rabinbach A. The human motor: energy, fatigue and the origins of modernity. New York: Basic Books, 1990.

53. Zeldin T. Intellect and pride. Oxford: Oxford University Press, 1980.

54. Wessely S. The history of the postviral fatigue syndrome. Br Med Bull 1991; 47:919–41.
55. Haller J. Neurasthenia: the medical profession and urban "blahs." NY State J Med 1970; 70:2489–97.
56. Ballet G, Proust A. The treatment of neurasthenia. London; Henry Kimpton, 1902.
57. Rankin G. Neurasthenia: the wear and tear of life. Br Med J 1903; 1:1017–20.
58. Ash E. Nervous breakdown: the disease of our age. Med Times 1909; 37:35–54.
59. Muscio B. Is a fatigue test possible? Br J Psychol 1921; 12:31–46.
60. Meyer A. Discontent—a psychobiological problem of hygiene. (1919). In: Winters E, ed. The collected papers of Adolf Meyer. Baltimore: Johns Hopkins Press, 1962:383–400.
61. Donley J. On neurasthenia as a disintegration of personality. J Abnorm Psychol 1906; 1:55–68.
62. Brock A. "Ergotherapy" in neurasthenia. Edinb Med J 1911; pp 430–4.
63. Glorieaux. Neurasthenia among the working classes. J Nerv Ment Dis 1906; 33:607.
64. Savill T. Clinical lectures on neurasthenia. London: Henry J Glaisher, 1906.
65. Pritchard W. The American disease: an interpretation. Can J Med Surg 1905; 18:10–22.
66. Sicherman B. The uses of a diagnosis: doctors, patients and neurasthenia. J Hist Med 1977; 32:33–54.
67. Gay P. The bourgeois experience. Victoria to Freud. volume 2; the tender passion. London: Oxford University Press, 1986.
68. Leubuscher P, Bibrowicz W. Die neurasthenie in arbeitkreisen. Dtsch Med Wochenscr 1905; 31:820–4.
69. Iscouesco. De la neurasthénie des pauvrès. Bull Méd 1905; 19:359. Reviewed by Feindel, Rev Neurol 1905; 2:732.
70. Charcot J. Leçons du mardi a la Salpêtrière. Progrès médical. Paris: Lecrosniew & Babe, 1889.
71. Jelliffe S, Clark L. The work of a neurological dispensary clinic. J Nerv Ment Dis 1903; 30:482–8.
72. Stedman H. The public obligations of the neurologist. J Nerv Ment Dis 1906; 33:489–99.
73. Schwab S. Neurasthenia among the garment workers. Bull Am Econ Assoc 1911; 4th series, no 2:265–70.
74. Burr C. Neurasthenia. The traumatic neuroses and psychoses. In: Osler W, McCrae T, eds. A system of medicine. London: Frowde, 1910:721–38.
75. Hurry J. The vicious circles of neurasthenia and their treatment. London: Churchill, 1914.
76. Freud S. (1895). On the grounds for detaching a particular syndrome from neurasthenia under the description "anxiety neurosis." standard edition, vol 3. Strachey J, ed. London: Hogarth Press, 87–115.
77. Berrios G. Obsessional disorders during the nineteenth century: terminological and classificatory issues. In: Bynum W, Porter R, Shepherd M, eds. The anatomy of madness; essays in the history of psychiatry. London: Tavistock, 1985:166–87.
78. Jones E. The life and work of Sigmund Freud. London: Penguin, 1961.

79. Starr M. The toxic origin of neurasthenia and melancholia. Boston Med Surg J 1901; 144:563.

80. De Fleury M. Les grands symptômes neurasthéniques (pathogénie et traitement). Paris: Germer Balliere, 1901.

81. Dana C. The partial passing of neurasthenia. Boston Med Surg J 1904; 60:339–44.

82. Kinnier-Wilson S. Medical Society of London: Discussion of neurasthenia. Lancet 1913; 2:1542–4.

83. Stoddart W. Mind and its disorders: a textbook for students and practitioners of medicine. 5th ed. London: H Lewis, 1926.

84. Walton O. Proceedings of the Boston Neurological Society. J Nerv Ment Dis 1906; 33:279.

85. Mitchell SW. The evolution of the rest treatment. J Nerv Men Dis 1904; 31:368–73.

86. Playfair W. Notes on the systematic treatment of nerve prostration and hysteria connected with uterine disease. Lancet 1881; 1:857–9, 949–50, 991–2, 1029–30.

87. Shorter E. Private clinics in Central Europe 1850–1933. Soc Hist Med 1990; 3:159–95.

88. Ziemssen H. Neurasthenia and its treatment. In: Clinical lectures on subjects connected with medicine and surgery. London: New Sydenham Society, 1894:53–86.

89. Wood A. The fashionable diseases: women's complaints and their treatment in nineteenth century America. J Interdisciplinary Hist 1973; 4:25–52.

90. Cayleff S. Prisoners of their own feebleness: women, nerves and Western medicine—a historical overview. Soc Sci Med 1988; 26:1199–208.

91. Dutil A. Neurasthénie. In: Ballet G, ed. Traite de pathologie mentale. Paris: Octave Doin, 1903:842–50.

92. Drummond D. The mental origin of neurasthenia, and its bearing on treatment. Br Med J 1907; 2:1813–6.

93. Waterman G. The treatment of fatigue states. J Abnorm Psychol 1909; 4:128–39.

94. Earnest E. S Weir Mitchell: novelist and physician. Philadelphia: University of Pennsylvania Press, 1950:180.

95. Dutil A. Neurasthénie, ou la maladie de Beard. In: Charcot J, Bouchard E, Brissaud E, eds. Traite de médicine. vol 6. Paris: G Masson, 1894:1281–301.

96. Arndt R. Neurasthenia. In: Tuke D, ed. Dictionary of psychological medicine. vol 2. London: J Churchill, 1892:840–50.

97. Taylor J. Management of exhaustion states in men. Int Clin 1907; 17:36–50.

98. Hall H. The systematic use of work as a remedy in neurasthenia and allied conditions. Boston Med Surg J 1905; 152:29–31.

99. Henderson D. The evolution of psychiatry in Scotland. Edinburgh: Livingstone, 1964:250.

100. Weisenburg T. The Weir Mitchell rest cure forty years ago and today. Arch Neurol Psychiatry 1925; 14:384–9.

101. Menninger K. The abuse of rest in psychiatry. JAMA 1944; 125:1083–7.

102. Browning W. Is there such a disease as neurasthenia? A discussion and classification of the many conditions that appear to be grouped under that head. NY State J Med 1911; 11:7–17.

103. Diller T. The psychoneuroses: how shall we look at them today? JAMA 1917; 69:956–8.
104. Peterson F. Neurasthenia. In: Cecil R, ed. A textbook of medicine. Philadelphia: WB Saunders, 1927:1419–26.
105. Fourness-Brice J. Medical etiquette on board ship. Br Med J 1880; 1:238;
106. Crichton Browne J. Dr Beard's experiments in hypnosis. Br Med J 1881; 2:378–9.
107. Clark A. Some observations concerning what is called neurasthenia. Lancet 1886; 1:1–2.
108. Playfair W. Some observations concerning what is called neurasthenia. Br Med J 1886; 2:853–5.
109. Gowers W. A manual of diseases of the nervous system. volume 2. 2nd ed. London: Churchill, 1888:960.
110. Gowers W. A manual of diseases of the nervous system. vol 1. 3rd ed. London: Churchill, 1899:668.
111. Ireland W. Review of "the treatment of neurasthenia; Proust and Ballet." J Men Sci 1907; 48:548–9.
112. The definition and treatment of neurasthenia. Lancet 1913; 2:1557–8.
113. Gosling F, Ray J. The right to be sick. J Soc Hist 1986; 20:251–67.
114. Althaus J. On failure of brain power (encephalasthenia); its nature and treatment. 5th ed. London: Longmans, Green & Co, 1898.
115. Mitchell Clarke J. Hysteria and neurasthenia. London: The Bodley Head, 1905.
116. Playfair W. Neurasthenia—treatment. In: Tuke D, ed. Dictionary of psychological medicine. London: J Churchill, 1892:850–7.
117. Brill A. Diagnostic errors in neurasthenia. Med Rev 1930; 36:122–9.
118. Reynolds E. Hysteria and neurasthenia. Br Med J 1923; 2:1193–5.
119. Mott F. War neuroses and shell shock. London: Hodder & Stoughton, 1919.
120. Risien Russell J. The treatment of neurasthenia. Lancet 1913; 2:1453–6.
121. Hallock F. The sanatorium treatment of neurasthenia and the need of a colony sanatorium for the nervous poor. Bost Med Surg J 1911; 44:73–7.
122. Review of Otto Binswanger: the pathology and treatment of neurasthenia. Br Med J 1897; 1:920–1.
123. Madden H. On nervousness. Mon Homeopath Rev 1868; 12:211–21.
124. Nerves and nervousness. Spectator 1894; 72:11–2.
125. Edes R. The New England invalid. Boston Med Surg J 1895; 133:53–7.
126. Myerson A. Anhedonia. Am J Psychiatry 1922; 2:87–103.
127. Ross T. The common neuroses. 2nd ed. London: Edward Arnold, 1937.
128. Blumer G. The coming of psychasthenia. J Nerv Ment Dis 1906; 33:336–53.
129. Bleuler E. Textbook of psychiatry. (Brill A, trans). New York: Macmillan, 1924:557–9.
130. Tinel J. Conceptions et traitement des états neurasthéniques. Paris: JB Bailliere et Fils, 1941.
131. Adams R, Victor M. Principles of neurology. 3rd ed. New York: McGraw-Hill, 1985.
132. Buzzard E. The dumping ground of neurasthenia. Lancet 1930; 1:1–4.
133. Tredgold A. Neurasthenia and insanity. Practitioner 1911; 86:84–95.
134. Gosling F. Before Freud: neurasthenia and the American medical community, 1870–1910. Springfield: University of Illinois Press, 1987.

135. Cronin A. Adventures in two worlds. London: Victor Gollancz, 1952.
136. Grob G. The inner world of American psychiatry; 1890–1940. New Brunswick, NJ: Rutgers University Press, 1985.
137. Culpin M. Recent advances in the study of the psychoneuroses. London: Churchill, 1931.
138. Dicks H. Neurasthenia: toxic and traumatic. Lancet 1933; 2:683–6.
139. Kleinman A. Neurasthenia and depression: a study of somatisation and culture in China. Cult Med Psychiatr 1982; 6:117–90.
140. Paul O. Da Costa's syndrome or neurocirculatory asthenia. Br Heart J 1987; 58:306–15.
141. MacKenzie J. Soldier's heart. Br Med J 1916; 1:117–20.
142. Wood P. Diseases of the heart and circulation. 3rd ed. London: Eyre & Spottiswoode, 1968:1075.
143. Rosen S, King J, Wilkinson J, Nixon P. Is chronic fatigue syndrome synonymous with effort syndrome? J R Soc Med 1990; 83:761–4.
144. Singer M, Arnold C, Fitzgerald M, Madden L, von Legat C. Hypoglycaemia: a controversial illness in US society. Med Anthropol 1984; 8:1–35.
145. Straus S. History of chronic fatigue syndrome. Rev Infect Dis 1991; 13 (suppl 1):82–7.
146. Stewart D. The changing face of somatisation. Psychosomatics 1990; 31:153–8.
147. Stewart D. Emotional disorders misdiagnosed as physical illness: environmental hypersensitivity, candidiasis hypersensitivity and chronic fatigue syndrome. Int J Ment Health 1990; 19:56–68.
148. Crook W. Chronic fatigue syndrome and the yeast connection. Jackson, TN: Professional Books, 1992.
149. Black D, Raithe A, Goldstein R. Environmental illness: a controlled study of 26 subjects with "20th century disease." JAMA 1990; 264:3166–70.
150. Bennett R. Searching for the yeast connection. N Engl J Med 1990; 323:1766–7.
151. Young P. Two cases of neurasthenia of long standing successfully treated by the Weir Mitchell method. Edinb Clin Pathol J 1884; 47:905–9.
152. Craig M. Nerve exhaustion. London: J Churchill, 1922:141.
153. Lane C. The mental element in the etiology of neurasthenia. J Nerv Ment Dis 1906; 33:463–6.
154. Streckler E. Review of Robertson: the infective factors in neurasthenia. Arch Neurol Psychiatr 1920; 3:449.
155. Reiter H. Uber eine bisher unerkannte spirochateninfection (spirochaetosis arthritica). Dtsch Med Wochenschr 1916; 42:1535–47.
156. Benjamin J, Hoyt R. Disability following postvaccinal (yellow fever) hepatitis: a study of 200 patients manifesting delayed convalescence. JAMA 1945; 128:319–24.
157. Frank J. Emotional reactions of American soldiers to an unfamiliar disease. Am J Psychiatry 1946; 102:631–40.
158. Evans C. Chronic brucellosis. JAMA 1934; 103:665.
159. Evans C. Brucellosis in the United States. Am J Public Health 1947; 37:139–51.
160. Spinks W. What is chronic brucellosis? Ann Intern Med 1951; 35:358–74.

161. Cluff L, Trever R, Imboden J, Canter A. Brucellosis. II. Medical aspects of delayed convalescence. Arch Intern Med 1959; 103:398–405.
162. Imboden J, Canter A, Cluff L. Brucellosis. III. Psychologic aspects of delayed convalescence. Arch Intern Med 1959; 103:406–14.
163. Eisenberg L. The social construction of mental illness. Psychol Med 1988; 18:1–9.
164. A new clinical entity? Lancet 1956; 1:789–90.
165. Parish J. Early outbreaks of "epidemic neuromyasthenia." Postgrad Med J 1978; 54:711–7.
166. Hyde B. A bibliography of ME/CFS epidemics. In: The clinical and scientific basis of ME. Ottawa: The Nightingale Research Foundation, 1992:176–186.
167. Aronowitz R. From myalgic encephalitis to yuppie flu: a history of chronic fatigue syndromes. In: Rosenberg C, Golden J, eds. Framing disease. New Brunswick, NJ: Rutgers University Press, 1992:155–81.
168. Crowley N, Nelson M, Stovin S. Epidemiological aspects of an outbreak of encephalomyelitis at the Royal Free Hospital. J Hyg 1957; 55:102–22.
169. Acheson E. The clinical syndrome variously called benign myalgic encephalomyelitis, Iceland disease and epidemic neuromyasthenia. Am J Med 1959; 26:569–95.
170. Bigler M, Nielsen J. Poliomyelitis in Los Angeles in 1934: neurologic characteristics of the disease in adults. Bull LA Neurol Soc 1937; 2:47–58.
171. McEvedy C, Beard A. Royal Free epidemic of 1955: a reconsideration. Br Med J 1970; 1:7–11.
172. McEvedy C, Beard A. Concept of benign myalgic encephalomyelitis. Br Med J 1970; 1:11–5.
173. Hare M. Epidemic malaise. Br Med J 1970; 1:299.
174. Mausner J, Gezon H. Report on a phantom epidemic of gonorrhoea. Am J Epidemiol 1967; 85:320–31.
175. Paul J. A history of poliomyelitis. New Haven: Yale University Press, 1971.
176. Daikos G, Garzonis S. Paleologue A, Bousvaros G, Papadoyannakis N. Benign myalgic encephalomyelitis: an outbreak in a nurses' school in Athens. Lancet 1959; 1:693–6.
177. Ramsay A. Encephalomyelitis in northwest London. An endemic infection simulating poliomyelitis and hysteria. Lancet 1957; 2:1196–200.
178. Hill R, Cheetham R, Wallace H. Epidemic myalgic encephalomyelopathy: the Durban outbreak. Lancet 1959; 1:689–93.
179. May P, Donnan S, Ashton J, Ogilvie M, Rolles C. Personality and medical perception in benign myalgic encephalomyelitis. Lancet 1980; 2:1122–4.
180. Jenkins R. Introduction. In: Jenkins R, Mowbray J, eds. Post-viral fatigue syndrome. Chichester: John Wiley & Sons, 1991:3–34.
181. Hope Pool J, Walton J, Brewis E, Uldall P, Wright A, Gardner P. Benign myalgic encephalomyelitis in Newcastle upon Tyne. Lancet 1961; 1:733–7.
182. McEvedy C, Beard A. A controlled follow up of cases involved in an epidemic of "benign myalgic encephalomyelitis." Br J Psychiatry 1973; 122:141–50.
183. Briggs N, Levine P. Neurologic manifestations of chronic fatigue syndrome: contemporary implications of an historic perspective. Paper presented at International CFS/ME Conference, Albany, New York, Oct 3–4th, 1992.

184. Dowsett E, Ramsay A, McCartney R, Bell E. Myalgic encephalomyelitis—a persistent enteroviral infection? Postgrad Med J 1990; 66:526–30.
185. Poskanzer D. Epidemic malaise. Br Med J 1970; 2:420–1.
186. Howells B. Epidemic malaise. Br Med J 1970; 1:300.
187. Ramsay A. Benign myalgic encephalomyelitis. Br J Psychiatry 1973; 122:618–9.
188. Macy J, Allen E. Justification of the diagnosis of chronic nervous exhaustion. Ann Intern Med 1933–34; 7:861–7.
189. Alvarez W. What is wrong with the patient who feels tired, weak and toxic? N Engl J Med 1935; 212:96–104.
190. Allan F. The clinical management of weakness and fatigue. JAMA 1945; 127:957–60.
191. Wilbur D. Clinical management of the patient with fatigue and nervousness. JAMA 1949; 141:1199–204.
192. Ware N. Suffering and the social construction of illness: the delegitimation of illness experience in chronic fatigue syndrome. Med Anthropol Quart (in press).
193. Jones J, Ray C, Minnich L, Hicks M, Kibler R, Lucas D. Evidence for active Epstein–Barr virus infection in patients with persistent, unexplained illnesses; elevated anti-early antigen antibody. Ann Intern Med 1985; 102:1–7.
194. Straus S, Tosato G, Armstrong G, et al. Persisting illness and fatigue in adults with evidence of Epstein–Barr virus infection. Ann Intern Med 1985; 102:7–16.
195. Tobi M, Morag A, Ravid Z, et al. Prolonged atypical illness associated with serological evidence of persistent Epstein–Barr infection. Lancet 1982; 1:61–64.
196. Tobi M, Straus S. Chronic Epstein–Barr disease: a workshop held by the National Institute of Allergy and Infectious Diseases. Ann Intern Med 1985; 103:951–2.
197. Straus S. The chronic mononucleosis syndrome. J Infect Dis 1988; 157:405–12.
198. Jones J, Straus S. Chronic Epstein–Barr virus infection. Annu Rev Med 1987; 38:195–209.
199. Charatan F. Chronic fatigue in the US. Br Med J 1990; 301:1236.
200. Chronic fatigue: all in the mind? Consumer Rep 1990; Oct:671–5.
201. A mysterious illness receives recognition. Awake 1992; Aug 22.
202. Holmes G, Kaplan J, Gantz N, et al. Chronic fatigue syndrome: a working case definition. Ann Intern Med 1988; 108:387–9.
203. Lloyd A, Wakefield D, Boughton C, Dwyer J. What is myalgic encephalomyelitis? Lancet 1988; 1:1286–7.
204. Sharpe M, Archard L, Banatvala J, et al. Chronic fatigue syndrome: guidelines for research. J R Soc Med 1991; 84:118–21.
205. Wookey C. Myalgic encephalomyelitis, post-viral fatigue syndrome and how to cope with it. London: Chapman & Hall, 1988.
206. Franklin M, Sullivan J. The new mystery fatigue epidemic. ME What is it? Have you got it? How to get better. London: Century, 1989.
207. Smith D. Understanding ME. London: Robinson Publishing, 1989.
208. Feiden K. Hope and help for chronic fatigue syndrome. New York: Prentice Hall, 1990.
209. Johnson H. Journey into fear. The growing nightmare of Epstein Barr virus. Rolling Stone, 1987; Jul 30.
210. Wessely S. Mass hysteria: two syndromes? Psychol Med 1987; 17:109–20.

211. Stevens G. The 1934 epidemic of poliomyelitis in Southern California. Am J Public Health 1934; 12:1213–4.

212. Holmes G, Kaplan J, Stewart J, Hunt B, Pinsky P. Schonberger S. A cluster of patients with a chronic mononucleosis-like syndrome. Is Epstein–Barr virus the cause? JAMA 1987; 257:2297–303.

213. Boly W. Raggedy Ann town. Hippocrates 1987; Jul/Aug:31–40.

214. Digon A, Goicoechea A, Moraza M. Chronic fatigue syndrome. J Neurol Neurosurg Psychiatry 1992; 55:85.

215. Ramsay A. "Epidemic neuromyasthenia" 1955–1978. Postgrad Med J 1978; 54:718–21.

216. Holt G. Epidemic neuromyasthenia: the sporadic form. Am J Med Sci 1965; 98–112.

217. Price J. Myalgic encephalomyelitis. Lancet 1961; 1:737–8.

218. Compston N. An outbreak of encephalomyelitis in the Royal Free Hospital group, London, 1955. Postgrad Med J 1978; 554:722–4.

219. Behan P, Behan W. The postviral fatigue syndrome. CRC Crit Rev Neurobiol 1988; 42:157–78.

220. Sharpe M, Hawton K. Seagroatt V, Pasvol G. Follow up of patients with fatigue presenting to an infectious diseases clinic. Br Med J 1992; 305:347–52.

221. Behan P, Behan W, Bell E. The postviral fatigue syndrome—an analysis of the findings in 50 cases. J Infect 1985; 10:211–22.

222. Miller N, Carmichael H, Calder B, Behan P, Bell E, McCartney R, Hall F. Antibody to Coxsackie B virus in diagnosing postviral fatigue syndrome. Br Med J 1991; 302:140–3.

223. Gow J, Behan W, Clements G, Woodall C, Riding M, Behan P. Enteroviral RNA sequences detected by polymerase chain reaction in muscle of patients with postviral fatigue syndrome. Br Med J 1991; 302:692–6.

224. Yousef G, Bell E, Mann G, et al. Chronic enterovirus infection in patients with postviral fatigue syndrome. Lancet 1988; 1:146–50.

225. Merry P. Management of symptoms of myalgic encephalomyelitis. In: Jenkins R, Mowbray J, eds. Postviral fatigue syndrome. Chichester: John Wiley & Sons, 1991:281–96.

226. de la Torre J, Borrow P, Oldstone M. Viral persistence and disease: cytopathology in the absence of cytolysis. Br Med Bull 1991; 47:838–51.

227. White P. Fatigue syndrome: neurasthenia revived. Br Med J 1989; 298:1199–200.

228. Greenberg D. Neurasthenia in the 1980s: chronic mononucleosis, chronic fatigue syndrome and anxiety and depressive disorders. Psychosomatics 1990; 31:129–37.

229. Wessely S. Old wine in new bottles; neurasthenia and "ME." Psychol Med 1990; 20:35–53.

230. Abbey S, Garfinkel P. Neurasthenia and chronic fatigue syndrome: the role of culture in the making of a diagnosis. Am J Psychiatr 1991; 148:1638–46.

231. Ware N, Kleinman A. Culture and somatic experience: the social course of illness in neurasthenia and chronic fatigue syndrome. Psychosom Med 1992; 54:546–60.

232. Shepherd C. Living with ME: a self-help guide. London: Heinemann, 1989.

233. Steincamp J. Overload: beating ME. London: Fontana, 1989.

234. Dawes B, Downing D. Why M.E.? A guide to combatting post-viral illness. London: Grafton, 1989.

235. Payer L. Medicine and culture; varieties of treatment in the United States, England, West Germany and France. New York: Henry Holt, 1988.
236. Allen J. Myalgic encephalomyelitis. Homeopathy 1992; 42:152–4.
237. Iverson M, Presse C. CFIDS and AIDS; facing facts. CFIDS Chron, 1990; spring/summer:159–162; Christopher Street; Issue 131; Volume 11, No 11.
238. Regush N. AIDS, words from the front. Spin 1990; 6:69–70.
239. MacIntyre A. ME: post-viral fatigue syndrome: how to live with it. London: Unwin, 1989.
240. La fatigue: une vraie maladie. Nouvel Observ, 1992; 13–19 Feb.
241. Althaus J. On cerebrine alpha and myelin alpha in the treatment of certain neuroses. Lancet, 1893; Dec 2.
242. Goldstein J. Chronic fatigue syndrome: the struggle for health. A diagnostic and treatment guide for patients and their physicians. Beverley Hills: Chronic Fatigue Syndrome Institute, 1990.
243. Hilgers A, Krueger G, Lembke U, Ramon A. Postinfectious chronic fatigue syndrome; case history of thirty-five patients in Germany. In Vivo 1991; 5:201–6.
244. Could your back hold the clue to "Yuppie flu"? Daily Mail 1992; Dec 2.
245. Karno M, Hoffman R. The pseudoanergic syndrome. In: Kiev A, ed. Somatic manifestations of depressive disorders. Amsterdam: Excerpta Medica 1974; 352:55–85.
246. Eichner E. Chronic fatigue syndrome: searching for the cause and treatment. Physician Sports Med 1989; 17:142–52.
247. See for example the reviews in the St Louis Clin Rec (1880; 7:92–4); Am J Insanity (1880; 36:520–6); St Louis Clin Rec (1881; 8:122–4); J Nerv Men Dis (1881; 8:773–7); Med Rec (1881; 20:296–7); Boston Med Surg J (1881; 105:162–3).
248. La psychothérapie chez les neurasthénique. Encephale 1907; 2:266–7; Pathogenie des état neurasthénique. Encephale 1908; 3:525–31.
249. Allan F. The differential diagnosis of weakness and fatigue. N Eng J Med 1944; 231:414–8.
250. Lechky O. Life insurance MDs sceptical when chronic fatigure syndrome diagnosed. Can Med Assoc J 1990; 143:413–5.
251. Ostrom N. It's a dirty little war: proponents of a "psychoneurotic" cause of CIDS try again. Christopher Street 1989; 1:32–3.
252. Collee J. A doctor writes. Observer, 1991; 25 Aug.
253. Brodsky C. Depression and chronic fatigue in the workplace. Primary Care 1991; 18:381–96.
254. Urquhart A. Austrian retrospect: review of the writings of Professor Benedikt of Vienna. J Ment Sci 1889; 34:276–81.
255. Yellowlees H. Abnormal fatigability. In: Early mental disease. Lancet (extra number) 1912; no 2.
256. Beevor C. Diseases of the nervous system: a handbook for students and practitioners. London; H K Lewis, 1898.
257. Mitchell J. Diagnosis and treatment of neurasthenia. Johns Hopkins Hosp Bull 1908; 19:41–3.
258. Experiences of antidepressants. Interaction; J ME Action 1993; 12:37.

2

Defining Chronic Fatigue Syndrome

Dedra Buchwald
University of Washington and Harborview Medical Center,
Seattle, Washington

> Disease is very old and nothing about it has changed. It is we who change as we learn to recognize what was formerly imperceptible.
>
> J. M. Charcot

Numerous diseases have appeared for the first time in the last century. New causes for old problems also have been recognized, ranging from iatrogenic to environmental. However, for most diseases, Charcot's astute observation still rings true. Rather, it is clinicians and researchers who recognize similarities and differences, define syndromes, and begin to understand disease processes that were previously imperceptible. The evidence presented in this chapter suggests that, although formal diagnostic criteria have been only recently formulated, chronic fatigue syndrome (CFS) is unlikely to be a new entity. Several clinical syndromes, both sporadic and epidemic, have been described previously by clinicians and researchers that, in retrospect, appear to share certain features. These include neurasthenia, benign myalgic encephalomyelitis, and chronic Epstein–Barr virus (EBV) infection. The purpose of this chapter is, first, to review the history of chronically fatiguing illnesses and, second, to summarize, compare, and contrast the three case definitions for CFS currently in use around the world.

It has been said that "interest in fatigue is as old as medicine itself" [1]. Indeed, one of the first descriptions of a chronically fatiguing illness was penned by practitioners of traditional Chinese medicine almost 2000 years ago. In the classic Chinese medical text, *Shang Han Lun*, a condition resembling CFS known as Shao Yin illness (including a hot and cold subtype) is described [2]. In traditional Chinese medicine, the body is viewed as a system of dynamic interactions between intrinsic body parts and the extrinsic environment, conceptualized as Yin and Yang. Shao Yin illness is viewed as one of many causes of fatigue. The hallmark of patients with Shao Yin illness is their "tendency to always fall asleep" and a feeble, weak pulse. Other symptoms characteristic of Shao Yin illness that have a remarkable resemblance to CFS are sore throat, agitation, fear of cold, body aches, painful joints, "heaviness" in the body, abdominal distension, constipation, and insomnia. In more recent times a similar illness, known in Western terminology as neurasthenia, has reemerged in Chinese medicine [3].

NEURASTHENIA

In the United States and Europe, great interest in fatigue was spawned in the late 1880s with George Beard's description of neurasthenia or "nervous exhaustion" [4,5]. Beard, an American neurologist and himself a sufferer, popularized the concept of neurasthenia as an organic illness [4,5]. Although he never proposed a case definition in the epidemiological sense, Beard described five essential components of neurasthenia. These five characteristics were first, an overwhelming exhaustion affecting both the body and mind. Second, it was an organic condition, meaning that the condition derived from problems with the body and not of the mind. Third, the major form of treatment was rest. Fourth, neurasthenia was more likely to occur in the educated, higher socioeconomic classes and, lastly, it resulted primarily from environmental causes. As in CFS today, Beard [4] and others noted that physical signs were "conspicuous by their absence" [6]. Somatic symptoms were ubiquitous; those involving cardiac and gastrointestinal function, temperature regulation, alterations of sensory functions, paresthesias, cognitive dysfunction, and pain syndromes were particularly prominent [4,5]. In a fashion reminiscent of the current tendency to categorize types of CFS (e.g., postviral versus insidious onset, mental versus physical fatigue), Beard further defined subtypes of neurasthenia based on symptomatology [4]. *Cerebrasthenia*, or cerebral exhaustion, was typified by physical or emotional symptoms, such as scalp tenderness, sensory disorders, and emotional distress. In contrast, *myelasthenia*, or spinal exhaustion, was characterized by musculoskeletal symptoms, sensitivity to temperature and climatic changes, and sexual difficulties.

Despite Beard's widespread influence, within several decades of its appearance in the medical vocabulary, neurasthenia virtually disappeared as a diagnosis and as an area worthy of scientific inquiry [1]. In a series of intriguing analyses, contemporary scholars have examined the popularity and eventual decline of diagnoses such as neurasthenia in the context of cultural and psychosocial factors, social change, and contemporary attitudes of mental illness [1,7–9]. These authors also observed parallels between neurasthenia and modern-day fatigue syndromes, including similarities in social setting, symptoms, and treatment. Despite its relegation to relative diagnostic obscurity, neurasthenia continued to be in the medical lexicon through the publication of the *Diagnostic and Statistical Manual of Mental Disorders*, 2nd edition (*DSM-II*) in 1968. Since the publication of the third edition in 1980, neurasthenia has been replaced by three diagnoses: panic disorder, generalized anxiety disorder, and dysthymia [10].

CHRONIC POSTINFECTIOUS ILLNESSES

In the middle of this century, several chronically fatiguing illnesses were attributed to persistent infections. Cases of sporadic onset usually followed acute illnesses with known pathogens. Isaacs and others reported patients who complained of symptoms that persisted following acute infectious mononucleosis [11–13]. These patients were generally felt to have recurrent or "chronic mononucleosis" although many did not satisfy existing clinical, hematological, or serological criteria for infectious mononucleosis, either at presentation or during their prolonged convalescence [11,12]. Likewise, nonspecific symptoms persisting after documented brucellosis, occasionally in conjunction with elevated brucella titers, were attributed to "chronic brucellosis" [14]. This diagnosis was cast into doubt by an elegant study of 24 subjects recovering from brucellosis in which Imboden and colleagues observed that delayed recovery following acute brucellosis was strongly associated with psychological distress and socioeconomic status [14].

In addition to these sporadic cases of fatiguing illnesses, there were at least 23 so-called epidemics of fatiguing illnesses from around the world reported from 1934 to 1958 [reviewed in 15]. These outbreaks had as many manifestations as names: Icelandic disease, Akureyri disease, Royal Free disease, epidemic neuromyesthenia, benign myalgic encephalomyelitis, epidemic vegetative neuritis, acute infective encephalomyelitis, and so on. However, the signs and symptoms of these epidemic fatiguing illnesses are, in many respects, similar to contemporary descriptions of CFS.

Perhaps, the most notorious of these epidemics occurred in 1955 at the Royal Free Hospital and resulted in the labeling of a supposedly new disease entity called benign myalgic encephalomyelitis (or myalgic encephalomyelitis [ME], as it is known in the United Kingdom) [16], although several similar epidemics had occurred previously (reviewed in 17–19). The original literature concerning the Royal Free Hospital outbreak, as well as the predecessors and successors to that outbreak, described an acute disease that was presumably infectious and contagious. Although the onset of illness was extremely variable, it was often preceded by a gastrointestinal or upper respiratory infection. The initial constitutional symptoms commonly evolved into neurological ones, with features reminiscent of acute poliomyelitis. Pain the the back, neck, and extremities; motor weakness; and muscle spasm were frequent and usually were not associated with the loss of deep tendon reflexes or muscle wasting characteristic of polio. The spectrum of presentation ranged from a mild systemic illness, to a meningoencephalitic one, with ocular palsies and upper motor neuron signs. Fatigue was common, but did not hold the prominent position among symptoms that it does in CFS. Many patients exhibited a prolonged convalescence characterized by depression, fatigue, autonomic disturbances, and a propensity to relapse [17–19].

Despite their apparent similarities, it is not possible to conclude unequivocally that each of these epidemic fatiguing illnesses represent the same pathophysiological process, or even a single syndrome. This is, in part, because the clinical syndromes were rarely, if ever, defined in any rigorous fashion. Rather, they were reported descriptively across decades and continental borders, without the benefit of a case definition. Acheson reviewed 14 epidemics and acknowledged the "difficulties in defining a disorder from which no deaths have occurred, and for which no causative infective or toxic agent has been discovered" [20]. He asserted that recognition had to depend on clinical and epidemiological patterns. Thus, although not strictly a case definition, he retrospectively noted that the outbreaks reported in his day shared the following clinical and epidemiological features: (1) headache; (2) myalgia; (3) paresis; (4) symptoms or signs other than paresis suggestive of damage to the brain, spinal cord, or peripheral nerves; (5) mental symptoms; (6) low or absent fever; and (7) no mortality. In addition, the tendency to affect women, a predominantly normal cerebrospinal fluid, and a relapsing course were present in virtually every outbreak. Thus, the various epidemics shared clinical and demographic features that permitted their inclusion under the rubric of "benign myalgic encephalomyelitis," despite the lack of a formal case definition that could have been applied prospectively to individual outbreaks.

Several facts concerning these outbreaks suggest that at least some cases would not meet current criteria for CFS. For example, an intriguing aspect of Henderson's work is that of the 23 outbreaks he reviewed, only in 10 was fatigability or malaise noted [15]. Likewise, only in eight of the outbreaks was protracted disability prominent enough to deserve comment. Still, Henderson remarked that the ". . . apparent similarity in the courses of illness, the common nature of most symptoms and signs, the remarkable paucity of abnormal laboratory determinations and the similar epidemiologic characteristics suggest a nosologic, if not etiologic, association among outbreaks" [15].

In 1970, two psychiatrists reexamined the case notes of patients from the Royal Free Hospital outbreak and reviewed reports of other similar outbreaks [21,22]. Their provocative conclusion was that there was a strong element of mass hysteria in many of these outbreaks. Subsequent to that work, with the exception of a widely publicized outbreak in the Lake Tahoe, Nevada, area in the mid-1980s [23], there have been virtually no published reports of epidemic forms of benign myalgic encephalitis or similarly fatiguing illnesses.

CHRONIC EPSTEIN–BARR VIRUS INFECTION

Interest in sporadic illnesses characterized by persistent fatigue was reawakened in the mid-1980s. In 1985, a pair of articles by Jones and Straus and their colleagues [24,25] in the *Annals of Internal Medicine* garnered much attention from the scientific and clinical community, as well as the media and patients. These reports described in great detail the clinical and laboratory features of a syndrome that appeared to bear some relation to mononucleosis. Symptoms included persistent or recurrent fatigue, sleep disturbances, headache, myalgia, depression, decreased memory, confusion, inability to concentrate, lymphadenopathy, and sore throat. Many patients were disabled. Although serological findings thought to be consistent with reactivation of EBV were frequent, few patients had any objective physical findings. Both investigators were cautious in interpreting their results, suggesting that the apparent viral reactivation might well represent an epiphenomenon.

Nevertheless, the lay press, as well as patients and physicians everywhere, seized on the diagnosis of chronic EBV infection and the belief the syndrome could be reliably diagnosed by viral serological tests. Elevated EBV titers, in particular antibodies to early antigens and the viral capsid antigen IgG, rapidly became the serological hallmark of chronic EBV infection. Subsequent studies, however, failed to confirm the association of elevated EBV antibody levels with chronic fatigue. Evidence from seroepidemiological studies indicated that elevated antibody levels were present in healthy, nonfatigued individuals [26,27]. Likewise, clinic-based investigations failed to support the association of EBV with chronic fatigue. For example, several studies failed to document differences in antibody levels to EBV antigens between fatigued and age- and sex-matched nonfatigued patients [28,29]. Finally, in a study comparing fatigued patients with and without elevated EBV titers, no significant differences were found in a variety of clinical factors [30].

Public awareness and interest in chronic fatigue were fueled further by media coverage and the report, in 1987, of a cluster of patients in the Lake Tahoe area of Nevada and California, with a mononucleosislike syndrome [31]. To determine the role of viruses, in particular EBV, Holmes and co-workers tested over 100 patients and a smaller number of control subjects for antibodies to EBV and other herpesviruses. Although a small group of the most severely affected patients appeared to have higher antibody titers against several herpesviruses, they concluded that EBV serological studies were not a reliable method for identifying patients. In fact, the serological associations between other viruses tested were as strong or stronger than that for EBV. Despite this additional evidence against the usefulness of EBV serological tests as a means of detecting cases, the illness only became more controversial. The chronic EBV syndrome continued to be diagnosed, often based on little more than the presence of detectable (not elevated) serum EBV antibody titers [32].

CENTERS FOR DISEASE CONTROL CASE DEFINITION

The current definition of CFS used in the United States grew out of the controversies arising from the publications in the *Annals of Internal Medicine* and the initial reports of the epidemic in the Lake Tahoe, Nevada, area. In 1987, an informal working group of public health epidemiologists, academic researchers, and clinicians was convened by the Centers for Disease Control (CDC) to develop a consensus statement on the salient clinical characteristics of the syndrome [32]. This group proposed a working case definition designed to improve the comparability and reproducibility of clinical research and epidemiological studies and to provide a rational basis for evaluating patients with chronic fatigue of unknown cause. Furthermore, they proposed that chronic EBV infection be renamed CFS, thereby removing the implication that EBV is the causal agent and emphasizing the syndrome's most striking feature.

The case definition consists of 2 major and 14 minor criteria—11 symptom and 3 physical criteria (Table 1). A case of CFS must fulfill both major criteria and either 8 of 11 minor symptom criteria or 6 of 11 symptom criteria and at least 2 physical criteria. No laboratory studies are required to make the diagnosis of CFS. The CDC CFS criteria is not empirically based and has never been subjected to rigorous scrutiny.

Problems in Interpretation and Modifications

Among the first problems encountered by researchers in attempting to use the CDC criteria was the difficulty in distinguishing CFS from psychiatric disorders. This difficulty results from the enormous overlap between the symptoms of CFS and those of affective, anxiety, and somatization disorders. For example, a patient reporting fatigue, clearly a prerequisite for CFS, is simultaneously endorsing a symptom of major depression. Symptoms approximating the prerequisite 6 months of fatigue, with a 50% reduction in activity, appear in three *DSM-III-R* diagnoses. Likewise, the 11 minor symptoms of CFS, occur in 23 individual queries and contribute to 4 *DSM-III-R* diagnoses. Thus, patients endorsing symptoms characteristic of CFS are often simultaneously endorsing symptoms of psychiatric disorders. The similarity of CFS symptoms to those of major depression, and the apparently high rate of preexisting psychiatric disorders in patients with CFS, have led some authors to suggest that CFS is simply depression or the modern reincarnation of neurasthenia [1,8,9].

There also has been confusion over the psychiatric exclusion criterion imposed

Table 1   The Centers for Disease Control Working Case Definition of Chronic Fatigue
Syndrome

Both major and either eight minor symptoms *or* six minor symptoms *and* at least two
  physical examination criteria must be present to fulfill the case definition.

Major Criteria

  1. Persistence of relapsing fatigue or easy fatigability that does not resolve with bed
     rest and is severe enough to reduce average daily activity by at least 50% for at
     least 6 months
  2. Other chronic conditions have been satisfactorily excluded, including chronic
     psychiatric illness

Minor Symptom Criteria

  1. Mild fever (37.5°–38.6°C [99.5°–101.4°F] orally) or chills
  2. Sore throat
  3. Posterior cervical, anterior cervical, or axillary lymph node pain
  4. Unexplained generalized muscle weakness
  5. Muscle discomfort or myalgia
  6. Prolonged (at least 24 h) generalized fatigue following previously tolerable levels
     of exercise
  7. New, generalized headaches
  8. Migratory noninflammatory arthralgias
  9. Neuropsychiatric symptoms, photophobia, transient visual scotoma, forgetful-
     ness, excessive irritability, confusion, difficulty thinking, inability to con-
     centrate, depression
  10. Sleep disturbance (hypersomnia or insomnia)
  11. Patient's description of initial onset of symptoms as acute or subacute

Physical Examination Criteria

Must be documented by a physician on at least two occasions, at least 1 month apart:

  1. Low-grade fever (37.6°–38.6°C [99.6°–101.4°F] orally or 37.8°–38.8°C [100.1°–
     101.8°F] rectally)
  2. Nonexudative pharyngitis
  3. Palpable or tender anterior cervical, posterior cervical, or axillary lymph nodes
     (< 2 cm in diameter)

Source: Ref. 32.

by the CDC case definition. This criterion is not explicit and does not identify
clearly which patients and which disorders should be excluded. Until recently,
some investigators excluded only patients with current psychiatric disorders,
others eliminated those with a premorbid history of a psychiatric disorder, and
still other researchers required the absence of any (either current or lifetime)
psychiatric diagnosis to make the diagnosis of CFS.

These problems have resulted in a series of proposed modifications to the CDC case definition in the years since its publication. First, in a letter to the *Annals of Internal Medicine*, several of its original authors suggested that CFS could be diagnosed in the presence of a mood disorder, if patients otherwise met the case definition and if the mood disorder developed after the onset of the chronic fatigue [33]. A further modification was later proposed stating that a history of a psychiatric diagnosis that long predated the onset of fatigue should not necessarily exclude the diagnosis of CFS [34]. This recommendation was based on clinical observations of patients with long-standing mood disorders who went on to develop CFS, some of whom had objective findings, such as abnormal laboratory tests or persistent fevers.

In 1991, a workshop was held at the National Institutes of Health (NIH) to address critical issues in CFS research, including the CDC case definition [35]. The group found, perhaps not surprisingly, that the case definition was not being uniformly applied. Several investigators reported that strict application of the psychiatric history criteria exclusion did not identify a discrete group with CFS. Likewise, patients excluded solely for an insufficient number of symptoms also did not appear to differ in any way from "true" CFS cases. The meeting concluded that a major revision in the CDC criteria was needed, but should not be undertaken until such an effort could be empirically based. Modifications to the psychiatric exclusion, however, were recommended. The revised criteria do not absolutely exclude patients with major depression, panic, generalized anxiety, or somatization disorders. It recommends screening for psychiatric distress and disorders such that patients can be clearly identified in subsequent stratified analyses. Disorders that continue to be grounds for exclusion are schizophrenia, bipolar disorder, psychotic depression, and substance abuse.

In contrast to the controversy surrounding the inclusion or exclusion of patients with psychiatric disorders in the CDC case definition, there has been little discussion of its other exclusions. For example, the classification of patients initially diagnosed with CFS who subsequently develop medical conditions (which would have initially excluded the diagnosis of CFS) has not been adequately addressed in the United States.

Does the Centers for Disease Control Case Definition Work?

There has been relatively little formal evaluation of the CDC case definition. The existing data, although limited, suggest that the case definition does not identify a unique patient group. Komaroff and colleagues examined 204 patients with debilitating fatigue of at least 6-months duration [36]. Signs and symptoms that are not part of the case definition, as well as laboratory tests, were compared in subjects who met the CDC case definition (39%) with findings in those who did not do so (61%). More common among subjects meeting the CDC's criteria

($p < 0.01$) were abdominal pain, nausea, dry mouth, and night sweats. However, for every other sign, symptom, and laboratory test abnormality compared, the rates in the two groups were not significantly different. Moreover, the CDC criteria did not identify a subgroup of patients more likely to have objective evidence of disease. The authors concluded that restricting studies of patients with chronic fatigue to only those fully meeting the CDC criteria may be unwise. Their results suggest that patients with some, but not all, features of the CDC criteria could be included in studies. In such instances, formal analyses should consider them as a separate subset of patients.

In another study, Bates and colleagues examined the results of inexpensive, readily available laboratory studies performed in over 800 patients with chronic fatigue, presenting to an urban tertiary care facility in Boston and an urban county hospital in Seattle, and compared these results with healthy control subjects [37,38]. Cases were more likely than control subjects to have higher than normal levels of immune complexes, immunoglobulin (Ig) G, antinuclear antibodies, and alkaline phosphatase and cholesterol. The presence of immune complexes or elevated immunoglobulin levels identified 48% of patients with CFS and only 6% of control subjects. Similar findings were observed in patients with chronic fatigue of unknown cause not meeting the CDC criteria, suggesting that the more inclusive case definitions may be superior.

In a cross-sectional study, Katon and colleagues compared patients with chronic fatigue with those with rheumatoid arthritis for a variety of measures of psychosocial distress and disability [39]. By using a strict interpretation of the CDC criteria that excluded patients with current psychiatric disorders as well as those taking any medication that could cause fatigue, patients with CFS were indistinguishable from those with chronic fatigue not meeting the CDC criteria. Both groups differed from patients with rheumatoid arthritis on several psychosocial and functional status measures. A second study by these investigators demonstrated that chronically fatigued patients with the highest number of medically unexplained physical symptoms had the most psychiatric morbidity. On the basis of these two investigations, the authors recommended that the case definition for CFS be modified to include patients with fewer physical symptoms, and conversely, to consider excluding those with many unexplained physical complaints [40]. It was their contention that the requirement for many somatic symptoms in the CDC case definition biases subject inclusion toward a higher proportion of individuals with psychiatric illnesses, particularly somatization disorder.

BRITISH CASE DEFINITION

In 1990, researchers and clinicians convened in Oxford, England, to pursue a consensus on guidelines for the future study of CFS [41]. Represented at the meeting were authorities in biochemistry, virology, psychology, neurology, psychiatry, muscle physiology, general practice, immunopathology, magnetic resonance imaging, and anthropology. The British committee tackled a problem unaddressed by prior attempts at defining fatigue syndromes: the meaning of *fatigue* itself. An appropriate research glossary was prepared describing and defining terms that may carry different meanings, but that are often used interchangeably. This thesaurus of fatigue includes symptoms, such as exhaustion, languor, and lassitude. This was a crucial first step, since patients and clinicians alike often do not make subtle, yet important distinctions between weakness, exhaustion, muscle discomfort, sleepiness, and so on. Mental and physical fatigue are both defined as subjective sensations. *Mental fatigue* is characterized by lack of motivation and diminished alertness. In contrast, *physical fatigue* is a lack of energy or strength often perceived to be in the muscles. This subjective definition of physical fatigue is to be distinguished from *physiological fatigue* in which failure to sustain muscle force or power can be objectively measured. Furthermore, it was recommended that for each symptom of interest, information should be collected on its description, relation to exertion, its differential diagnosis, and its severity or frequency rating.

The primary aim of the meeting, however, was to seek agreement among British researchers on recommendations for the conduct and reporting of future studies of patients with chronic fatigue. Specifically, issues addressed included which patients should be considered eligible, how such studies should be approached, and the minimal data that should be reported. The case definition generated by this meeting requires four conditions to be met for inclusion and also specified four exclusionary conditions (Table 2). Similar to the CDC criteria, 6 months of fatigue are required. Symptoms, such as myalgia, mood, and sleep disturbances, may be present, but are not required for the diagnosis. In addition, a postinfectious subtype is distinguished from CFS with other patterns of onset (see Table 2). It is characterized by definite evidence of infection at onset of presentation. Patients' reports are unlikely to be sufficiently reliable. Investigators should state clearly which syndrome is being reported. Affective and anxiety disorders are not grounds for exclusion, although all patients should be assessed for psychiatric morbidity and the results reported. Finally, in contrast with the CDC and Australian criteria, an attempt should be made to measure and state the degree of disability. Specific methods for assessing disability in CFS, however, are not proposed.

AUSTRALIAN CASE DEFINITION

In addition to the differing criteria for CFS currently used in the United States and Britain, still another case definition exists in Australia [42,43]. As in the other definitions, 6 months of fatigue is the principal symptom of the illness. In

Table 2 British Case Definition of Chronic Fatigue Syndrome

To meet criteria an illness must

1. Have fatigue as its principal symptom
2. Be of definite onset (not lifelong)
3. Be severe, disabling, and affect physical and mental functioning
4. Be present at least 50% of the time for at least 6 months

Patients with the following conditions are excluded:

1. Medical conditions known to produce chronic fatigue
2. Current diagnoses of schizophrenia, manic depressive illness, substance abuse, eating disorder, or proved organic brain disease

For the postinfectious subtype to be present, the following conditions are necessary:

1. The illness is present for more than 6 months after onset of infection or after resolution of clinical signs associated with acute infection
2. The infection has been corroborated by clinical signs or laboratory evidence

Source: Ref. 41.

general, the other symptom requirements are similar to those found in the British definition and are not as numerous as those mandated by the CDC criteria (Table 3). One notable exception is the requirement for neuropsychological symptoms, such as impaired memory and concentration of new onset. These mandatory symptoms might be expected to select for a group of individuals with a higher frequency of affective disorders. In contrast with the CDC and British criteria, consideration is given to the presentation of the psychiatric symptoms. For example, a primary depression, rather than CFS, is suggested by certain symptoms, such as weight loss, hopelessness, suicidal ideation, and loss of motivation or pleasure. Likewise, a recurrent history of psychiatric illness in a patient presenting with chronic fatigue may suggest the current symptoms are the result of a recurrence of the psychiatric disorder, not CFS. Schizophrenia, other psychotic illnesses, and bipolar affective disorder are exclusions, and drug or alcohol dependence make CFS very unlikely. A long and complex medical and psychiatric history, with resultant disability that is more severe than would be expected, suggests somatization disorder.

Three subclassifications of CFS are recognized by Australian researchers: a postinfective type, a form of CFS with neurocognitive impairment, and one associated with fibromyalgia. Postinfective cases are characterized by a definite history of an acute onset following an infectious illness. The diagnosis of the preceding illness is based on past records from a physician and an appropriate evaluation. When fatigue occurs following such a well-documented infection, Australian investigators feel the diagnosis of CFS can be made with greater

Table 3 The Australian Case Definition of Chronic Fatigue Syndrome

To be considered a case, the patient must have an illness that is

1. Characterized by disabling and prolonged feelings of physical tiredness or fatigue, exacerbated by physical activity.
2. Present for at least 6 months.
3. Unexplained by an alternative diagnosis reached by history, laboratory, or physical examinations.
4. Accompanied by the new onset of neuropsychological symptoms including impaired short-term memory and concentration, decreased libido, and depressed mood. These symptoms usually have their onset at the same time as the physical fatigue, but are typically less severe, and less persistent than those seen in classic depressive illness.

Patients are excluded if

1. They have a chronic medical condition that may result in fatigue.
2. There is a history of schizophrenia, other psychotic illnesses, or bipolar affective disorder.

In addition, drug or alcohol dependence makes CFS very unlikely.

Source: Ref. 42.

confidence. Although this subtype is presumed (but not proved) to have a higher rate of spontaneous remission, Australian researchers favor the consideration of immunological interventions in patients with postinfective fatigue.

The second subtype recognized by the Australian research group is CFS accompanied by concurrent neuropsychological disturbances. This presentation of CFS would warrant consideration of psychotropic medications, such as tricyclic antidepressants or monoamine oxidase inhibitors, or nonpharmacological, psychological interventions. Finally, in patients with concurrent fibromyalgialike symptoms, such as prominent musculoskeletal complaints, the combination of low-dose nonsteroidal anti-inflammatory agents and tricyclic antidepressants is recommended.

HOW DO THE CENTERS FOR DISEASE CONTROL, BRITISH, AND AUSTRALIAN CASE DEFINITIONS COMPARE?

Since the vast majority of published research in the area of CFS has emanated from the United States, Britain, and Australia, and different case definitions are applied on each of the three continents, it would be very helpful to know how the three case definitions compare in identifying possible CFS patients. Although all three criteria require chronic, debilitating fatigue of at least 6 months duration, they differ in many other respects (Table 4). Unfortunately, very few studies have examined the important question of comparability of case definitions. In Bates's study, the results of inexpensive, readily available laboratory studies in over 800 patients with chronic fatigue presenting to urban hospitals in Boston and Seattle were examined and compared with findings in normal control subjects [38]. In addition, the investigators applied the CDC, British, and Australian criteria to ascertain the effect on prevalence of CFS and patient identification resulting from the use of different case definitions. The proportion of patients meeting the CDC, British, and Australian case definitions were similar in the Boston and Seattle cohorts, as were the distributions of age, gender, and laboratory abnormalities. Overall, the percentage meeting the CDC, British, and Australian criteria was 44, 62, and 82%, respectively. Despite these substantial differences, similar laboratory abnormalities were found in all groups defined by one of the case definitions (Table 5). In another study, 1000 consecutive patients were surveyed in a hospital-based primary care clinic to determine the prevalence and etiology of fatigue of at least 6 months duration [44]. Twenty-two patients completed the protocol and remained with no diagnosis after a review of their medical records, a physical examination, and laboratory testing. Of these 22 patients, 3 met the CDC criteria, 4 the British, and 10 the Australian case definition for CFS. One patient met the British, but had too few minor symptoms to meet the CDC criteria. Six patients were included as an Australian, but not a British or CDC case, because the onset of illness was not acute. Thus, a conservative estimate of the point prevalence of CFS ranged from 0.3 to 1.0%,

Table 4 Comparison of Requirements of the Three Case Definitions of Chronic Fatigue Syndrome

Requirement	CDC	British	Australian
Fatigue duration	>6 mo	>6 mo	>6 mo
Fatigue severity	50% decrease	Severe and disabling, present 50% of time	Disabling, disruptive of daily activities
Fatigue onset	New onset	Definite	Not specified
New impairment of short-term memory or concentration	Not required, may be present	Must "affect" mental function	Required
Medical conditions associated with fatigue	Excluded	Excluded	Excluded
Specific somatic symptoms required	Required	Not required	Not required
Postinfectious subtype	No	Yes	Yes
Physical examination findings	May be present	Not required	Not required
Laboratory abnormalities	None	None	None

Source: Ref. 44.

Table 5 Comparison of Laboratory Abnormalities in the Three Case Definitions of Chronic Fatigue Syndrome

Parameters	CDC	British	Australian	None	Controls	
N =	352 (44%)	500 (62%)	660 (82%)	145	50	97
Immune complexes >23	35%	36%	35%	33%	2%	
IgG > 1250	24%	24%	24%	34%	4%	
Alkaline phosphatase >89	18%	18%	19%	24%		5%
Cholesterol >200	47%	49%	50%	48%		33%

Source: Ref. 38.

depending on the case definition used. Given these scant data, it is premature to state that these three definitions are interchangeable or even comparable.

CONCLUSION

The study of chronic fatigue has been hampered in at least three ways. First, there is a lack of a consistent, specific definition for the symptom of fatigue itself. Second, an adequate method for its quantification has yet to be discovered. Third, none of the three case definitions for CFS has been empirically derived or prospectively tested.

Despite these obvious obstacles, international agreement on a uniform definition is desirable. Such consensus would allow direct comparisons of studies as well as facilitating collaboration and cooperation among different research groups. The reality is, however, that researchers have only begun to examine rigorously the three case definitions and, as of yet, too little data exist to offer intelligent, empirically based recommendations for change in the criteria for CFS. Even if a single definition is agreed on, the ultimate success of such a case definition is not assured. As one reporter commented: "It is impossible to forecast whether the consensus recommendations will help researchers and clinicians get to grips [with myalgic encephalitis/chronic fatigue syndrome] but the requirements set for the conduct of future studies should make it more likely that they pick up the same scent" [45].

REFERENCES

1. Wessely S. Old wine in new bottles: neurasthenia and "ME." Psychol Med 1990; 20:35–53.
2. Zhang Z. Shao Yin disease. In: Treatise on febrile diseases caused by cold. Beijing: New World Press, 1986.
3. Kleinman A. Neurasthenia and depression: a study of somatization and culture in China. Cultural Med Psychiatry 1982; 6:117–90.

4. Beard G. A practical treatise on nervous exhaustion (neurasthenia). New York: William Wood, 1880.

5. Beard G. American nervousness. New York: GP Putnam, 1881.

6. Savill T. Clinical lectures on neurasthenia. London: Henry J Glaisher, 1906.

7. Ware N, Kleinman A. Culture and somatic experience: the social course of illness in neurasthenia and chronic fatigue syndrome. Psychosom Med 1992; 54:546–60.

8. Greenberg D. Neurasthenia in the 1980's: chronic mononucleosis, chronic fatigue syndrome, and anxiety and depressive disorders. Psychosomatics 1990; 31:129–37.

9. Abbey SE, Garfinkel PE. Neurasthenia and the chronic fatigue syndrome: the role of culture in the making of a diagnosis. Am J Psychiatry 1991; 148:1638–46.

10. American Psychiatric Association diagnostic and statistical manual of mental disorders. 3rd ed, revised (DSM-III-R). Washington, DC: American Psychiatric Association, 1987.

11. Isaacs R. Chronic mononucleosis. Blood 1948; 3:858–61.

12. Kaufman RE. Recurrences in infectious mononucleosis. Am Pract 1950; 1:673–6.

13. Bender CE. Recurrent mononucleosis. JAMA 1962; 182:954–6.

14. Imboden JB, Canter A, Cluff LE, Trevor RW. Brucellosis III: psychological aspects of delayed convalescence. Arch Intern Med 1959; 103:406–14.

15. Henderson DA, Shelekov A. Epidemic neuromyasthenia—clinical syndrome? N Engl J Med 1959; 260:757–64.

16. Medical staff of the Royal Free Hospital. An outbreak of encephalomyelitis in the Royal Free Hospital group, London, in 1955. Br Med J 1957; 2:895–904.

17. Parish J. Early outbreaks of "epidemic neuromyasthenia." Postgrad Med J 1978; 54:711–7.

18. Parish J. Worldwide outbreaks. Nurs Times 1978; 74:699–701.

19. Behan P, Behan W. The postviral fatigue syndrome. Crit Rev Neurobiol 1988–1989; pp 157–78.

20. Acheson ED. The clinical syndrome variously called benign myalgic encephalomyelitis, Icelandic disease and epidemic neuromyasthenia. Am J Med 1959; 26:569–95.

21. McEvedy CP, Beard AW. Concept of benign myalgic encephalomyelitis. Br Med J 1970; 1:11–5.

22. McEvedy CP, Beard AW. Royal Free epidemic of 1955: a reconsideration. Br Med J 1970; 1:7–11.

23. Buchwald D, Cheney PR, Peterson DL, et al. A chronic illness characterized by fatigue, neurologic and immunologic disorders: association with human herpesvirus-6. Ann Intern Med 1992; 116:103–13.

24. Jones JF, Ray CG, Minnich LL, Hicks MJ, Kibler R, Lucas DO. Evidence for active Epstein–Barr virus infection in patients with persistent, unexplained illness: elevated anti-early antigen antibodies. Ann Intern Med 1985; 102:1–7.

25. Straus SE, Tosato G, Armstrong G, et al. Persisting illness and fatigue in adults with evidence of Epstein–Barr virus infections. Ann Intern Med 1985; 107:7–16.

26. Lamy ME, Favart AM, Cornu E, et al. Study of Epstein–Barr virus (EBV) antibodies: IgG and IgM anti-VCA, IgG anti-EA and IgG anti-EBNA obtained with an original microtiter technique: serological criterions of primary and recurrent EBV

infections and follow-up of infectious mononucleosis: seroepidemiology of EBV in Belgium based on 5178 sera from patients. Acta Clin Belg 1982; 37:281–98.

27. Horowitz C, Henle W, Henle G, Rudnick H, Latts E. Long term serological follow-up of patients for Epstein–Barr virus after recovery from infectious mononucleosis. J Infect Dis 1985; 151:1150–3.

28. Buchwald D, Sullivan J, Komaroff A. Frequency of "chronic active Epstein-Barr virus infection" in a general medical practice. JAMA 1987; 257:2303–7.

29. Kroenke K, Wood DR, Mangelsdorff D, Meier NJ, Powell JB. Chronic fatigue in primary care. JAMA 1988; 260:929–34.

30. Hellinger W, Smith T, Van Scoy R, Spitzer P, Forgacs P, Edson R. Chronic fatigue syndrome and the diagnostic utility of Epstein–Barr virus early antigen. JAMA 1988; 260:971–3.

31. Holmes GP, Kaplan JE, Stewart JA, Hunt B, Pinsky PF, Schonberger L. A cluster of patients with a chronic mononucleosis-like syndrome: is Epstein–Barr virus the cause? JAMA 1987; 257:2297–2302.

32. Holmes GP, Kaplan JE, Gantz NM, et al. Chronic fatigue syndrome: a working case definition. Ann Intern Med 1988; 108:387–89.

33. Holmes CP, Schonberger LB, Straus SE, et al. Definition of the chronic fatigue syndrome [letter]. Ann Intern Med 1988; 109:512.

34. Komaroff AL, Straus SE, Gantz NM, Jones JF. The chronic fatigue syndrome [letter]. Ann Intern Med 1989; 110:407–8.

35. Schleuderberg A, Straus S, Peterson P, et al. Chronic fatigue syndrome research. Ann Intern Med 1992; 117:325–31.

36. Komaroff AL, Geiger A. Does the CDC working case definition of chronic fatigue syndrome identify a distinct group? Clin Res 1989; 37:778A.

37. Bates DW, Buchwald D, Lee J, et al. Laboratory abnormalities in patients with the chronic fatigue syndrome [abstract]. Clin Res 1992; 40:552A.

38. Bates DW, Buchwald D, Lee J, Kornish J, Doolittle T, Komaroff AL. A comparison of case definitions of chronic fatigue syndrome [abstract]. Clin Res 1992; 40:434A.

39. Katon WJ, Buchwald DS, Simon GE, Russo JE, Mease PJ. Psychiatric illness in patients with chronic fatigue and rheumatoid arthritis. J Gen Intern Med 1990; 6:277–85.

40. Katon W, Russo J. Chronic fatigue syndrome criteria. A critique of the requirement for multiple physical complaints. Arch Intern Med 1992; 152:1604–9.

41. Sharpe MC, Archard LC, Banatvala JE, et al. A report—chronic fatigue syndrome: guidelines for research. J R Soc Med 1991; 84:12118–21.

42. Hickie I, Wakefield D. Diagnosing CFS: principles and pitfalls for the patient, physician, and researcher. CFIDS Chron 1992; Sept.

43. Lloyd AR, Wakefield D, Boughton C, Dwyer J. Prevalence of chronic fatigue syndrome in an Australian population. Med J Aust 1990; 153:522–8.

44. Bates DW, Schmitt W, Buchwald D, Ware N, Lee J, Thoyer E, Kornish RJ, Komaroff AL. Prevalence of fatigue and chronic fatigue syndrome in a primary care practice. Arch Intern Med (in press).

45. Dawson J. Consensus on research into fatigue syndrome. Br Med J 1990; 300:832.

3

Clinical Presentation and Evaluation of Fatigue and Chronic Fatigue Syndrome

Anthony L. Komaroff
Harvard Medical School and Brigham and Women's Hospital, Boston, Massachusetts

FATIGUE

The Experience of Fatigue

Fatigue is a universal human experience. Many people probably experience intermittent periods of unusual fatigue that are not apparently explained by the intellectual, emotional, or physical challenges of the previous days. Sometimes the cause for this can be identified, sometimes not.

A substantial minority of persons describe themselves as *chronically* fatigued: in one British survey, 20% of adults said that during the preceding month they "always felt tired" [1]. The pace of life in the late 20th century is escalating. Far from evolving toward a "leisure society," we are working increasingly longer hours, with less time for relaxation [2]. Moreover, many citizens of the developed nations may suffer from a chronic state of sleep deprivation [3].

Although chronic fatigue is not uncommon, only a small fraction of people who experience this disorder perceive it as a medical problem and seek medical attention. Nevertheless, this small fraction of individuals in society at large constitutes a relatively large fraction of persons seen in a physician's office. Chronic fatigue is a common problem in general medical practice [4–9], accounting for 10–15 million office visits per year in the United States.

The Frustrations of Fatigue

Fatigue is one of the most frustrating problems for a physician to deal with, for several reasons. First, the complaint of "fatigue" does not mean the same thing to all persons. For one person, it is an increased need to sleep. For another, it is trouble finding the energy to start new tasks. For others, it is difficulty concentrating. Still others mean that their muscles are weak, or easily become tired.

Another reason that the complaint of fatigue is a frustrating one for the physician is that patients who seek medical care for fatigue are often the "worried well." A physician may naturally respond by thinking: "You're tired? Well join the club!" Physicians know that many patients "medicalize" symptoms and experiences that have no pathological implications, and some physicians prefer not to deal with patients who do so. Fatigue is also a frustrating complaint for the physician, because the diagnosis is often obscure, and no physician likes to feel defeated in making a diagnosis. Although there may be hints of an underlying psychological or physical disorder, the evidence is often inconclusive. Finally, fatigue is frustrating because attempts at treatment are frequently unsuccessful [10]. This is especially discouraging, since patients with chronic fatigue often have remarkable degrees of functional impairment, often being as restricted in their levels of activity as patients with well-characterized major medical disorders [4].

The Differential Diagnosis of Fatigue

Some causes of fatigue sufficient to bring a patient to a physician's office are summarized in Table 1. Lifestyle (e.g., the pace of life, substance abuse) along with primary psychiatric disorders are thought to be the most common causes of fatigue. Most systematic studies of the complaint of fatigue in a primary care practice [4–8] indicate that well-characterized organic diseases, such as those in Table 1, explain the complaint of fatigue in fewer than 10% of patients. Thus, the physician's dilemma: numerous diseases (each of which may require many different diagnostic tests to help establish the diagnosis) *may* be present, yet the odds are that none are present.

In our experience, many organic diseases that produce fatigue can be easily recognized from history, physical examination, or simple laboratory testing. For example, fatigue caused by cardiac or respiratory insufficiency is generally accompanied by clear physical signs, is predictably reproduced by exercise and relieved by rest, and becomes progressively more severe over time. Infectious, neoplastic, and hematological diseases that are sufficiently severe to produce fatigue usually also produce weight loss, fever, pallor, lymphadenopathy, and other findings.

Depression and Fatigue

It is widely held that primary psychological disorders are the most common causes of chronic fatigue. We agree. Indeed, in the patient whose presenting

Table 1   Some Causes of Fatigue[a]

Physiological	*Endocrine disorders*
Increased physical exertion	Hyperparathyroidism
Inadequate rest	Hypothyroidism
Sedentary lifestyle	Apathetic "hyperthyroidism"
Environmental stress (noise, vibra-	Adrenal insufficiency
tion, heat)	Cushing syndrome
New physical disability, recent ill-	Hypopituitarism
ness, surgery, trauma	Diabetes mellitus
Habit patterns	*Syndromes of uncertain etiology*
Caffeine habituation	Chronic fatigue syndrome
Alcoholism	Fibromyalgia (fibrositis)
Other substance abuse	Sarcoidosis
	Wegener granulomatosis
Psychosocial	
Depression	*Occult malignancy*
Dysthymia and grief	
Anxiety-related disorders	*Hematological problems*
Stress reaction	Anemia
	Myeloproliferative syndromes
Pregnancy	
	Hepatic disease
Autoimmune disorders	Alcoholic hepatitis or cirrhosis
Systemic lupus erythematosus	
Multiple sclerosis	*Cardiovascular disease*
Thyroiditis (with or without thyroid	Low-output states
dysfunction)	Silent myocardial infarction
Rheumatoid arthritis	Bradycardias
Myasthenia gravis	Mitral valve dysfunction
Sleep disorders	*Metabolic disorders*
Sleep apnea	Hyponatremia
Narcolepsy	Hypokalemia
	Hypercalcemia
Infectious diseases	
Mononucleosis	*Renal disease*
Human immunodeficiency virus in-	Chronic renal failure
fection	
Chronic hepatitis B or C virus infec-	*Respiratory disorders*
tion	Chronic obstructive pulmonary dis-
Lyme disease	ease
Fungal disease	
Chronic parasitic infection	*Miscellaneous*
Tuberculosis	Medications
Subacute bacterial endocarditis	Autonomic overactivity
	Reactive hypoglycemia

[a]This list is not meant to be an exhaustive catalogue of every illness that can cause chronic fatigue. Rather, it is intended to highlight some of the illnesses that most commonly do so.
Source: Adapted from Ref. 97.

complaint is chronic fatigue, the first three diagnoses on the differential diagnosis list are: depression, depression, and depression [11–16]. At the same time, the physician can too easily be led to label the patient with fatigue as depressed when the initial clinical and laboratory evaluation is inconclusive.

The question of the role that psychological disorders play in patients with the complaint of chronic fatigue, and in those who meet criteria for the chronic fatigue syndrome (CFS), are discussed in more detail in Chapter 10; here, we present our views only briefly.

Making the diagnosis of depression can be difficult because the patient may find that diagnosis stigmatizing. This may lead sophisticated patients to consciously or subconsciously suppress certain aspects of their condition (such as the feeling of sadness or the experience of crying). Rather, they present with physical symptoms: headache, myalgias, abdominal pain, fatigue, and other symptoms. They express their suffering by somatizing it. As a consequence, physicians (other than psychiatrists) do not do a good job of identifying and treating depression [17,18]. Even if the diagnosis is recognized, it may be difficult for many patients to accept the doctor's suggestion that depression is playing a role in their fatigue, and this may generate conflict with the patient. Particularly if the patient will not accept a diagnosis of depression, the complaint of fatigue will also be frustrating because it will be hard to treat.

Fatigue That Is Neither Clearly Organic nor Psychiatric

Unfortunately, even after careful assessment, a substantial fraction of patients seeking medical care for fatigue do not have clear evidence of either organic or psychiatric causes for it. Kroenke and his colleagues performed a systematic evaluation of patients seeking medical care for chronic fatigue, including assessment of organic and psychiatric illness, in several hundred patients [4]. Despite an extensive evaluation, a substantial fraction of the patients fell into a gray zone in which some features of their illness suggested organic or psychiatric diseases, but they did not meet established diagnostic criteria for any organic or psychiatric disease.

Organic Illness That Presents in Obscure Fashion

Most organic illnesses become recognizable and definitively diagnosable only when they are at their most severe. For example, although multiple sclerosis (MS) and systemic lupus erythematosus (SLE) are well-recognized organic illnesses, it can be very difficult to make the diagnosis of either disease when it is less than full-blown. Indeed, in many patients with mild MS or SLE, the preponderant symptom for which they seek medical care is not a focal neurological deficit, a malar rash, or other characteristic manifestation of the illness; instead, the presenting symptom is fatigue. Sometimes such mild cases of MS and SLE progress over time to the point at which the diagnosis becomes clear; in other cases, the illness remains in a gray zone where clinicians cannot make a definitive diagnosis, or where different clinicians make different diagnoses.

In our own experience caring for and studying patients with CFS, we have seen many patients who have been given absolutely contradictory diagnoses by different, highly competent physicians. Indeed, on one occasion we saw a patient who had arranged to be evaluated by two neurologists on the faculty of our medical school on the same day; after her examination, one neurologist concluded that the patient definitely had MS (although a "mild case"), whereas the other concluded that there was no sign of MS. In one recent study, it was found that, in a group of 60 consecutive patients, in whom MS was finally diagnosed, the average time that had elapsed between the first symptom of the disease and the diagnosis was 43 months [19]. Had these patients experienced two or more unambiguous focal neurological deficits, separated in space and time, the diagnosis of MS would have been apparent to any neurologist and probably any physician. But their disease did not present this way.

Lupus also can be difficult to diagnose. Schur writes of this difficulty and of its effect on patients and doctors, in describing the experience of many patients with SLE:

> Patients . . . are often labeled as hysterical. . . . They often present their symptoms in a dramatic manner; have incorporated the symptoms into their daily life; fly from doctor to doctor seeking explanations, convinced that their symptoms cannot be explained by known biologic processes; and hang on to any positive laboratory test to confirm their suspicions. This pattern is often initiated and perpetuated by episodes of stress with which the individual cannot deal appropriately or adequately. Patients often relate . . . a long history of frustration in obtaining the proper diagnosis. Unfortunately, physicians often dislike [such] patients. . . . On the other hand, many of the symptoms turn out to be the first signs of organic disease. [20]

It is hard not to recognize the parallels between this description and the description of patients with other fatiguing illnesses of obscure etiology, such as CFS.

THE CHRONIC FATIGUE SYNDROME FAMILY OF ILLNESSES

Before discussing the clinical evaluation of patients with fatigue and with suspected CFS, it is important to briefly discuss some illnesses that have been described in the medical literature of the last 150 years and that resemble CFS in many important respects.

Neurasthenia

Neurasthenia (or neurocirculatory asthenia) was first described in the mid-19th century [21]. It was typically (but not exclusively) an affliction of young adults, usually women, characterized by chronic malaise that had often started with symptoms of an acute "infectious" illness. In the early 20th century, the illness was ascribed to weakness of the nervous system and cardiovascular system. When no characteristic objective deficits of the neurological or cardiovascular system were identified, however, physicians stopped using neurasthenia as a diagnostic label.

Myalgic Encephalomyelitis

Myalgic encephalomyelitis is a very similar chronic fatiguing illness that typically has been described as occurring in epidemic form, affecting hundreds of individuals living in small towns or numerous co-workers; outbreaks have been reported from many developed nations [22–28]. These outbreaks have been studied by national public health organizations, such as the United States Centers for Disease Control (CDC), and described in the medical literature. Myalgic encephalomyelitis has also gone by a variety of other names, including epidemic neuromyasthenia, Akureyri disease, and Icelandic disease.

Typically the illness begins with symptoms of acute respiratory infection, followed by months or years of profound fatigue, muscular weakness and twitching, muscular pain (especially in the neck, shoulder girdle, low back, and thighs), pharyngitis, nausea, vomiting, abdominal cramps, swelling in the fingers and feet, cognitive problems, emotional instability, depression, insomnia, paresthesias, and a tendency to transpose words. Often the symptoms worsen in damp weather or in the premenstrual period. Although the physical examination may be entirely unremarkable, a substantial number of individuals have been reported to suffer from low-grade fevers, adenopathy (especially in the posterior cervical chain), splenomegaly, and nystagmus. Past outbreaks have led to disability and work loss lasting many months or years. The few long-term follow-up studies that have been done suggest gradual improvement in the following years, although many patients continue to experience mild, but similar, episodes of illness. No particular viral agent has been definitively associated with these syndromes.

Fibromyalgia

Fibromyalgia, originally called fibrositis, is a very common cause of chronic musculoskeletal pain and fatigue. It is discussed in more detail in Chapter 12. Up to 5% of patients at a general medical clinic and 12% of new patients seen by rheumatologists may have fibromyalgia [29–33]. Indeed, some rheumatologists believe that primary fibromyalgia is the most common rheumatological condition seen in their practice, particularly in women younger than 50 [29–33]. It has been estimated that 3–6 million persons in the United States suffer from fibromyalgia [29,34,35].

In fibromyalgia there also is morning stiffness and increased tenderness at specific sites known as *tender points*. A large, systematic study of fibromyalgia conducted by the American College of Rheumatology has demonstrated that the tender points occur at characteristic locations, and that tenderness is not elicited at other "control" points [36]. Along with the musculoskeletal pain, fibromyalgia is also characterized by poor sleep, headaches, irritable bowel syndrome, and fatigue. Partial or total work disability is common [37,38].

Recent research suggests that patients with fibromyalgia often have the symptoms characteristic of chronic fatigue syndrome (described later), particularly the sudden onset of their syndrome with an infectiouslike illness, chronic fevers, sore throat, cough, and adenopathy [39]. Moreover, patients with chronic fatigue syndrome have detectable tender points with a frequency approaching that seen in fibromyalgia, and much more often than in healthy control subjects [40].

In fibromyalgia a disturbance in stage 4 deep sleep is reported in many patients, in which alpha waves (typical of the awake, alert state) intrude on the delta-wave electroencephalographic (EEG) pattern characteristic of deep sleep; moreover, repeatedly interrupting sleep as healthy volunteers slip into stage 4 sleep produces symptoms and the tender point findings on examination that are consistent with fibromyalgia [17]. One study found this alpha-wave intrusion in most patients studied with chronic fatigue syndrome [41]. The alpha-wave intrusion pattern is not characteristically seen in depression. Conversely, the shortened latency before rapid-eye movement (REM) sleep that is often seen in depression [42] is not characteristically seen in fibromyalgia or in CFS.

Epstein–Barr Viral Infections

Chronic Epstein–Barr Virus Infection Syndrome

Infection with Epstein–Barr virus (EBV) is ubiquitous and permanent: over 90% of adults in the developed nations are infected. This chronic infection is not associated with illness in the vast majority of individuals. The virus is generally dormant: the viral DNA takes up residence in B lymphocytes and other cells, but the virus is not reproducing itself. In the mid-1980s, several studies found increased levels of antibodies to particular Epstein–Barr virus antigens in a pattern suggesting that the virus had been reactivated from its normally dormant state in patients with probable CFS [43–50]. The authors were careful to say that this did not mean that the syndrome was caused by reactivation to EBV. However, newspaper and television stories about the research suggested a causal connection. Subsequent research indicated that reactivation of EBV (associated with modest elevations of EBV viral capsid antigen [VCA] IgG and antiearly antigens, such as had been noted in the patients with chronic fatigue) is not uncommon in healthy individuals [51]. The syndrome originally misnamed chronic Epstein–Barr virus infection syndrome is better called chronic fatigue syndrome, because there is no convincing evidence that the illness is caused by EBV, except perhaps in a handful of cases, as described next.

Chronic Mononucleosis

Chronic mononucleosis [52,53] may be an example of a chronic, fatiguing illness associated with EBV. First described 40 years ago, chronic mononucleosis starts with classic acute infectious mononucleosis (caused in most cases by a new, primary infection with EBV), characterized by distinctive clinical, hematological, and serological features [54]. However, instead of recovering, these patients remain ill for years. Some of them have serological evidence of persistently active EBV infection (persistent heterophil antibody or clearly elevated antibodies to EBV), although, in our experience, there are some patients who remain chronically ill, but whose EBV serological studies become unremarkable. For this reason, although this chronic illness clearly begins with a well-characterized acute viral infection with EBV, the role of this virus or other organic factors in producing the chronic fatiguing illness remains uncertain.

Severe chronic active EBV infection [45,55] is a very rare illness that can produce chronic fatigue. This illness often, but not always, follows acute infectious mononucleosis, as does chronic mononucleosis. Indeed, it may represent the most severe form of chronic mononucleosis. By definition, these patients have strikingly abnormal levels of antibodies against EBV, particularly IgG antibodies to the viral capsid antigen and viral early antigens. Many of these patients also have evidence of major organ involvement, such as recurrent interstitial pneumonia, persistent non-A, non-B hepatitis (most reports predate the discovery of hepatitis C virus), splenomegaly and adenopathy, pancytopenia, or selective cytopenia. Again, the parsimonious explanation is that these patients have an illness related to EBV infection, in which immunological containment of EBV is impaired.

CLINICAL PRESENTATION OF CHRONIC FATIGUE SYNDROME
Case Definitions

As summarized in Chapter 3, the illness now called chronic fatigue syndrome (CFS) is described in a case definition developed by the Centers for Disease Control (CDC) [56]. Somewhat less restrictive case definitions also have been developed by British [57] and Australian [58] investigators. The CDC case definition relies entirely on a combination of symptoms and signs (not laboratory data), and on the exclusion of chronic active organic or psychiatric illnesses that can produce chronic fatigue.

Symptoms

The symptoms and signs associated with CFS have been previously mentioned in this chapter, in the discussion of the various syndromes that are like CFS, and in other chapters. Rather than make more general descriptive remarks, we will highlight the most interesting results from our own studies.

Table 2 summarizes the symptoms (and signs) reported by 320 patients we have studied. These patients were selected for study from a group of about 2000 subjects who have sought care in our practice. Participants were selected in large measure *because* they indicated that their condition was substantially interfering with their lives; thus, these patients are a highly selected, unusually sick group, who may not be representative of the universe of patients with this syndrome. About 70% of the 320 patients summarized in Table 2 meet the CDC criteria, and those who do not generally come close to doing so.

Of the 320 patients in our series, the mean and median ages at onset of the illness are 33.5 and 31.8, respectively. Women constitute 73% of the sample, and 63% are college graduates. The mean and median durations of illness as of April 1992 were 7.3 and 6.5 years, respectively.

Each patient completed the same detailed questionnaire concerning symptoms. The data in Table 2 indicate how frequently patients stated that the symptoms were *recurrently* and *frequently* present: symptoms that were experienced occasionally, for brief periods, were not counted. Also, all patients were asked to indicate whether the symptoms had been experienced chronically *before* versus *after* the onset of their chronic fatigue. Only the data on symptoms experienced after the onset of the illness are included in Table 2; the frequency of each symptom in the years before the onset of illness was much lower, typically being reported by fewer than 5% of the patients (data not shown).

The degree of fatigue was severe in this selected group of patients: 50% were periodically bedridden or shut-in, 15% were unable to work at all, and 53% were unable to work full-time. Of those able to work, 46% stated that their work performance had suffered. Ninety percent reported having to cut down on social or recreational activities, and 71% stated that they were less able to fulfill their responsibilities to their families. Many patients described feeling that their friends, co-workers, and families—after initially being sympathetic about their illness—have subsequently become unsympathetic or even hostile, as the patients' debility continued, but no clear diagnosis emerged.

The symptoms most commonly described by patients indicate involvement of the respiratory tract, musculoskeletal system, and nervous system, along with systemic symptoms and a few miscellaneous symptoms (see Table 2). Patients were also asked, for each symptom, whether it constituted a *serious* problem: in general the neuropsychological symptoms (particularly problems with cognitive ability and sleep) were considered the most disruptive symptoms (data not shown). It has been our clinical impression that neuropsychological symptoms are also the most persistent over the course of years; formal study of longitudinal questionnaire data addressing this question is underway.

In 85% of our patients, the chronic fatiguing illness began suddenly with a

Table 2 Frequency of Symptoms and Signs in Chronic Fatigue Syndrome[a]

Symptom/sign	Frequency (%)
Fatigue	100
Intermittently bedridden/shut-in	50
Regularly bedridden/shut-in	19
Systemic symptoms/signs	
Night sweats, frequent and recurrent	50
Unintentional weight loss (median, 10 lb)	49
Unintentional weight gain (median, 15 lb)	63
Low-grade fever (by self-report), frequent and recurrent	36
Temperature $>99.3°F$, by examination[a]	30
Temperature $<97.0°F$, by examination[a]	20
Respiratory tract symptoms/signs	
Sudden onset with flulike illness	85
Swollen lymph glands in neck, frequent and recurrent	58
Sore throat, frequent and recurrent	51
Cough, frequent and recurrent	27
Palpable posterior cervical nodes[a]	54
Musculoskeletal symptoms	
Muscles hurt, frequent and recurrent	89
Postexertional malaise, frequent and recurrent	88
Joints painful but not red or swollen, frequent and recurrent	75
Generalized muscle weakness, frequent and recurrent	70
Morning stiffness, frequent and recurrent	58
Gelling, after sitting for hours, frequent and recurrent	56
Digits turn blue/white with cold, then red when warm	21
Neuropsychological symptoms/signs	
Awaken most mornings unrested	87
Difficulty concentrating, frequent and recurrent	83
Headaches, new or different in character, frequent and recurrent	76
Unusually forgetful, frequent and recurrent	71
Depression, by self-report	
Following onset of CFS	68
Before onset of CFS	6
Anxiety, by self-report	
Following onset of CFS	65
Before onset of CFS	12
Alcohol regularly makes symptoms worse	59
Tingling/numbness in extremities, frequent and recurrent	57
Bright lights hurt eyes, frequent and recurrent	56

Table 2 Continued

Symptom/sign	Frequency (%)
Dizzy when move head suddenly, frequent and recurrent	51
Visual blurring, frequent and recurrent	50
Impaired tandem gait, by examination[a]	23
Abnormal Romberg test, by examination[a]	22
Impaired serial 7s test, by examination[a]	40
Miscellaneous symptoms	
Premenstrual exacerbation of fatigue, frequent and recurrent	61
Nocturia, frequent and recurrent	46
Nausea, frequent and recurrent	44
Sudden rapid heartbeat, frequent and recurrent	44

[a]As detected on at least one physical examination.
Source: Summarized from formal studies of 320 patients, as of April 1992 [Komaroff AL, unpublished data].

"flulike" illness, characterized by fever, malaise, respiratory tract symptoms, myalgias, gastrointestinal symptoms, or combinations thereof. Without prompting, most of these patients stated that they had been feeling well and functioning very well in meeting their responsibilities at work and at home until "one day" they became acutely ill, never regaining full health or function thereafter. Essentially or actually, this large fraction of patients have stated that "it all started with that flu." This history was given just as often by patients seen in our practice before 1987, when media coverage of CFS became extensive and could have "educated" patients about the clinical features of CFS.

In our judgment, another striking aspect of the illness has been the number of patients who describe postexertional malaise (88%). After the onset of the illness, these patients have noted that even modest physical exertion (e.g., walking half a mile, raking the leaves for 15–30 min) typically produces a worsening of their illness. The worsening fatigue does not typically occur during the exercise or immediately after, but 1–2 days afterward. Also, not only do the muscles used in the exercise feel more tender and weak (compatible with deconditioning), but exercise also regularly provokes new or worse fevers (26% of patients), new or worse swelling of lymph nodes in the neck (33%), new or worse sore throat (36%), and increased difficulty with concentration (59%). Virtually all of the patients explicitly deny any such postexertional symptoms in the years before they became ill. Interestingly, before the onset of their illness, the patients state that they were unusually physically vigorous: 57% state that they were more "full of energy than most people" they knew, and 88% state that they had regularly engaged in modest or vigorous exercise.

Another striking aspect of the illness is the frequency with which patients describe regular night sweats. After the onset of the illness, 50% of patients report experiencing recurrent night sweats; before the onset of the illness, only 1% of the patients reported experiencing recurrent night sweats. Typically, the night sweats are drenching, requiring changes of bedclothes or sheets. In some patients this occurs several times a week, in others less frequently. In some it can be a nightly phenomenon when other symptoms are more severe, but then remits when other symptoms improve. Whatever the pattern, it is a new experience since the onset of the illness. Only a few patients have taken their temperatures during these night sweats and, in most cases, unusually low (rather than elevated) temperatures have been noted.

By patient self-report, psychological disorders were quite uncommon in the years before the onset of the illness: anxiety was reported by 12% and depression by 6% (see Table 2). Extensive psychiatric evaluations are now underway, including formal interviews of patients with the Diagnostic Interview Survey (DIS), to more clearly define a past history of psychological disorders. Our cumulative data indicates that patients may be underreporting a past history of psychological illness: scorable psychiatric disorders are being found in approximately 30% of patients, on at least one occasion, in the years before they became ill.

Altogether, our experience generally seems consonant with that of other investigators who have described these patients in the literature [43–45,47–50]. Although we have not studied children with this illness, others have done so [49,59]. Of our patients, 11% were older than age 50 when their illness began; these patients were just as likely to note an acute onset of the illness with a flulike syndrome.

A few patients with this disorder have had transient acute neurological events, typically in the first 6 months of the illness: primary seizures; acute, profound ataxia; focal weakness; transient blindness; and unilateral paresthesias (not in a dermatomal distribution). The seizures have been witnessed by reliable observers; the ataxia, focal weakness, and unilateral sensory deficits (that sometimes accompany the paresthesias) have been documented by physicians and neurologists; the blindness has never been documented, in our experience. Similar acute and transient neurological events have also been reported occasionally in outbreaks of myalgic encephalomyelitis, as well.

Many patients report that certain factors regularly worsen their illness: physical exertion and the premenstrual period often do so. In addition, our patients report that humid weather (66% of patients), hot weather (44%), changes in weather (38%), drinking alcoholic beverages (59%), and "stress" (88%) regularly worsen the symptoms of the illness.

Past Medical History

Although most elements of the past medical history are unremarkable in patients with CFS, there is a strikingly high frequency of atopic or allergic illness: 60–80%

of patients with CFS have long-standing atopic disorders, versus a point prevalence of approximately 20% in the general US population [60–63].

Physical Examination

A few "abnormal" findings may be present on physical examination more often in CFS than in healthy subjects: fevers; unusually low basal body temperature (below 97°F); posterior cervical adenopathy; and abnormal tests of balance (Romberg and tandem gait) (see Table 2). Whether such findings would be seen less often in control subjects remains to be determined from controlled studies with blinded observers. The tender points described in patients with fibromyalgia are frequently seen in chronic fatigue syndrome [40]. Therefore, the finding of a significant number of tender points, along with the absence of tenderness at control sites, is evidence in favor of the diagnosis of CFS (or fibromyalgia, which also is associated with a prominent chronic fatigue). The absence of tender points, however, does not rule out the diagnosis of CFS, in our view.

Standard Laboratory Testing

Standard laboratory testing is generally unremarkable in CFS [64]. Controlled studies have demonstrated that a few abnormalities may occur more frequently in CFS than in healthy control subjects of similar age and sex: relative lymphocytosis; atypical lymphocytosis; elevated alkaline phosphatase levels; elevated total cholesterol levels [65]. However, none of these abnormalities are seen in more than 50% of patients with CFS; thus, none constitutes a sufficiently sensitive diagnostic test. Moreover, each can be seen in other disorders; thus, none is a sufficiently specific test.

Immunological Testing

A large and growing literature reports immunological abnormalities in patients with CFS [64,66]. This will be discussed in detail in Chapter 8; here, we will discuss only those findings that may have relevance in a typical office practice. Most of the studies reported thus far are expensive or are experimental tests, performed reliably in only a few laboratories. As such, they are not currently indicated in the evaluation of possible CFS.

Several investigators reported T-lymphocyte dysfunction, as reflected by skin test anergy or reduced T-cell lymphoproliferative responses after stimulation with various mitogens and antigens [67–69]. In our view, testing for skin test anergy is a reasonable diagnostic procedure, although it has not yet been established how useful such testing is among patients in the developed nations of the Northern Hemisphere, as most of the reported experience is from Australia and New Zealand.

Several groups found low levels of circulating immune complexes [50,65] in patients with CFS. These patients are without evidence of immune complex-mediated disease. Our group formally compared the presence of immune complexes in patients with CFS and in healthy control subjects [65]. We found that the relative risk of immune complexes in patients with CFS was remarkably high, after adjusting for age and gender: the odds ratio was 28:1 (95% CI 4-313, $p <$ 0.000001). A very sensitive radiolabeled C1q-binding assay was employed, because less-sensitive assays did not detect as striking a difference between cases and controls. One hypothesis is that the immune complexes represent some chronic immunological response to antigens that are perceived by the immune system as foreign, including antigens from one or more infectious agents.

We have also found [65] that elevated levels of IgG are present more often in patients with CFS than in healthy control subjects: the adjusted odds ratio was 9:1 (95% CI 2-38, $p <$ 0.000001). In a handful of individuals, IgG levels have been below the normal range in our laboratory but, unlike others [48], we have not found frequent hypogammaglobulinemia. In a few patients, we also have found remarkably elevated levels of IgM (two to five times higher than the top of the normal range and always polyclonal); however, IgM values for the entire group of patients we have studied with CFS are no greater than for healthy control subjects. In a small, highly selected group of patients, one-fourth had IgG subclass deficiencies [70].

Again, unfortunately, none of these abnormalities are seen more frequently than in 50% of patients with CFS. Therefore, none constitutes a sensitive diagnostic test by itself. Also, none is specific to CFS.

Neurological Studies

We conducted a study of patients from one geographic area (northern California and Nevada) who had an illness that closely resembles CFS and myalgic encephalomyelitis; most of the patients became ill within a relatively narrow window of time, and in many cases family members or co-workers also were affected. In this one group, we found areas of abnormal signal in the white matter of the central nervous system by magnetic resonance imaging (MRI); such areas of abnormal signal were seen in 79% of patients with CFS versus 20% of healthy control subjects of similar age and sex ($p < 10^{-8}$) [66]. However, in our studies of patients in New England we have found such areas of high signal in the white matter less frequently (in about 40% of cases). Thus, MRI also appears to be a relatively insensitive diagnostic test. Given that it also is nonspecific and very expensive, we do not believe that routine use of MRI is indicated in patients with suspected CFS. When the history or physical examination suggest the possibility of MS (as in some patients with CFS), MRI may be useful.

Studies of other neurologic tests of the brain are underway—particularly evoked potentials, cognitive evoked potentials, BEAM-scanning, and single-photon emission positron tomography (SPECT)—because of preliminary data suggesting abnormalities of these tests in patients with CFS. Currently, these expensive modalities must also be considered experimental and should not be routinely used in patients with suspected CFS.

Neuroendocrine Studies

As will be discussed in Chapter 11, an abnormality of the hypothalamic–pituitary–adrenal (HPA) axis has been demonstrated in CFS. The data are consistent with the hypothesis that diminished secretion of corticotropin-releasing hormone (CRH) by the hypothalamus leads to diminished secretion of corticotropin (adrenocorticotropic hormone; ACTH) by the pituitary and, thereby, to diminished production of cortisol by the adrenal glands [71]. Although these findings are of great interest, HPA axis studies currently should also be regarded as experimental and not for routine use in patients with suspected CFS. Also, the value of random morning cortisol levels, or of cosyntropin (Cortrosyn) stimulation tests, has not been established in CFS. Moreover, these findings do not provide evidence that CFS should be treated with low-dose steroid replacement. Such treatment is currently under study.

Infectious Disease Studies

Although CFS can apparently begin following a variety of stressful noninfectious events (e.g., major surgery, accidents, and severe allergic reactions), it typically begins suddenly with an infectiouslike illness. However, in most cases of CFS, the infectiouslike illness that has allegedly initiated the chronic illness has not been carefully studied. Therefore, some observers are skeptical that CFS is associated with infection.

Yet an illness such as CFS can follow in the wake of very well-characterized primary infection with Epstein–Barr virus. Several groups have reported associations of CFS with enteroviruses [72–75] and with human herpesvirus-6 [66]. However, chronic infection with these viruses is common, and their etiological role in CFS has not been established. One group has reported an association with a putative novel retrovirus [76]; this finding has not yet been confirmed by another group, and some nonconfirmatory evidence has been reported [77]. Routine testing for any of the foregoing viruses is not currently indicated in patients with suspected CFS.

Chronic fatigue syndrome, or an illness much like it, also has been seen following documented influenza virus infection [78], acute parvovirus infection [79], and a variety of other acute infections [46,80–84]. It has also been found in patients with proved Lyme disease who have received adequate antibacterial treatment, and in whom the cardinal manifestations of Lyme disease (e.g., arthritis, carditis) have resolved [85]. These associations between specific infectious agents and CFS are as yet anecdotal case reports. It is unclear how frequently these infectious agents may trigger CFS. But these instances document that an acute infection can trigger a chronic illness, even though the nature of the chronic illness, including the ongoing role of the triggering agent, remains obscure. Therefore, we do not recommend routine testing for these infectious agents.

What are the implications of these findings for the practicing physician? Surely, there is no reason to routinely test for various infectious agents in patients with suspected CFS, since their etiological relation to CFS remains unestablished. In our practice, we obtain an antibody profile to EBV (IgG and IgM to the viral capsid antigens, IgG to the early antigens, and IgG to the Epstein–Barr nuclear antigen) in those patients whose chronic illness has begun with what was a classic case of acute infectious mononucleosis. We obtain serological tests for Lyme disease when there is a likelihood of exposure and a history of symptoms suggesting Lyme disease (not simple fatigue), given that this is the one treatable infectious agent that has been suggested as a trigger for some cases of CFS.

Psychological Studies

As stated at the outset, most patients seeking medical care for chronic fatigue probably are suffering from depression and/or anxiety disorders or somatization disorder. Moreover, most patients seeking medical care for chronic fatigue probably do not have CFS [4,86].

A detailed discussion of the role of psychological disorders in CFS is found in Chapter 10. I will summarize here my own views. Although some of the symptoms of CFS are also characteristic of depression, generalized anxiety disorder, and somatization disorder (e.g., headaches, myalgias, sleep disturbance, difficulty with concentration), other symptoms are not (e.g., the sudden onset, recurrent fevers, adenopathy, arthralgias, photophobia). Moreover, several investigators have argued that the fact that these symptoms typically started abruptly in the context of an acute infectious-type illness also suggests that the symptoms are not likely to be due exclusively to a psychiatric disorder.

Most studies of the question have found that most patients with CFS *become* depressed and anxious following the (usually sudden) onset of their disorder [87–91]. For many patients the depression and anxiety become the most debilitating parts of their illness, and it is imperative that they be recognized and treated. At the same time, it should be noted that these studies also indicate that a substantial fraction of patients with CFS (25–40%) have no evidence of any active psychiatric disorder since the onset of CFS.

By and large, there appears to be a higher past history of psychiatric disorders in patients with CFS than in the population at large: the average across all studies is about 30% (range, 20–50%) of CFS patients [87–92]. Although this past history of psychiatric disorders is greater than is found in the general population (range, 5–10%); despite extensive psychiatric evaluation no evidence of a preexisting psychiatric disorder can be found in most patients with CFS.

In my view, the present evidence leads to several conclusions for the practicing physician. First, the presence of an underlying psychological disorder must always be sought in patients with the presenting complaint of chronic fatigue. Whether this should be done with a formal screening instrument, such as the General Health Questionnaire, or whether the physician can elicit comparable information through more flexible interviewing of the patient, is uncertain. Second, the process of making the psychiatric diagnosis can make the patient aware of how his or her feelings relate to the symptoms, an essential first step in management. Thus, the patient's emotional status is explored while the medical history is being obtained. A simple interviewing technique can be based on the biopsychosocial approach developed by Engel [93] and the medical interviewing techniques developed by Bird and Cohen-Cole [94,95]. In attempting to elicit submerged information, it is important to remember that occult alcohol abuse (and other forms of substance abuse) often produces chronic fatigue, either directly as a result of chronic intoxication, or indirectly through its disruptive effects on sleep or its production of inflammatory disease of the liver.

In sum, the clinician should be vigilant in looking for evidence of psychological disorders and should have a low threshold for having patients formally evaluated for such disorders. The same principles apply even when the patient fully meets criteria for CFS, given that psychological disorders can often be present in CFS and can be the most disabling part of the illness.

LABORATORY TESTING IN PATIENTS WITH FATIGUE

In the patient with fatigue of modest severity and relatively short duration (e.g., 1–3 months)—who probably is most typical of patients seeking medical care for fatigue—no laboratory testing may be warranted. This is particularly true when the patient clearly has many lifestyle features that are likely to explain fatigue, when a psychological disorder is deemed likely, and when no other symptoms suggest an organic abnormality.

In patients with fatigue of a longer duration (6 months or more) or severity (significantly interfering with their ability to work or maintain their responsibilities at home), a modest screening evaluation is warranted to look for evidence of an underlying organic disorder. A panel of tests recently recommended by a 1991 National Institutes of Health conference is shown in Table 3. Although not all these tests are highly sensitive for organic disease, nor highly specific for any particular disease, they serve as a useful screen for organic illness. The various immunological, neurological, and virological tests mentioned in the discussion

Table 3 Case-Finding Laboratory Tests

Complete blood count

Manual differential white blood cell count (unless automated counts accurately determine atypical lymphocytes)

Erythrocyte sedimentation rate (Westergren technique)

Chemistry panel including assessment of renal and hepatic function, glucose, electrolytes, calcium, phosphate, total cholesterol, albumin, and globulin levels

Thyroid function tests (highly sensitive TSH is sufficient)

Antinuclear antibodies and rheumatoid factor, if there are prominent arthralgias and myalgias

Urinalysis

Source: Adapted from Ref. 96.

of chronic fatigue sydrome should be considered experimental and not yet appropriate for general use.

The history obtained for a patient with severe chronic fatigue should include questions that screen for the many conditions that can cause chronic fatigue, some of which are summarized in Table 1. Extensive testing for all of these conditions is definitely *not* to be routinely performed in patients with chronic fatigue. Rather, such testing should be reserved for cases in which any of these conditions is suggested by the history or physical examination, according to the clinical judgment of the examining physician.

The role of sleep laboratory testing is particularly uncertain at this time. Such testing is clearly indicated when the patient has a history of prominent snoring (particularly if snoring was not frequent or prominent before the chronic fatigue), or witnessed apneic periods during sleep, frequent jerking movements of the legs during sleep, or an overwhelming urge to sleep during the day. Recent unpublished studies have suggested that important sleep disorders—not only the alpha-intrusion pattern mentioned earlier—may be reasonably common in patients with severe chronic fatigue and CFS, even though these patients may not experience the foregoing symptoms [Buchward D, personal communication]. However, because it is not clear that these conditions respond to treatment in patients with CFS, and because sleep laboratory testing is very expensive, the role of such testing now remains uncertain.

MEDICAL FOLLOW-UP IN PATIENTS WITH FATIGUE

There have been no reported longitudinal studies of patients with chronic fatigue, including CFS. Therefore, there are no empiric data on which to base recommendations for the medical follow-up of patients with fatigue. When a patient continues to have a debilitating chronic fatigue that significantly interferes with his or her life, and no organic or psychological cause of the fatigue has been uncovered, it is appropriate to obtain an interval history, and to repeat the physical examination and the panel of tests shown in Table 3, every 6–12 months.

REFERENCES

1. Cox B, Blaxter M, Buckle A, Fenner NP, Golding JF, Gore M, Huppert FA, Nickson J, Roth M, Stark J, Wadsworth MEJ, Whichelow M. The health and lifestyle survey. London: Health Promotion Research Trust, 1987:61–2.
2. Schor JB. The overworked American. The unexpected decline of leisure. New York: Basic Books, 1992.
3. Dement W. The sleepwatchers. Stanford, CA: Stanford University Press, 1992.
4. Kroenke K, Wood DR, Mangelsdorff AD, Meier NJ, Powell JB. Chronic fatigue in primary care. Prevalence, patient characteristics, and outcome. JAMA 1988; 260:929–34.
5. Allan FN. The differential diagnosis of weakness and fatigue. N Engl J Med 1944; 231:414–8.
6. Morrison JD. Fatigue as a presenting complaint in family practice. J Fam Pract 1980; 10:795–801.
7. Katerndahl DA. Fatigue of uncertain etiology. Fam Med Rev 1983; 1:26–38.
8. Nelson E, Kirk J, McHugo G, Douglass R, Ohler J, Wasson J, Zubkoff M. Chief complaint fatigue: a longitudinal study from the patient's perspective. Fam Pract Res J 1987; 6:175–88.
9. Solberg LI. Lassitude. A primary care evaluation. JAMA 1984; 251:3272–6.
10. Kroenke K, Arrington ME, Mangelsdorff AD. The prevalence of symptoms in medical outpatients and the adequacy of therapy. Arch Intern Med 1990; 150:1685–9.
11. Stoeckle JD, Zola IK, Davidson GE. The quantity and significance of psychological distress in medical patients. J Chronic Dis 1964; 17:959–70.
12. Reifler BV, Okimoto JT, Heidrich FE, Inui TS. Recognition of depression in a university-based family medicine residency program. J Fam Pract 1979; 9:623–8.
13. Hoeper EW, Nycz GR, Cleary PD, Regier DA, Goldberg ID. Estimated prevalence of RDC mental disorder in primary medical care. Int J Ment Health 1979; 8:6–15.
14. Nielsen ACI, Williams TA. Depression in ambulatory medical patients. Arch Gen Psychiatry 1980; 37:999–1004.
15. Kessler LG, Cleary PD, Burke JD. Psychiatric disorders in primary care. Arch Gen Psychiatry 1985; 42:583–7.
16. Barsky AJI. Hidden reasons some patients visit doctors. Ann Intern Med 1981; 94:492–8.
17. Moldofsky H, Scarisbrick P. Induction of neurasthenic musculoskeletal pain syndrome by selective sleep stage deprivation. Psychosom Med 1976; 38:35–44.
18. Littlejohn GO, Weinstein C, Helme RD. Increased neurogenic inflammation in fibrositis syndrome. J Rheumatol 1987; 14:1022–5.

19. Scheinberg LC, Kalb RC, Larocca NG, Giesser BS, Slater RJ, Poser CM. The doctor–patient relationship in multiple sclerosis. In: Poser CM, Paty DW, Scheinberg LC, McDonald WI, Ebers GC, eds. The diagnosis of multiple sclerosis. New York: Thieme-Stratton, 1984:205–15.

20. Schur PH. Clinical features of SLE. In: Kelley WN, Harris ED, Ruddy S, Sledge CB, eds. Textbook of rheumatology. Philadelphia: WB Saunders, 1989:1101–29.

21. Paul O. DaCosta's syndrome or neurocirculatory asthenia. Br Heart J 1987; 58:306–15.

22. Sigurdsson B, Sigurjonsson J, Sigurdsson JHJ, Thorkelsson J, Gudmundsson KR. A disease epidemic in Iceland simulating poliomyelitis. Am J Hyg 1950; 52:222–38.

23. Sigurdsson B, Gudmundsson KR. Clinical findings six years after outbreak of Akureyri disease. Lancet 1956; 1:766–7.

24. Shelokov A, Habel K, Verder E, Welsh W. Epidemic neuromyasthenia: an outbreak of poliomyelitislike illness in student nurses. N Engl J Med 1957; 257:345–55.

25. Poskanzer DC, Henderson DA, Kunkle EC, Kalter SS, Clement WB, Bond JO. Epidemic neuromyasthenia: an outbreak in Punta Gorda, Florida. N Engl J Med 1957; 257:356–64.

26. Medical staff of the Royal Free Hospital. An outbreak of encephalomyelitis in the Royal Free Hospital group, London, in 1955. Br Med J 1957; 2:895–904.

27. Acheson ED. The clinical syndrome variously called benign myalgic encephalomyelitis, Iceland disease and epidemic neuromyasthenia. Am J Med 1959; 4:569–95.

28. Henderson DA, Shelokov A. Epidemic neuromyasthenia—clinical syndrome. N Engl J Med 1959; 260:757–64.

29. Yunus M, Masi AT, Calabro JJ, Miller KA, Feigenbaum SL. Primary fibromyalgia (fibrositis): clinical study of 50 patients with matched normal controls. Semin Arthritis Rheum 1981; 11:151–71.

30. Goldenberg DL. Fibromyalgia syndrome: an emerging but controversial condition. JAMA 1987; 257:2782–803.

31. Wolfe F, Cathey MA, Kleinheksel SM. Fibrositis (fibromyalgia) in rheumatoid arthritis. J Rheumatol 1984; 11:814–8.

32. Dinerman H, Goldenberg DL, Felson DT. A prospective evaluation of 118 patients with the fibromyalgia syndrome: prevalence of Raynaud's phenomenon, sicca symptoms, ANA, low complement, and Ig deposition at the dermal–epidermal junction. J Rheumatol 1986; 13:368–73.

33. Felson DT, Goldenberg DL. The natural history of fibromyalgia. Arthritis Rheum 1986; 29:1522–6.

34. Wolfe F, Cathey MA. Prevalence of primary and secondary fibrositis. J Rheumatol 1983; 10:965–8.

35. Campbell SM, Clark S, Tindall ES, Forehand ME, Bennett RM. Clinical characteristics of fibrositis. I. A "blinded" controlled study of symptoms and tender points. Arthritis Rheum 1983; 26:132–7.

36. Wolfe F, Smythe HA, Yunus MB, Bennett RM, Bombardier C, Goldenberg DL, Tugwell P, Campbell SM, Abeles M, Clark P, Fam AG, Farber SJ, Fiechtner JJ, Franklin CM, Gatter RA, Hamaty D, Lessard J, Lichtbroun AS, Masi AT, McCain GA, Reynolds J, Romano TJ, Russell IJ, Sheon RP. The American College of Rheumatology 1990 criteria for the classification of fibromyalgia. Report of the multicenter criteria committee. Arthritis Rheum 1990; 33:160–72.

37. Cathey MA, Wolfe F, Kleinheksel SM, Hawley DJ. Socioeconomic impact of fibrositis. Am J Med 1986; 81:578–84.
38. Wolfe F, Cathey MA. Assessment of functional ability in patients with fibromyalgia. Arch Intern Med 1990; 150:460.
39. Buchwald D, Goldenberg DL, Sullivan JL, Komaroff AL. The "chronic, active Epstein–Barr virus infection" syndrome and primary fibromyalgia. Arthritis Rheum 1987; 30:1132–6.
40. Goldenberg DL, Simms RW, Geiger A, Komaroff AL. High frequency of fibromyalgia in patients with chronic fatigue seen in a primary care practice. Arthritis Rheum 1990; 33:381–7.
41. Whelton CL, Salit I, Moldofsky H. Sleep, Epstein–Barr virus infection, musculo-skeletal pain, and depressive symptoms in chronic fatigue syndrome. J Rheumatol 1992; 19:939–43.
42. Thase ME, Frank E, Kupfer DJ. Biological processes in major depression. In: Beckham EE, Leber WR, eds. Handbook of depression: treatment, assessment and research. Homewood, IL: Dorsey Press, 1985:816–913.
43. Tobi M, Morag A, Ravid Z, Chowers I, Feldman-Weiss V, Michaeli Y, Ben-Chetrit E, Shalit M, Knobler H. Prolonged atypical illness associated with serological evidence of persistent Epstein–Barr virus infection. Lancet 1982; 1:61–4.
44. Ballow M, Seeley J, Purtilo DT, St Onge S, Sakamoto K, Rickles FR. Familial chronic mononucleosis. Ann Intern Med 1982; 97:821–5.
45. Edson CM, Cohen LK, Henle W, Strominger JL. An unusually high-titer human anti-Epstein Barr virus (EBV) serum and its use in the study of EBV-specific proteins synthesized in vitro and in vivo. J Immunol 1983; 130:919–24.
46. Salit IE. Sporadic postinfectious neuromyasthenia. Can Med Assoc J 1985; 133:659–63.
47. Hamblin TJ, Hussain J, Akbar AN, Tang YC, Smith JL, Jones DB. Immunological reason for chronic ill health after infectious mononucleosis. Br Med J 1983; 287:85–8.
48. DuBois RE, Seeley JK, Brus I, Sakamoto K, Ballow M, Harada S, Bechtold TA, Pearson G, Purtilo DT. Chronic mononucleosis syndrome. South Med J 1984; 77:1376–82.
49. Jones JF, Ray CG, Minnich LL, Hicks MJ, Kibler R, Lucas DO. Evidence for active Epstein–Barr virus infection in patients with persistent, unexplained illnesses: elevated anti-early antigen antibodies. Ann Intern Med 1985; 102:1–7.
50. Straus SE, Tosato G, Armstrong G, Lawley T, Preble OT, Henle W, Davey R, Pearson G, Epstein J, Brus I, Blaese RM. Persisting illness and fatigue in adults with evidence of Epstein–Barr virus infection. Ann Intern Med 1985; 102:7–16.
51. Horwitz CA, Henle W, Henle G, Rudnick H, Latts E. Long-term serological follow-up of patients for Epstein–Barr virus after recovery from infectious mononu-cleosis. J Infect Dis 1985; 151:1150–3.
52. Komaroff AL. The "chronic mononucleosis" syndromes. Hosp Pract 1987; 22:71–5.
53. Straus SE. The chronic mononucleosis syndrome. J Infect Dis 1988; 157:405–12.
54. Isaacs R. Chronic infectious mononucleosis. Blood 1948; 3:858–61.
55. Schooley RT, Carey RW, Miller G, Henle W, Eastman R, Mark EJ, Kenyon K, Wheeler EO, Rubin RH. Chronic Epstein–Barr virus infection associated with fever and interstitial pneumonitis. Clinical and serologic features and response to antiviral chemotherapy. Ann Intern Med 1986; 104:636–43.

56. Holmes GP, Kaplan JE, Gantz NM, Komaroff AL, Schonberger LB, Straus SE, Jones JF, DuBois RE, Cunningham-Rundles C, Pahwa S, Tosato G, Zegans LS, Purtilo DT, Brown N, Schooley RT, Brus I. Chronic fatigue syndrome: a working case definition. Ann Intern Med 1988; 108:387–9.

57. Sharpe MC, Archard LC, Banatvala JE, Borysiewicz LK, Clare AW, David A, Edwards RHT, Hawton KEH, Lambert HP, Lane RJM, McDonald EM, Mowbray JF, Pearson DJ, Peto TEA, Preedy VR, Smith AP, Smith DG, Taylor DJ, Tyrrell DA, Wessely S, White PD. A report–chronic fatigue syndrome: guidelines in research. J R Soc Med 1991; 84:118–21.

58. Lloyd AR, Hickie I, Boughton CR, Spencer O, Wakefield D. Prevalence of chronic fatigue syndrome in an Australian population. Med J Aust 1990; 153:522–8.

59. Bell KM, Cookfair D, Bell DS, Reese P, Cooper L. Risk factors associated with chronic fatigue syndrome in a cluster of pediatric cases. Rev Infect Dis 1991; 13(suppl 1):S32–8.

60. Olson GB, Kanaan MN, Gersuk GM, Kelley LM, Jones JF. Correlation between allergy and persistent Epstein–Barr virus infections in chronic active Epstein–Barr virus-infected patients. J Allergy Clin Immunol 1986; 78:308–14.

61. Olson GB, Kanaan MN, Kelley LM, Jones JF. Specific allergen-induced Epstein–Barr nuclear antigen-positive B cells from patients with chronic-active Epstein–Barr virus infections. J Allergy Clin Immunol 1986; 78:315–20.

62. Straus SE, Dale JK, Wright R, Metcalfe DD. Allergy and the chronic fatigue syndrome. J Allergy Clin Immunol 1988; 81:791–5.

63. Salvaggio JE. Allergic rhinitis. In: Wyngaarden JB, Smith LH Jr, Bennett JC, eds. Cecil textbook of medicine. Philadelphia: WB Saunders, 1992:1457–62.

64. Buchwald D, Komaroff AL. Review of laboratory findings for patients with chronic fatigue syndrome. Rev Infect Dis 1991; 13:S12–8.

65. Bates DW, Buchwald D, Lee J, Doolittle T, Kornish J, Rutherford C, Churchill WH, Schur P, Wybenga D, Winkelman J, Komaroff AL. Laboratory abnormalities in patients with the chronic fatigue syndrome. Clin Res 1992; 40:552A.

66. Buchwald D, Cheney PR, Peterson DL, Henry B, Wormsley SB, Geiger A, Ablashi DV, Salahuddin SZ, Saxinger C, Biddle R, Kikinis R, Jolesz FA, Folks T, Balachandran N, Peter JB, Gallo RC, Komaroff AL. A chronic illness characterized by fatigue, neurologic and immunologic disorders, and active human herpesvirus type 6 infection. Ann Intern Med 1992; 116:103–13.

67. Murdoch JC. Cell-mediated immunity in patients with myalgic encephalomyelitis syndrome. NZ Med J 1988; 101:511–2.

68. Lloyd AR, Wakefield D, Boughton CR, Dwyer JM. Immunological abnormalities in the chronic fatigue syndrome. Med J Aust 1989; 151:122–4.

69. Klimas NG, Salvato FR, Morgan R, Fletcher M. Immunologic abnormalities in chronic fatigue syndrome. J Clin Microbiol 1990; 28:1403–10.

70. Komaroff AL, Geiger AM, Wormsley S. IgG subclass deficiencies in chronic fatigue syndrome. Lancet 1988; 1:1288–9.

71. Demitrack MA, Dale JK, Straus SE, Laue L, Listwak SJ, Kruesi MJP, Chrousos GP, Gold PW. Evidence for impaired activation of the hypothalamic–pituitary–adrenal axis in patients with chronic fatigue syndrome. J Clin Endocrinol Metab 1991; 73:1224–34.

72. Yousef GE, Bell EJ, Mann GF, Murugesan V, Smith DG, McCartney RA, Mowbray JF. Chronic enterovirus infection in patients with postviral fatigue syndrome. Lancet 1988; 1:146–50.

73. Archard LC, Bowles NE, Behan PO, Bell EJ, Doyle D. Postviral fatigue syndrome: persistence of enterovirus RNA in muscle and elevated creatine kinase. J R Soc Med 1988; 81:326–9.

74. Cunningham L, Bowles NE, Lane RJM, Dubowitz V, Archard LC. Persistence of enteroviral RNA in chronic fatigue syndrome is associated with the abnormal production of equal amounts of positive and negative strands of enteroviral RNA. J Gen Virol 1990; 71:1399–402.

75. Gow JW, Behan WMH, Clements GB, Woodall C, Riding M, Behan PO. Enteroviral RNA sequences detected by polymerase chain reaction in muscle of patients with postviral fatigue syndrome. Br Med J 1991; 302:692–6.

76. DeFreitas E, Hilliard B, Cheney PR, Bell D, Kiggundu E, Sankey D, Wroblewska Z, Palladino M, Woodward JP, Koprowski H. Retroviral sequences related to human T-lymphotropic virus type II in patients with chronic fatigue immune dysfunction syndrome. Proc Natl Acad Sci USA 1991; 88:2922–6.

77. Gunn WJ, Komaroff AL, Levine SM, Connell DB, Bell DS, Cheney PR. Inability of retroviral tests to identify persons with chronic fatigue syndrome. MMWR 1992; 1993; 42:183–90.

78. Imboden JB, Canter A, Cluff LE. Convalescence from influenza. Arch Intern Med 1961; 108:393–9.

79. Leventhal LJ, Naides SJ, Freundlich B. Fibromyalgia and parvovirus infection. Arthritis Rheum 1991; 34:1319–24.

80. Benjamin JE, Hoyt RC. Disability following postvaccinal (yellow fever) hepatitis. JAMA 1945; 128:319–24.

81. Lawton AH, Rich TA, McLendon S, Gates EH, Bond JO. Follow-up studies of St Louis encephalitis in Florida: reevaluation of the emotional and health status of the survivors five years after acute illness. South Med J 1970; 63:66–71.

82. Rosene KA, Copass MK, Kastner LS, Nolan CM, Eschenbach DA. Persistent neuropsychological sequelae of toxic shock syndrome. Ann Intern Med 1982; 96:865–70.

83. Cluff LL, Trever RW, Imboden JB, Canter A. Brucellosis II: medical aspects of delayed convalescence. Arch Intern Med 1959; 103:393–405.

84. Imboden JB, Canter A, Cluff LE, Trever RW. Brucellosis III: psychologic aspects of delayed convalescence. Arch Intern Med 1959; 103:406–14.

85. Coyle PK, Krupp LB. *Borrelia burgdorferi* infection in the chronic fatigue syndrome. Ann Neurol 1990; 28:243–4.

86. Manu P, Lane TJ, Matthews DA. The frequency of the chronic fatigue syndrome in patients with symptoms of persistent fatigue. Ann Intern Med 1988; 109: 554–6.

87. Taerk GS, Toner BB, Salit IE, Garfinkel PE, Ozersky S. Depression in patients with neuromyasthenia (benign myalgic encephalomyelitis). Int J Psychiatry Med 1987; 17:49–56.

88. Kruesi MJP, Dale J, Straus SE. Psychiatric diagnoses in patients who have chronic fatigue syndrome. J Clin Psychiatry 1989; 50:53–6.

89. Wessely S, Powell R. Fatigue syndromes: a comparison of chronic "postviral" fatigue with neuromuscular and affective disorders. J Neurol Neurosurg Psychiatry 1989; 52:940–8.

90. Hickie I, Lloyd A, Wakefield D, Parker G. The psychiatric status of patients with the chronic fatigue syndrome. Br J Psychiatry 1990; 156:534–40.

91. Gold D, Bowden R, Sixbey J, Riggs R, Katon WJ, Ashley R, Obrigewitch R, Corey L. Chronic fatigue: a prospective clinical and virologic study. JAMA 1990; 264:48–53.

92. Robins LN, Helzer JE, Weissman MM, Orvaschel H, Gruenberg E, Burke JD, Regier DA. Lifetime prevalence of specific psychiatric disorders in three sites. Arch Gen Psychiatry 1984; 41:949–58.

93. Engel GL. The need for a new medical model: a challenge for biomedicine. Science 1977; 196:129–36.

94. Bird J, Cohen-Cole SA, Boker J, Freeman A. Teaching psychiatry to non-psychiatrists: I. The application of educational methodology. Gen Hosp Psychiatry 1983; 5:247–53.

95. Cohen-Cole SA, Bird J. Teaching psychiatry to nonpsychiatrists: II. A model curriculum. Gen Hosp Psychiatry 1984; 6:1–11.

96. Schluederberg A, Straus SE, Peterson P, Blumenthal S, Komaroff AL, Spring SB, Landay A, Buchwald D. Chronic fatigue syndrome research: definition and medical outcome assessment. Ann Intern Med 1992; 117:325–31.

97. Komaroff AL. Chronic fatigue. In: Branch WJ Jr, ed. Office practice of medicine. 3rd ed. Philadelphia: WB Saunders (in press).

4

An Anthropological Approach to Understanding Chronic Fatigue Syndrome

Norma C. Ware
Harvard Medical School, Boston, Massachusetts

An extensive, multidisciplinary research literature confirms the influence of social factors on the onset and course of particular illnesses, as well as on longevity and general well-being.

Social epidemiologists and life events researchers have identified relationships between negative life events (and long-term difficulties) and illness onset in multiple sclerosis [1,2], myocardial infarction [3–7], and depression [8,9]. There is also evidence to suggest that the risk-producing effects of life events vary by social class [10,11]. Chronic stress ensuing from lifestyle incongruity (i.e., the discrepancy between material consumption and other behaviors conveying prestige on the one hand, and social status as indicated by occupational class on the other) has been linked to hypertension in several studies [11–14]. Other research on chronic stress has shown that social role conflicts and ongoing minor concerns ("daily hassles") contribute to depressive symptoms [15,16].

The influence of expressed emotion (criticism, hostility, overinvolvement) by family members on relapse in schizophrenia has been documented in a large number of investigations [see 17, for review]. Less consistent, but still very suggestive, is data indicating that life events trigger psychotic episodes in schizophrenic patients [18,19]. Cross-cultural research on the course of schizophrenia being carried out by the World Health Organization reveals a significantly higher proportion of "favorable courses" in developing, compared with developed, countries [20]. Reduction in long-term difficulties and the occurrence of "neutralizing" or "fresh start" events have been associated with recovery from clinical depression in a recent investigation by Brown et al. [21].

Recent research in medical anthropology also points to the interaction of body and society in illness. Kleinman's study of the social origins of neurasthenia in contemporary China shows how the trauma of the Cultural Revolution as well as core principles of Chinese culture are reflected in the patterning of symptoms and illuminate their meaning [22,23]. His recent [24] work with chronic pain patients details the impact of microlevel interpersonal processes on the exacerbation and alleviation of distress over time.

In a study of illness course in schizophrenia, Corin [25] posed the question: How do schizophrenic patients' relations to the world—their "ways of being" in the social environment—affect their ability to sustain independent living outside the hospital? Her findings, based on a combination of qualitative and quantitative methodologies, suggest that independent living is associated with the development of a "distancing-and-relating" style of interacting, a life stance she terms "positive withdrawal."

The impact of illness meanings on clinical outcomes is also the subject of current research in medical anthropology. In a study of hip fracture patients' narrative accounts of their experiences, Borkan et al. [26] found that those individuals who viewed their situation as a problem external to themselves were more mobile at 3- and 6-month follow-up than patients who interpreted their condition as somehow internal or "organic." Perceived causes of medical illness were shown to be related to depression in a study of leprosy and mental health in India, recently reported by Weiss et al. [27].

Two aims animate the discussion to follow. The first is to focus attention on the importance of social context for understanding chronic fatigue syndrome by using data from a recent anthropological interview study. The second is to point out the culturally constituted nature of the mind–body dichotomy, and the implications of mind–body dualism for research and illness experience in CFS.

DESCRIPTION OF RESEARCH

Fifty individuals from the more than 350 chronic fatigue patients being followed by Anthony Komaroff were participants in the study. Initially, these patients sought help for a debilitating fatigue that significantly interfered with their work or home responsibilities. Approximately 60% met criteria for the Centers for Disease Control (CDC) working case definition of chronic fatigue syndrome [28]. The study sample was similar in age, sex, and educational background to the larger group, but tended to have fewer objective abnormalities on laboratory tests.

Subjects were interviewed using a semistructured, open-ended interview schedule designed to elicit narrative data on life history and illness experience.

Interviews were tape-recorded and transcribed. Most interviews took place in the participants' homes.

Eighty percent ($N = 40$) of the study participants were women; 92% were white. They ranged in age from 23 to 66 years at the time of data collection; the mean age of the sample was 39. Almost half (48%) of the group had left formal education before completing the bachelor's degree; nearly a quarter (22%) had only secondary education or less. Fifty percent of subjects had been ill for 5 years or more at the time the interview took place; the mean length of illness was 5.7 years.

Social Worlds, Meaning, and Experience

Interviewees' descriptions of the months and years before their illness began suggest that they saw themselves as extremely *busy* people. Their accounts overflow with references to how intensely involved they were in the wide range of activities that defined the scope of their lives. Men and women who were employed devoted up to 80 hours a week to their jobs. Mothers who worked at home began their days early and stayed up late to complete chores after the children were in bed.

Not content to focus on just one or two responsibilities, respondents reported being involved in "a million things at once." They piled part-time on top of full-time employment; combined jobs with child-rearing, volunteer work, and demanding exercise programs; cared for sick or ageing parents; and prided themselves on maintaining active social lives. Coping with this number and variety of responsibilities meant they had to move fast; thus days were spent racing from one activity to another in a constant, frantic effort to "keep up." The following excerpts from study interviews are illustrative.

> I wouldn't do just *one* thing. I'd do six or seven at the same time! Put in a load of wash, work on a load in the dryer, hang out a load on the line. Just get it all done while I'm sewing, while I'm cleaning up the kitchen, while I'm vacuuming, while I'm washing the floor. I'd even put a child in the bathtub and take the wallpaper off the wall! Take the wallpaper off the wall and give the child a bath. Just don't stop until you get it all done. And I'd put in 14–16 h a day. I'd hear somebody else saying, "I've put in a 14-h day, or a 70-h week," and I'd think, "I've been doing that for years!"

> I was an extremely energetic sort of person. Physically I was in very very good shape. I was working 12–13 h a day, including weekends, going to school nights, and teaching. I had a husband, children, kept up with the laundry, cooked on weekends for the week. Until recently, I hadn't had a vacation in years.

Life history data from the interviews reveal evidence of considerable distress (Table 1). Negative life events in the form of serious injury, divorce, job loss, or death of a family member or close friend were reported as occurring before the onset of CFS by a large proportion of the sample. Chronic difficulties, such

Table 1 Life History Data for Individuals with
Chronic Fatigue Syndrome ($N = 50$)

History	n	$\%^d$
Negative life event(s)[a]	21	42
Chronic life difficulties[b]	20	40
Evidence of family psychiatric history[c]	26	52
Abuse, low self-esteem, family tension in childhood	22	44

[a]Serious injury, divorce, job loss, death of family member or close friend.
[b]Serious illness in immediate family, troubled or failing marriage, persistent work problems.
[c]Depression, anxiety, alcohol or other drug abuse, or physical violence in parents or other close family members.
[d]These categories are not mutually exclusive; thus the total exceeds 100%.

as serious illness in the immediate family, a troubled or failing marriage, or persistent problems at work, were also described by many. Approximately half of the subjects represented their childhoods in terms that suggested the presence of significant depression or anxiety, alcohol or other drug abuse, or physical violence in parents or other close family members. Physical, sexual, or verbal abuse, low self-esteem, and chronic tension or fighting in the family were other recurring childhood themes. As these data emerged as part of spontaneous reports made in the context of a life history narrative (i.e., the interview did not include specific questions about these events), the percentages in Table 1 may actually be conservative estimates.

The character of these local social worlds is reflected in the meaning and experience of CFS for this study sample.

For example, many interviewees explicitly attributed the onset of their illness to events in those worlds—what they referred to as "stress." Stress was cited as either a contributing factor or the single probable cause of CFS by almost half of the interviewees, who used the term to mean sensations of being overwhelmed by obligations and commitments, experiences of loss, fears of displeasing others, or feelings of loneliness and isolation. Most often, stress was represented as the instigating factor in a chain reaction leading to "weakened immune system" and resulting viral infection—a "biopsychosocial model" of CFS (Table 2).

The symbolism of fatigue as a symptom also deserves recognition here. What, if not exhausting, are the hectic pace, the myriad responsibilities, the unrelenting activity, that these individuals describe? In this as in other forms of distress, the social world inscribes itself in symbolic language on the body. Although it may

Table 2 Attributions of Illness Onset in
CFS ($N = 50$)

Attributed to	n	$\%$
Stress only[a]	4	8
Virus only	13	26
Biopsychosocial model[b]	18	36
Other psychosocial[c]	5	10
Other[d]	8	16
No information	2	4

[a]Feeling overwhelmed by obligations or commitments,
experiences of loss, fears of displeasing others, feelings
of loneliness or isolation.
[b]Stress leading through immune dysfunction to viral
infection.
[c]Trauma, overwork, depression, anxiety, sorcery.
[d]For example, contagion, contamination, illness as
punishment or "test."

have other meanings as well, fatigue is emblematic of the local social worlds of
these CFS patients.

Local worlds of experience mediate and reflect macro-order sociocultural
processes. Since the 1970s in the United States, pressured, overcommitted
lifestyles have served as an index of success for women straining to meet
feminism's challenge to "have it all" by combining a demanding career with a
rich and fulfilling family life. In the 1980s, "baby boomers" of both sexes found
themselves forced into efforts to work longer, and do better, than their peers to
land jobs in a competitive labor market. Once employed, they had to advance
quickly enough to keep pace with escalating inflation.

Others [29] have noted the parallels between the rapid social change and
increasing life pace that surrounded the rise of neurasthenia in the 19th century
and the emergence of CFS in recent years. What is added here is an empirical
association between CFS and a stressful, fast-paced lifestyle.

Attributions of cause to social sources and the symbolic representation of
social experience in the core complaint of fatigue illustrate the connection of
CFS to local worlds and the larger social forces they mediate. These patterns
also exemplify some of the social meanings of the disorder and suggest that
social processes may play a role in its development and course. The symptoms
of CFS may represent the embodied experience and expression of social sources
of distress. This is not to deny the involvement of biological dysfunction. Rather,
it raises the question: how are society, mind, and body woven together in ways
that produce this illness?

CULTURAL ORIGINS OF MIND–BODY DUALISM: IMPLICATIONS

Illness episodes are customarily assigned to one of two basic categories. A given set of signs and symptoms is interpreted *either* as bodily disease, the result of some identifiable biological malfunction, *or* as psychiatric disorder, the product of invisible pathological processes inferred to be taking place in the mind. The taxonomy that guides diagnostic practice in professional medicine rests on a fundamental dichotomy that splits mind and body into separate, mutually exclusive, entities.

We are accustomed to thinking of the mind–body dichotomy as given in Nature, a reflection of empirical reality. Yet an anthropologically informed view reveals this concept to be a cultural and historical construct, one of a series of assumptions rooted in cartesian dualism that cast in opposition not only body and mind, but matter and spirit, subject and object, Nature and culture. The cultural specificity of mind–body dualism is thrown into relief through comparison with other epistemological traditions.

In traditional Chinese medicine, for example, psyche and soma converge. Physical and psychological complaints are considered different aspects of a single disorder. The locus of illness, in Chinese medical thought, is not body *or* mind, but rather a unified body–mind. In Chinese, as in many non-Western traditions, the body is considered mind*ful* and the mind, in the same way, *embodied* [22,30].

A nondualistic conception of mind–body relations has implications for the interpretation and classification of symptoms. Thus, emotional as well as physical symptoms are included in diagnostic definitions of neurasthenia in Chinese medicine. However, whereas in the case of CFS the presence of depression raises questions about whether the condition should be classified as medical or psychiatric, in neurasthenia psychological and somatic symptoms are seen as having a common organic origin. (Neurasthenia is also a diagnostic category in Chinese psychiatry, where its status has been the subject of considerable debate in recent years [for discussion, see 22 and 51].)

We see the mind–body dichotomy reflected in the social organization of research on CFS. Despite isolated appeals for "unifying hypotheses" [31] and "multifactorial" or "integrative" approaches [32,33], most empirical research has focused *either* on attempts to isolate various pathophysiological mechanisms— viral infections [34,35], immune dysfunction [36,37], disorders of muscle physiology [38]—or on the assessment of psychiatric disorder in CFS patients [39–42]. However, truly integrative approaches, in which pathophysiology and psychopathology are examined as part of the same research effort rather than in separate studies, are now beginning to appear [43,44].

The mind–body dichotomy is not, however, simply an organizing principle for disease classification and clinical research. It also symbolizes a set of "hidden values" in Western biomedicine [45] that imbue it with moral implications.

As a form of science, medicine subscribes to a world view in which Nature is primary and universal. Nature is seen as consisting of unchanging material substance organized in terms of "laws," which can be "discovered" through rational means. Rationality privileges observation over subjective experience as a way of knowing; hence in the naturalist paradigm only physical matter, the presence of which can be objectively verified, can be considered "real." In medicine, this means that the only true illnesses are those whose presence can be confirmed through the observation of physical abnormality. Conditions that cannot be traced to an abnormality in the body, which can only be inferred on the basis of patients' reports of experienced distress, are from a medical perspective, "not real" [46]. Mind–body dualism dictates that an illness that is not physical must be psychological; thus, CFS symptoms are defined as "psychosomatic."

CFS sufferers routinely find their experience of illness disconfirmed on these grounds. Participants in the study discussed earlier complained vociferously of repeatedly being told they were not sick because no objective evidence of disease could be found [47]. When clinical examinations and x-rays reveal nothing, when the results of every laboratory test come back negative, and because those affected by CFS often look perfectly healthy, many physicians (also colleagues and friends) conclude that the problem is psychological in origin. The following interview excerpt typifies patients' reported perceptions and experiences of "delegitimizing encounters":

> Even with doctors that I thought were basically good doctors, when I presented with all these symptoms, the feeling was, "Hmm, there are a lot of symptoms. Do you have a problem psychologically?" . . . It was like a dismissal. They would say things like, "You can't be experiencing what you are experiencing. You need to see a psychologist. You're not as sick as you think you are."

> *How did that make you feel?*

> Furious! I feel like I learned a lot in the process because it helped me be much more assertive. Because in our family we didn't go to doctors unless we were *so* sick! Then to get hit with, "You're not as sick as you think you are" made me furious. Not only was I paying all that money and they weren't helping me. *This* is what I get!

Sometimes the attribution of psychogenic origins included an intimation that patients were causing their own distress:

> The first doctor I saw said it's probably me. Probably I was hiding something. Probably I was very nervous—high-strung. I probably had all these dreadful problems, and that was causing me to make myself sick. That I was giving myself headaches, that I was making myself tired, because I was maybe depressed.

What was your reaction to that?

I got real mad. Once I calmed down, I said, "I have to play this thing out. If I don't go through all these tests that he wants, then I'm not going to prove to him that he's wrong. He's not going to believe me just because I sit here and yell at him and tell him he's crazy." So I went through all these things to show him, and I answered them all truthfully. I wanted him to see there was something else wrong, and we had to take this a step further. So after he reached that point himself, then we went on. But even when we were done with all that, he could find no physical cause, so he still went back to saying it was something I was doing to myself.

A frequent response to experiences of delegitimation was outrage, as these citations illustrate. Some respondents reported having temporarily accepted a psychogenic interpretation, going on then to contemplate the implications of being, as they put it, "crazy," or having an illness that was "all in their heads." Sooner or later, however, nearly everyone rejected a psychosomatic definition of their condition, instead arguing with considerable vigor that theirs was a physical and not a psychological illness.

Consistent with naturalism's emphasis on observable material evidence as the criterion for "real disease," wherever possible these arguments took the form of pointing to signs of physical pathology—fevers, swollen glands, muscle weakness that, as one person reported with obvious relief, "showed up on this little graph." Where observable evidence was lacking, subjectively experienced physical symptoms or severity of impairment was invoked. The number and intensity of somatic complaints and the level of incapacitation they involved could not, according to this line of reasoning, be produced by the mind. As one participant put it:

There were times when I thought it might be all in my head, but then the physical symptoms in my body were telling me it's not in my head. You can't have all these symptoms and get to the point where you're bedridden and you're laying on the couch all the time and have it be psychological. I know something psychological can't bring on all these symptoms. Maybe if I'd only had a few, maybe then I would have gone to a counselor or to talk to somebody different, but all these symptoms?

The often fierce resistance to psychological interpretations of CFS observed here and by other investigators [48] stems from the stigma attached to disorders of mind. This same stigma can lead patients with psychological and physical complaints to selectively perceive and report somatic symptoms, as students of somatization have observed [22,49].

But why is the stigma of psychiatric illness, compared with most physical conditions, particularly intense?

Mind and body, as Kirmayer [45] reminds us, symbolize a set of fundamental contrasts in Western metaphysics. Mind is the seat of reason and volition, body the locus of "natural" biological processes that lie largely outside the realms of rationality, agency, and intention. The task and the challenge of mind is to exercise dominance over the body, to bring it under rational control.

With control and volition, come responsibility. We are held accountable for what we command or intend. Thus, paradoxically, sickness of mind ("loss of reason") signifies not only failure of will and loss of control, but a failure of will and loss of control we *brought on ourselves*. It follows that we are responsible; psychological disorder is "our own fault."

Physical illness, in contrast, is not something we do to ourselves, but something that happens to us. Because the body continually defies willful mastery, its disorders are seemingly random and accidental, often occurring for no apparent reason and leaving us asking "Why me?" The involuntary nature of disease frees us from responsibility. We are *not* responsible for what we *cannot* control.

It is responsibility and blame that make illness into a moral issue. Degree of culpability—more in disorders of mind, less in afflictions of the body—determines the amount of stigma attached.

Thus we see a culturally constituted mind–body dichotomy, and the naturalist scientific paradigm embedded in it, reflected in medical research and practice related to CFS. Researchers have tended to look at either the bodies or the minds of those affected by the illness, only recently beginning to merge these two lines of investigation into a single unified endeavor. Medical practice informed by naturalism results in objectively verifiable complaints being accorded legitimacy as "real," whereas others are discounted. The real somatic distress experienced by CFS sufferers is thus relegated to the realm of the psychosomatic, where the stigma of moral reprehensibility quickly makes itself felt.

CONCLUSION

An anthropological perspective points out the advantages of placing the study of chronic fatigue syndrome in social and cultural context.

Evidence of links between symptoms and the quality of life in local social worlds suggests that social factors play a role in the development and course of CFS. Yet social influences have received almost no research attention to date, despite the fact that social contributors to onset and chronicity might be effectively addressed through behavioral interventions and psychotherapy. This seems especially important, given the absence, at present, of a truly effective medical treatment for this illness.

The observation that mind–body dualism is part of culture, not Nature, offers a critical distance on familiar ways of proceeding and smooths the path toward constructive change in our thinking about chronic fatigue syndrome. One such change is the recent recommendation to include selected psychiatric disorders in a revised working case definition [50], a recommendation that should help promote future efforts to integrate psyche and soma in empirical research. The development of a critical perspective on naturalistic definitions of what constitutes "real disease" is, however, a task that still lies ahead for mainstream medicine. Restructuring the standard paradigm to legitimate subjectively experienced symptoms that remain unverifiable through clinical or laboratory assessment is certain to reduce the suffering of CFS and other patients whose distress has no apparent medical explanation.

An anthropological perspective also reaches beyond the transcendence of mind–body dualism to propose a conceptualization of illness that connects interpersonal experience to psychological distress, felt bodily sensation, and observable or unobservable biological change. Thus, chronic fatigue syndrome is envisioned, not as physical, psychological, *or* social, but as physical, psychological, *and* social in an anthropological view. The challenge for those seeking to understand CFS is to identify the mediating mechanisms through which events in the social world are realized as experienced distress in the body and the mind. It is a challenge that calls for the combined efforts of social scientists, psychiatrists, and medical researchers.

ACKNOWLEDGMENTS

The research discussed here was conducted while the author was a postdoctoral fellow in an NIMH-sponsored research training program in clinically relevant medical anthropology (grant 5T32MH18006). A grant from the Robert Wood Johnson Foundation (13984) provided additional support. The guidance of Arthur Kleinman, MD, in designing and completing the study is gratefully acknowledged. Thanks are extended also to Anthony Komaroff, MD, who referred participants, and, of course, to the participants themselves.

Correspondence may be directed to the author at the Department of Social Medicine, Harvard Medical School, 641 Huntington Avenue, Boston, MA, 02115.

REFERENCES

1. Grant I, McDonald I, Patterson T, Trimble MR. Multiple sclerosis. In: Brown GW, Harris TO, eds. Life events and illness. New York: Guilford Press, 1989:295–312.
2. Warren SA, Greenhill S, Warren KG. Emotional stress and the development of multiple sclerosis: case control evidence of a relationship. J Chronic Dis 1982; 35:821–31.
3. Cottington EM, Mathews KA, Talbott E, et al. Environmental events preceding sudden death in women. Psychosom Med 1980; 42:567–74.

4.   Engle GL. Sudden and rapid death during psychological stress. Ann Intern Med 1971; 74:771–82.

5.   Glass DC. Behavior patterns, stress and coronary disease. Hillsdale, NJ: Lawrence Erlbaum Associates, 1977.

6.   Neilson E, Brown GW, Marmot M. Myocardial infarction. In: Brown GW, Harris TO, eds. Life events and illness. New York: Guilford Press, 1989:313–42.

7.   Siegrist J, Dittman KH, Rittner K, Weber I. The social context of active distress in patients with early myocardial infarction. Soc Sci Med 1982; 16:443–54.

8.   Brown GW, Harris TO: Social origins of depression: a study of psychiatric disorder in women. London: Tavistock, 1978.

9.   Brown GW, Andrews B, Harris TO, et al. Social support, self-esteem and depression. Psychol Med 1986; 16:813–31.

10.   Kessler RC, Cleary PD. Social class and psychological distress. Am Sociol Rev 1980; 45:463–78.

11.   Dressler WW, Alfonso M, Chavez A, Viteri FE. Arterial blood pressure and individual modernization in a Mexican community. Soc Sci Med 1987; 24:679–87.

12.   Dressler WW. Hypertension and culture change: acculturation and disease in the West Indies. New York: Redgrave Publishing, 1982.

13.   Dressler WW, Santos IED, Gallagher PN Jr, et al. Arterial blood pressure and modernization in Brazil. Am Anthropol 1987; 89:389–409.

14.   Dressler WW. Lifestyle, stress and blood pressure in a southern black community. Psychosom Med 1990; 52:182–98.

15.   Pearlin LI. The social contexts of stress. In: Goldberger L, Breznitz S, eds. Handbook of stress: theoretical and clinical aspects. New York: Free Press, 1982.

16.   Kanner AD, Coyne JC, Schaefer C, Lazarus RS. Comparison of two modes of stress measurement: daily hassles and uplifts vs major life events. J Behav Med 1980; 4:1–39.

17.   Leff J, Vaughn CE. Expressed emotion in families: its significance for mental illness. New York: Guilford Press, 1985.

18.   Brown GW, Birley J. Crises and life changes in the onset of schizophrenia. J Health Soc Behav 1968; 9:217–44.

19.   Day R, Nielson J, Korten A, et al. Stressful life events preceding the acute onset of schizophrenia: a cross-national study from the World Health Organization. Cult Med Psychiatry 1987; 11:1–123.

20.   Sartorius N, Jablensky A, Ernberg G, et al. Course of schizophrenia in different countries: some results of a WHO international comparative follow-up study. In: Hafner H, Gatteiz WF, Janzarik W, eds. Search for the causes of schizophrenia. Berlin: Springer-Verlag, 1987:107–13.

21.   Brown GW, Adler Z, Bifulco A. Life events, difficulties, and recovering from depression. Br J Psychiatry 1988; 152:487–98.

22.   Kleinman A. Social origins of distress and disease. New Haven: Yale University Press, 1986.

23.   Kleinman A, Kleinman J. Remembering the Cultural Revolution: alienating pains and the pain of alienation. Paper presented at the Asian Studies Annual Meeting, New Orleans 1991, April 13.

24.   Kleinman A. Pain and resistance: the delegitimation and relegitimation of local

worlds. In: Good DelVecchio MJ, Brodwin PE, Good BJ, Kleinman A, eds. Pain as human experience: an anthropological perspective. Berkeley: University of California, 1992:169–97.

25. Corin EE. Facts and meaning in psychiatry: an anthropological approach to the lifeworld of schizophrenics. Cult Med Psychiatry 1990; 14:153–88.

26. Borkan JM, Quirk M, Sullivan M. Finding meaning after the fall: injury narratives from elderly hip fracture patients. Soc Sci Med 1991; 33:947–57.

27. Weiss MG, Doongaji DR, Wypij D, et al. The explanatory model interview catalogue (EMIC): contribution to cross-cultural research methods from a study of leprosy and mental health. Br J Psychiatry 1992; 160:819–30.

28. Holmes G, Kaplan JE, Gantz NM, et al. Chronic fatigue syndrome: a working case definition. Ann Intern Med 1988; 108:387–89.

29. Abbey SE, Garfinkel PE. Neurasthenia and chronic fatigue syndrome: the role of culture in the making of a diagnosis. Am J Psychiatry 1991; 148:1638–46.

30. Scheper-Hughes N, Lock M. The mindful body: prolegomenon to future work in medical anthropology. Med Anthropol Q 1987; 1:6–41.

31. Straus SE. The chronic mononucleosis syndrome. J Infect Dis 1988; 157:405–12.

32. David AS, Wessely S, Pelosi AJ. Postviral fatigue syndrome: time for a new approach. Br Med J 1988; 296:696–99.

33. Demitrack MA, Greden JF. Chronic fatigue syndrome: the need for an integrative approach. Biol Psychiatry 1991; 30:747–52.

34. DeFreitas E, Hilliard B, Cheney PR, et al. Retroviral sequences related to human T-lymphotropic virus type II in patients with chronic fatigue and immune dysfunction syndrome. Proc Natl Acad Sci USA 1992; 88:2922–26.

35. Gow JW, Behan WM, Clements GB, et al. Enteroviral RNA sequences detected by polymerase chain reaction in muscle of patients with postviral fatigue syndrome. Br Med J 1991; 302:692–96.

36. Lloyd AR, Wakefield D, Boughton C, et al. Immunological abnormalities in the chronic fatigue syndrome. Med J Aust 1989; 151:122–24.

37. Caligiuri M. Murray C, Buchwald D, et al. Phenotypic and functional deficiency of natural killer cells in patients with chronic fatigue syndrome. J Immunol 1987; 139:3306–13.

38. Edwards RHT, Helliwell TR, Clague JE, Gibson H. Muscle physiology and histopathology in CFS. In: Kleinman A, Straus SE, eds. Chronic fatigue syndrome (CIBA Foundation Symposium 173). Chichester: John Wiley & Sons, 1993:102–17.

39. Manu P, Matthews DA, Lane TJ. The mental health of patients with a chief complaint of chronic fatigue. Arch Intern Med 1988; 148:2213–17.

40. Kruesi MJP, Dale J, Straus SE. Psychiatric diagnoses in patients who have chronic fatigue syndrome. J Clin Psychiatry 1989; 50:53–6.

41. Katon WJ, Buchwald DS, Simon GE et al. Psychiatric illness in patients with chronic fatigue and those with rheumatoid arthritis. J Gen Intern Med 1991; 6:277–85.

42. Hickie I, Lloyd A, Wakefield D, Parker G. The psychiatric status of patients with the chronic fatigue syndrome. Br J Psychiatry 1990; 156:534–40.

43. Gold D, Bowden R, Sixbey J, et al. Chronic fatigue: a prospective clinical and virologic study. JAMA 1990; 264:48–53.

44. Bates DW, Schmitt W, Buchwald D, et al. Prevalence of fatigue and chronic fatigue syndrome in a primary care practice. Arch Intern Med (in press).

45. Kirmayer LJ. Mind and body as metaphors: hidden values in biomedicine. In: Lock M, Gordon DR, eds. Biomedicine examined. Dordrecht: Kluwer Academic, 1988:57–91.

46. Gordon DR. Tenacious assumptions in Western medicine. In: Lock M, Gordon DR, eds. Biomedicine examined. Dordrecht: Kluwer Academic, 1988:19–55.

47. Ware NC. Suffering and the social construction of illness: the delegitimation of illness experience in chronic fatigue syndrome. Med Anthropol Q 1992; 6:347–61.

48. Wessely SE, Powell R. Fatigue syndromes: a comparison of chronic "postviral" fatigue with neuromuscular and affective disorders. J Neurol Neurosurg Psychiatry 1989; 52:940–48.

49. Katon W. Depression: somatization and social factors. J Fam Pract 1988; 27:579–80.

50. Schluederberg A, Straus SE, Peterson P, et al. Chronic fatigue syndrome: definition and medical outcome assessment. Ann Intern Med 1992; 117:325–31.

51. Lin T. Neurasthenia revisited: its place in modern psychiatry. Cult Med Psychiatry 1989; 13:2:105–29.

II

INFECTION AND IMMUNITY

5

Infection and Chronic Fatigue Syndrome

Robert Fekety
University of Michigan Medical Center, Ann Arbor, Michigan

> This chapter is dedicated to those patients with chronic fatigue syndrome who have been told by their physicians that there is nothing wrong with them and they should learn to live with it and get on with their lives.

Many references to the relation between psychological or emotional factors and infectious diseases have been made in the past. These often indicate that patients undergoing psychological stress are more susceptible to certain infections, or that they may recover more slowly from them [1–4]. Tumulty noted that weakness was the most common symptom between acute attacks of recurrent malaria in soldiers during World War II, and that emotional stress had a significant influence on the severity of their weakness and fatigue [1]. Frank reported that many soldiers in World War II with schistosomiasis showed, during convalescence, a prolongation of fatigue and other symptoms of illness that was out of proportion to objective evidence of disease [2]. He felt the strangeness and uncertainty of schistosomiasis played an important role in the development of emotional reactions that impeded recovery. Such factors are undoubtedly important even today when newly recognized or unusual infectious diseases are followed by chronic fatigue syndrome (CFS).

In 1959, Greenfield and associates reported a correlation in patients with infectious mononucleosis between measured "ego strength" and duration of illness, defined by objective hematological criteria [3]. However, almost all studies dealing with delayed recovery from infectious diseases have, of necessity, been concerned with the subjective prolongation of symptoms, since it is difficult to quantify weakness and easy fatigability. The lack of objective measures of both fatigue and effort has hampered many investigations of CFS. Graham and co-workers reported that "major life event stress" was associated with more episodes and more symptom days during respiratory infection [4].

Cohen and colleagues reported elegant and well-controlled studies concerning the interaction of psychological stress and susceptibility to common colds induced experimentally with rhinovirus types 2, 9, or 14; respiratory syncytial virus or coronavirus type 220E [5]. The rates of both documented infection ($p < 0.005$) and clinical illness ($p < 0.02$) caused by all five viruses increased, in a dose–response manner, with increases in degree of psychological stress. Increases were entirely attributable to increased rates of infection, and not to an increased duration of symptoms after infection. Controlling for many demographic, social, immunological, and personality variables did not negate these interesting findings.

Extreme fatigue or prostration, sore throat, painful muscles, lymphadeno-pathy, headache, and symptoms of an emotional or psychological nature are the rule, rather than the exception in patients with CFS [6], and it is often difficult in individual patients to tell whether psychological factors precipitated CFS or whether they were the result of it. Since it is very common (but not universal) for CFS to begin with what appears to be a viral or flulike illness (although it is rarely proved to be such), it is not surprising that CFS often was thought to be caused by common and usually benign, self-limited infections that for some reason became chronic. Chronic fatigue syndrome has occurred in outbreaks or clusters, which has strengthened the putative association with infection. In addition, when studied extensively, most patients with CFS have one or more deviations (in either direction) from what is considered "normal" in various tests of immunological reactivity or competence. Even though the specific deviations vary widely from one patient to another, and no single immunological dysfunction has been found in all patients with CFS, it has been attractive to consider these immunological aberrations causally related to the prolongation of the infectious process and development of CFS. Despite a great deal of investigative effort by highly qualified scientists, "the cause" of CFS has not yet been determined. It is my belief that no single infectious etiology will be found; rather, that many different infections will be found to be capable of precipitating the syndrome. Nevertheless, recent investigations have yielded a great deal of interesting and important information that is leading to new concepts and hypotheses concerning the relation between CFS and infection [7]. Before considering these newer concepts, it is appropriate to review the observations and conclusions of previous investigators.

In this chapter, the terminology, clinical aspects, and diagnostic criteria for the many illnesses described in earlier times that resemble chronic fatigue syndrome (CFS) will be not be analyzed in detail. Figure 1 illustrates the results

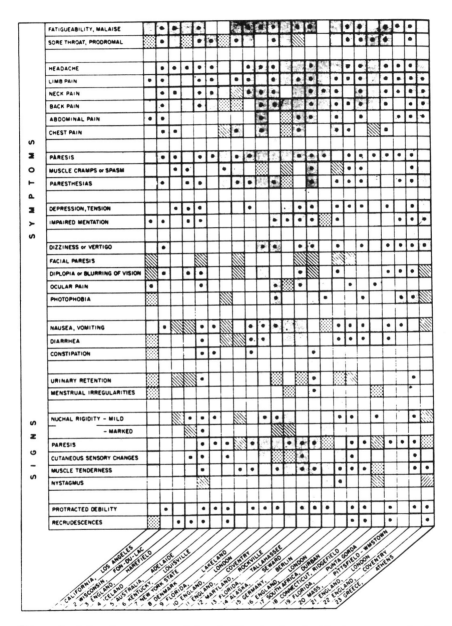

Figure 1   Selected symptoms and signs in 23 outbreaks of epidemic neuromyasthenia:
□ over 50% of cases; ▨ 25–50% of cases; ◪ under 25% of cases; ● frequency not stated.

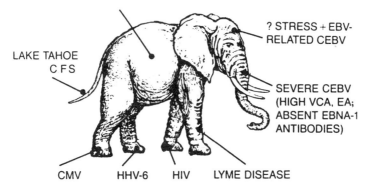

? STRESS + EBV-
RELATED CEBV

LAKE TAHOE
C F S

SEVERE CEBV
(HIGH VCA, EA;
ABSENT EBNA-1
ANTIBODIES)

CMV   HHV-6   HIV   LYME DISEASE

Figure 2   CFS: an elephantine enigma. CMV, cytomegalovirus; HHV-6, human herpesvirus type-6; HIV, human immunodeficiency virus. (From Ref. 9.)

Henderson and Shelokov obtained when they detailed the findings from numerous reports concerning an illness resembling CFS [8]. Our present understanding of etiology and pathogenesis of the illness does not justify considering entities, such as so-called chronic brucellosis, epidemic neuromyasthenia, benign myalgic encephalitis, chronic fatigue immune dysfunction syndrome, and CFS as separate and distinct. Although such specific names will be used when discussing the details of publications concerning what was believed at the time to be a new and unique syndrome, the reader is urged to consider it likely that they represented variations in time and place of the same entity, as conceptualized by Evans in Figure 2 [9]. In general, I prefer to use the (arguably) most popular name at present in the United States, the chronic fatigue syndrome or CFS, when discussing these illnesses. It should be emphasized that little attention will be given to whether the various entities discussed in this chapter qualify for the diagnosis of the chronic fatigue syndrome according to the Centers for Disease Control (CDC) criteria that were published in 1988 [6] and revised in 1992 [7].

CHRONIC BRUCELLOSIS

Some of the best studies of delayed recovery from infection were concerned with the entity known as chronic brucellosis, and it was probably the first well-documented example of the postinfectious chronic fatigue syndrome. Since it provides an excellent framework for evaluating more recent studies of the chronic fatigue syndrome, chronic brucellosis is worthy of presentation and consideration in detail.

Alice C. Evans, a bacteriologist at the National Institutes of Health, called attention to the condition she called chronic brucellosis in 1934 [10]. She described a chronic disabling form of brucellosis in humans that was associated with little or no fever, but was characterized by fatigue, myalgia, and irritability. During studies of slaughter house material, in which some animals were found to have viable brucellae in small abscesses, lymph nodes, spleen, and vertebral bones, she began to suspect that latent or subclinical brucellar infection was the cause of a unique, chronic illness in humans, many of whom had been diagnosed as having neurasthenia. She indicated that some patients referred to her with chronic active brucellosis had been diagnosed previously as having neurasthenia. She pointed out that the textbook definition of neurasthenia (exhaustion, insomnia, and complaints of aches and pains for which no objective signs could be found) also described chronic brucellosis. She also pointed out that it is a severe trial for a patient with chronic brucellosis who appeals for medical aid to be told that their illness is imaginary, and that all that is necessary for recovery is to acquire the proper mental attitude. In her opinion, the failure of physicians to appreciate the real diagnosis of chronic brucellosis contributed greatly to the mental depression characteristic of the disease, and there was no doubt in her mind that chronic brucellosis was often misdiagnosed as neurasthenia.

Evans wondered how often neurasthenia was caused by chronic brucellosis. She concluded that ordinary clinical studies would not yield the answer to this question, since neurasthenia was diagnosable only when no organic cause for the patient's symptoms could be found. In 1934, there were no reliable diagnostic laboratory tests for chronic brucellosis, and no specific or curative treatment. She also pointed out that positive cultures from blood, abscesses, or excretions are the one infallible proof of brucellar infection and that these cultures are frequently negative, even in acute brucellosis. At best, it was difficult to obtain appropriate material for culture from patients with chronic active brucellosis. Furthermore, she argued, negative serum antibody tests were of little significance in diagnosing chronic brucellosis because antibodies were often absent in severe, culture-positive cases, and were even less often present in mild cases. She rejected the usefulness of skin tests with brucellar antigens on the grounds that cutaneous reactivity to them may remain for long periods, even after recovery from the disease is complete. She concluded that a consideration of the combined results of all three tests (cultures, serological, and skin tests) was the best way then available to diagnose chronic brucellosis, and she expressed her hope that a fourth test, based on the opsonic power of the blood, would be definitive, although its practicality had not yet been confirmed.

This hope for a new and better diagnostic test has continued with monotonous regularity in subsequent studies of CFS. It is also of interest that brucellosis can present in many different ways; it can be mild or even subclinical, the organism may persist in the patient for long periods at occult sites, and the diagnosis is often one of exclusion.

Evans challenged "the right of physicians to make a diagnosis of neurasthenia—a diagnosis regarded as dishonorable by the patient and his family, his employer and his friends—without considering . . . the possibility of chronic brucellosis" [10].

Wesley Spink was, and still is, widely recognized as an expert in the epidemiology, pathogenesis, diagnosis, and management of brucellosis. Among his many contributions to our understanding of this disease was one concerning chronic brucellosis that was published in 1951 [11]. Spink pointed out there are enthusiasts who believe chronic brucellosis is a frequent cause of human disability, whereas there are skeptics who do not accept the criteria that are used for making that diagnosis. In relation to recent theories implicating cytokines produced during infection in the pathogenesis of CFS, it is noteworthy that brucellosis is an intracellular pathogen in which brucellae localize within mononuclear cells and other phagocytes of the reticuloendothelial system. Brucellae can actually multiply within these cells, where they are protected from the lethal action of many antibiotics. Thus, even with the best available therapy, viable brucellae might persist in tissues for long periods, with continued production of cytokines, and cause a chronic illness with frequent remissions and exacerbations. So, the idea of chronic brucellosis was a reasonable one, even in the light of present-day knowledge.

Spink reviewed the experience at his clinic at the University of Minnesota where brucellosis had been studied for many years, and where *Brucella abortus*, the least invasive species, caused most human brucellosis. About 75% of proved cases were in men, about 75% were due to direct contact with animals or their environment, and one-fourth were caused by ingestion of unpasteurized milk. Acute brucellosis in Minnesota occurred most frequently among farmers and meat-packing plant employees. The diagnosis of brucellosis was dependent on laboratory information. A positive intradermal test with brucellar antigens denoted previous tissue infection, but did not necessarily indicate active disease. In 1951, the skin test was frequently used as an aid in diagnosing suspected cases of chronic brucellosis, with a positive skin test tipping the scales in favor of the diagnosis. Spink cautioned that the scientific evidence weighed against this procedure and this interpretation. In Minnesota, about 20% of the healthy adult population in 1951 reacted positively to the intradermal injection of the brucellar antigen, and it was abandoned as an aid to diagnosis in Spink's clinic. The agglutination (serum antibody) reaction was the most reliable diagnostic test, aside from the actual isolation of the organism from blood or tissues, and it was extremely rare to recover organisms from the blood in the absence of agglutinins at a titer of less than 1:100. Even in those who recovered from brucellosis completely, a positive titer of agglutinins might persist for years.

In Spink's experience, patients suspected of having chronic brucellosis, or who were receiving therapy for it in absence of a definite diagnosis, usually had an ill-defined group of symptoms compatible with neurasthenia, psychoneurosis, or anxiety. Most of these patients were women, who often had a low-grade fever approaching 100°F. Blood cultures were sterile, and agglutinins were absent, even though the skin test was positive. Intensive antibiotic treatment for brucellosis was usually to no avail. These experiences revealed a pattern distinctly different from that seen with confirmed cases of brucellosis.

Spink and associates decided to study 65 patients with acute brucellosis, most of whom had been hospitalized, who had not been treated with antibiotics that are effective against brucella, and to observe them for several years to determine the consequences of the untreated infection. *Chronic brucellosis* was defined by them as an illness lasting for at least 1 year (the average in this study was 4.5 years). Of the 65 patients, there were only 12 women; 53 (77%) were men, a ratio similar to that of proved acute brucellosis, but the reverse of most studies with CFS. Most patients were between the ages of 20 and 50, and most had contracted the disease on farms or in meat-packing plants. About two-thirds had been proved by culture, and the remainder by clinical features and positive agglutinins. No patient died during the study, and it was difficult to determine with precision the duration of their illness.

There were four groups of patients. About 10 patients (16%) had acute brucellosis, but had recovered completely within 3 months; 25 patients (39%) had remained symptomatic for 3–12 months, during which time persistent bacteremia was often demonstrable in association with relapses. Chronic brucellosis was diagnosed in a group of 30 patients (46%) who had had ill health for more than 1 year; 17 of them had either definite relapsing disease, with positive blood cultures, or a focal complication. The final subgroup of 13 patients (about 20% of all cases) who had previously had acute brucellosis demonstrated no objective evidence of active disease at the time of the study, but still complained of ill health; some of them had lodged compensation claims. Although 30, or 46%, of all 65 patients complained of symptoms for more than 1 year, only 8 of the 30 (12%) were still disabled at the time of this study. In fact, 57% of all patients had been able to return to their usual routine at the end of 6 months, and 77% by 9 months.

Spink evaluated the effects of antibiotic therapy by comparing 61 treated cases of acute brucellosis with the 65 untreated cases just described. Although comparisons were difficult because the two groups were not strictly comparable, the outstanding difference (not surprisingly) between them was that the treated group tended to recover much more rapidly. Although 39% of the treated patients were still ill at 1 year, half of them (or about 20% of the total cases) complained of symptoms for which no cause could be found. Thus, the same percentage of patients with proved brucellosis complained of ill health without objective evidence of disease after 1 year, whether or not they had been treated with antibiotics.

Even though there is no way in retrospect to ascertain whether those individuals who were diagnosed with chronic brucellosis without objective evidence of disease would have met the criteria for the diagnosis of CFS, their symptoms appear very compatible with that diagnosis. Spink noted that with monotonous regularity they complained of weakness, vague aches and pains, easy fatigue, nervousness, and mental depression, despite that all cultures were sterile, and agglutinin titers had declined. Spink raised three possible explanations for their complaints. First, these patients may have had continued active brucellosis. Second, which was probably the correct explanation, they may have suffered from a disease process not caused by continued active infection, but because acute brucellosis had an impact on their nervous system (including the autonomic nervous system), as reflected in a reaction pattern that persisted long after the infection had subsided, such as an exaggeration or worsening of a preexisting personality disorder. And third, the symptoms may have been due to organic damage to the cerebral cortex.

Apter and associates suggested, in 1948, that cerebral impairment occurred in some patients with brucellosis and that damage to the cerebral cortex might explain many of the symptoms, psychiatric reactions, and changes in behavioral patterns seen in patients with chronic brucellosis [12]. They believed these symptoms needed to be distinguished from the rest of the disease complex, as they occurred so frequently in chronic brucellosis that a psychiatric label was often appended to the primary diagnosis. Seven of their ten patients exhibited clinical and laboratory evidence of organic brain disease, although definite neurological signs were elicited in only one patient. One of Apter's associates, W. C. Halstead, had developed a battery of 27 psychological indicators on which an "impairment index" of cortical functions and intelligence was based. They believed it provided an instrument to identify behavioral effects resulting from cortical damage. Apter and associates reported that patients with brucellosis and severe personality changes had measurable and sometimes severe impairment of "biological intelligence" and had organic brain disease, as measured by the Halstead index [12]. Furthermore, they had a "characteristic clinical picture" marked by headache, easy fatigability, inability to work, loss of former skills, insomnia without somnolence, decreased ability to adapt socially, intellectual defects, impoverished emotional expression, inability to plan for the future, and failure to establish ordinary rapport. Spink believed the issue of cerebral impairment or damage should be further explored in patients with chronic brucellosis.

Cluff and colleagues were able to do just that by studying 60 patients who accidentally acquired acute *B. melitensis* or *B. suis* infection from working in a large research laboratory where these organisms were being handled. They described the clinical [13], medical [14], and psychological aspects [15] of these infections in detail in three reports that appeared in 1959.

All 60 of their patients had acute brucellosis that was well documented by cultures or by serial agglutinin tests performed before, during, and after illness. Most patients were white males, with a mean age of 28 (range 20–49). The frequency of their symptoms and physical findings during the acute illness are shown in Table 1. The peripheral leukocyte count during the acute illness was normal in 2 of 58 patients, revealed leukopenia in 21, or leukocytosis up to 20,000 in 22; 5 patients had neutrophilia, 25 showed lymphocytosis, and 5 had monocytosis. Almost all patients had lymphocytosis or monocytosis during the early or late stages of their illness. Roentgenographic studies of bones and joints in several patients showed no abnormalities. Only 6 patients developed local complications, such as epididymitis, chronic synovitis, or chronic leg ulcers.

Twelve patients received no specific therapy during the acute illness, and the rest received sulfonamides, tetracyclines, or streptomycin alone or in combination with other antibodies.

Twenty-two patients (37% of the total) developed a chronic or recurrent illness, usually similar to, but milder than, the acute illness. None of the treatment regimens seemed more effective than the others in preventing persistence of symptoms for more than 6 months, and it was concluded that none of the regimens yielded consistently satisfactory results in the treatment of acute brucellosis.

Chronic brucellosis was defined for analytic purposes by these investigators as patients who complained of malaise, fatigue, myalgia, arthralgia, backache, or feverishness for a period of 1 year or longer beyond the acute illness,

Table 1 Symptoms and Physical Findings During Acute Brucellosis in 60 Patients

Symptoms	No.	Physical findings	No.
Headache	50	Fever	54
Fatigue	49	Pharyngitis	19
Feverish	48	Hepatomegaly	8
Myalgia	42	Rhinitis	7
Chills	34	Splenomegaly	6
Backache	28	Rales in lung	5
Arthralgia	24	Conjunctivitis	1
Nausea	21		
Cough	20		
Pharyngitis	17		
Chilliness	14		
Rhinitis	11		
Vomiting	10		
Diarrhea	7		
Chest pain	5		

Source: Ref. 13.

unassociated with bacteremia, changing serological titer, or abnormalities on physical examination. Twenty-four (40%) of the 60 patients with brucellosis met these criteria. Bacteremia was detected during the acute illness in 58% (14/24) of those who went on to develop chronic brucellosis and in 89% (32/36) of those who did not. There seemed to be no greater tendency for chronicity to follow infection by one species of the organism than by the other, and there were no characteristic serological patterns associated with chronic brucellosis, including the persistence of serum antibody titers of 1:100 or higher.

Cluff and associates were able to retrospectively study 24 of the 60 patients with acute brucellosis 4–8 years later [13–15]; 16 of the 24 had been diagnosed as having chronic brucellosis on the basis of persistence of symptoms for 1 year or longer after the acute illness. Ten of the 16 were still symptomatic at the time of study and were called the *chronic-symptomatic* group, whereas 6 (25%) with chronic brucellosis, who were by then asymptomatic, were called the *chronic-recovered* group. The remaining 8 patients had remained well since recovery from acute brucellosis, and were referred to as the *acute-recovered* group. The mean age of the 24 patients was about 35, and there were no significant differences between groups according to age, year of infection, or *Brucella* species. Other factors that did not differ included maximum temperature during the acute illness, frequency of febrile recurrences, height and pattern of agglutinin titers, nature and frequency of physical and laboratory abnormalities, and treatment regimen. In addition, the patients with chronic brucellosis were given additional courses of tetracycline before the study, but without benefit. A few were also given cortisone or hydrocortisone, with only transient improvement in their sense of well-being. None of them had important abnormal physical or neurological findings, and ordinary laboratory tests were essentially normal. Nine of the 24 patients had an abnormal electroencephalogram (EEG); 2 of them a history of head injury; and abnormal encephalograms in the remainder were distributed evenly between patients in the acute-recovered and chronic groups.

Patients who developed chronic brucellosis in this study tended to describe their illness as fluctuating in severity, with the principal symptoms being fatigue, headache, nervousness, depression, myalgia (either diffuse or in legs and back), and sexual impotence. Only two of them continued to have contact with *Brucella* species in the laboratory. There were no differences in the degree of delayed hypersensitivity skin test reactions to brucellergen between the groups, and none of the patients were anergic.

In short, the clinical and laboratory studies done on these three groups at the start of the study did not reveal any significant objective differences among them that would help distinguish between them, and there was no evidence of organic brain damage in patients with chronic brucellosis by the tests then available.

Reasons for the resemblance of the symptoms of chronic brucellosis to psychoneurosis and depression were the subject of the final paper in their series.

In it, Imboden and colleagues investigated the role of psychological factors in the pathogenesis of delayed convalescence from brucellosis [15]. They postulated that delayed resolution of illness could be the result either of enduring infection, or of a reduction in the patient's adaptive capacities (possibly because of organic brain damage or persistent susceptibility to infection), or to psychoneurosis. They explored the role of psychological or psychiatric factors in these patients by hospitalizing and further studying all 24 patients described in the previous section who had a history of acute brucellosis. Fourteen of them were healthy by then; 6 of them had recovered but had done so after 1 or more years from the onset of brucellar infection, and 10 were still symptomatic more than 2 years after the acute infection. All but 3 of the 14 recovered persons were professionals (bacteriologists or biochemists), whereas 6 of the 10 chronically symptomatic patients were nonprofessional employees.

Patients were evaluated by psychological tests of vocabulary, intelligence, memory, attention, recall, association, and efficiency; by the Bender–Visual–Motor–Gestalt test of visual motor coordination and perceptual confusion; by the empirically standardized Minnesota Multiphasic Personality Inventory (MMPI), designed to separate normal subjects into various clinical categories [hypochondriasis (Hs), depression (D), psychasthenia (Ps), hysteria (H)] and also to generate a neurotic index (AvN), which was an average of the clinical categories; and finally by additional personality tests called the Morale-Loss Index (ML) and a Self-Concept Scale (S-C) of the individual's perception of his or her worth. Subjects also underwent psychiatric interviews designed to determine their emotional and psychological condition. Importantly, the groups were also compared in terms of disturbed or troublesome life situations that existed at the time of the acute infection or the 1-year period before or after it.

Both of the recovered groups had a significantly higher mean intelligence level than the still-symptomatic one (fewer of whom were professionals), and there was no evidence of significant impairment of intellectual function or organic brain damage in any of the three groups.

In contrast, personality tests showed definite trends and differences among the groups (Table 2), and emotional disturbances were significantly more frequent at the time of the retrospective study in both chronic-symptomatic groups than in the acute-recovered group. The hypochondriasis score (reflecting somatization) was highest in the chronic-symptomatic group, whereas depression and psychasthenia scores, morale-loss index, and average neurotic index were significantly higher in both chronic groups than in the acute-recovered group. Depression was a prominent feature of the emotional disorders detected in both chronic groups. The acute-recovered group had significantly more positive self-concepts than the other two groups. Interestingly, patients in the chronic-symptomatic group tended to regard themselves as relatively normal emotionally. The chronic-recovered patients tended to have negative attitudes about their emotional health; indeed,

Table 2 Mean Scores of Patients on Personality Tests

	Hs	D	Pt	AvN	ML	S-C
Normal controls	48.2	49.4	48.2	50.5		
Acute-recovered	52.8	51.0	50.0	53.9	2.7	11.2
Chronic-recovered	54.8	64.0	62.8	58.7	8.2	64.3
Chronic-symptomatic	64.8	63.7	60.4	64.5	7.4	94.9

Hypochondriasis, Hs; depression, D; psychasthenia, Pt; average neurotic index, AvN; morale-loss index, ML; self-concept scale, S-C.
Source: Ref. 15.

psychological tests revealed evidence of emotional disturbance in that group. Chronic-symptomatic patients tended to be more resistant to a discussion of personal and emotional issues than the other two groups. Patients in the chronic-symptomatic group tended to believe they were emotionally healthy and believed they had an organic disease called "chronic brucellosis" that was capable of producing a wide variety of symptoms and disturbances in their sense of well-being. Both chronic groups were perceived as having more evidence of emotional disturbances, such as depression and anxiety, than the acute-recovered patients, who were also much less defensive. Most patients in all three groups viewed brucellosis as an acute infection that is often followed by a protracted illness.

It was the psychiatric interviewer's impression that patients in the two chronic groups showed considerably more evidence of emotional disturbance than those in the acute-recovered group. Most of the chronic patients were moderately depressed, often with symptoms of overt anxiety. Three of them appeared to be borderline schizophrenic, and hysterical features were present in several subjects.

Importantly, there was gross evidence of psychologic trauma during childhood in 11 of the 16 chronic patients and in only 2 of the 8 acute-recovered persons ($p < 0.05$). There were also significant differences in frequency of disturbed life situations during the period surrounding the acute infection; 11 of the 16 chronic patients experienced significant stresses during that period, as opposed to none of the 8 recovered patients. Factors commonly reported by chronic patients as occurring in relation to their acute illness were death or serious illness of a close family member (7 patients), conflictual interpersonal family situations (5), and serious failure or trouble in their work (2).

Thus, emotional disturbances, especially depression, were significantly more common in both the chronic groups than in the acute group. The authors believed it was unlikely that these emotional disturbances were the *consequence* of chronic brucellosis, because they were also seen in the chronic-recovered group and because they often occurred during childhood or concurrent with the acute brucellosis. They believed that chronic brucellosis was an emotional disorder that was critically related to the emotional state of the patient at the time of the acute infection or shortly thereafter, and that the symptoms of the emotional disorder merged in the minds of patients and their physicians with the syndrome of chronic brucellosis. Therefore, these psychological disturbances were perpetuated, intensified, and modified in these patients by the symptom pattern of the acute illness, which was often followed, even in those who recover uneventfully, by a period of lassitude or fatigue. It was also noted that the alleviation of symptoms in three of the six chronic-recovered patients occurred at the same time that personal difficulties in their lives were resolved.

Ten of the 16 chronically ill patients were still symptomatic an average of 5 years after the acute illness. This suggested that once the chronic illness was firmly established and labeled chronic brucellosis by a physician, other additional factors favored its perpetuation. The investigators thought it likely that traumatic early-life experiences rendered the chronically ill patient vulnerable to depressive reactions to interpersonal loss or its threat in adult life. They stated that "if the depressive reaction and the acute infection more or less coincide, the syndrome labelled chronic brucellosis is apt to ensue, and that if the temporal relationship is not close, it is far less likely that symptoms will be attributed to the infection." They also believed that neurotic symptoms tended to be intensified and modified by the pattern of the acute illness. The self-concept scores suggested these chronically ill patients thought of themselves as emotionally healthy, but physically ill; thus, their diagnosis of chronic brucellosis supported their self-esteem and favored the perpetuation of the disease as an explanation for a multitude of other problems. It was stressed by the authors that in no instance was there direct evidence in these patients that potential or actual financial compensation played a role in the persistence of their symptoms; especially since *all* the patients, including those who had recovered, would have been eligible for disability compensation.

The evidence strongly supports the concept that brucellar infection was the *cause* of the illness Imboden and associates called chronic brucellosis, and that it would now be called the chronic fatigue syndrome. It is also my belief that brucellar infection is certainly not the cause of any significant percentage of the illnesses called chronic fatigue syndrome in 1993, as brucellar infection is now very rare in the United States. If I am correct, then it must be that CFS may be caused by more than one infectious agent, and the observations of Imboden and associates in patients who developed CFS after brucellosis may be pertinent to patients who develop CFS after other infections or other inflammatory processes.

Imboden and his associates concluded in the final paper of their series that emotional disturbance constituted the essential feature of chronic brucellosis [15]. They also stressed that the emotional disturbances seen in chronic brucellosis were critically related to the personality structure and concurrent life situation of the patient at the time of the acute illness. However, since their conclusions were based on studies and analyses made *after* the syndrome of chronic brucellosis had developed, they acknowledged it was possible that the emotional disturbances were the *result* of the infectious process, and not because of important cofactors present before or at the onset of the infection. In an attempt to pursue this issue, they decided to collect psychological data prospectively on large numbers of employees at the research laboratory, *before* they accidentally contracted brucellosis, and to follow them subsequently for the development of chronic brucellosis. They planned to attempt to relate outcome to psychological factors existing before or during the acute illness. Because few employees developed brucellosis thereafter, their attention was directed to the course and outcome of other more prevalent or common infections occurring in the study population, especially influenza.

INFLUENZA

In August 1957, 600 employees (540 men and 60 women) at the same research facility in Maryland where Cluff et al. had studied patients with brucellosis [13–15] were asked to complete the Minnesota Multiphasic Personality Inventory (MMPI), the Cornell Medical Index Health Questionnaire (CMI), and a social questionnaire [16]. Hypochondriasis (Hs), morale-loss (ML), depression (D), and ego strength (ES) scores were derived from the MMPI while the employees were still well. They and the CMI results were used prospectively to objectively classify each individual's psychological vulnerability into one of three classes. Individuals were classed as *psychologically vulnerable* when their scores extended beyond the normal median in a pathological direction on any three of the four scores used. Conversely, individuals scoring similarly beyond the median in a healthy direction were classed as *nonvulnerable*, and evenly divided patterns placed subjects in an *intermediate* category. These results were kept confidential and had no bearing on employment status.

Three to six months after these tests were administered, an epidemic of Asian influenza began in the winter of 1957–1958 in the United States, and it affected many of the tested individuals. The opportunity for Imboden and his associates to delineate the importance of psychological factors in the expression and course of a common viral infection, influenza, was seized by them.

All employees had been required to report to the facility's medical dispensary in the event of any kind of illness. All persons reporting with an influenzalike illness during the winter epidemic of Asian influenza were followed for 3–6 weeks to evaluate their illness and to obtain specimens for diagnosis of influenza. Amantadine was not then available for prevention or treatment of influenza. Specimens included preillness, acute, and convalescent sera that were tested for antibodies to the prevalent influenza strain by hemagglutination-inhibition using a Japan 305-57 strain, complement fixation tests, and virus isolation from pharyngeal washings using embryonated eggs. A fourfold rise in serum antibody titers or the isolation of virus was required for diagnosing influenza.

The investigators reported the overall results of their studies on the total group in 1961 [16] and for a subgroup of men-only in 1966 [17]. Approximately six times as many persons developed serological evidence of recent influenza infection as were recognized to have symptomatic influenza. Twenty-six subjects (25 of whom were men) developed an illness proved to be Asian influenza during the epidemic; the attack rate for the disease was 4.3% in the 600 persons in this study [7], which was about the same as that for Maryland as a whole [16]. The incidence of documented *symptomatic* influenza was 11 of 96 (11.4%) in the vulnerable group, 11 of 306 (3.5%) in the nonvulnerable group ($p < 0.02$), and 4 of 78 (5.0%) in the intermediate group [17]. Forty-two percent of the known symptomatic influenza occurred in the 20% of subjects who were classed as vulnerable. Thus, psychological vulnerability appeared to increase the risk of illness 2.4 times above that of the nonvulnerable group. Influenza vaccination provided before or during the epidemic appeared to provide little protection against the infection. Vulnerable employees were no more or less likely to have been vaccinated before the outbreak than were those in the other groups. When vaccinated individuals were excluded from analysis, serological evidence of the rate of influenza infection was slightly higher in the vulnerable group than in the nonvulnerable group, but not significantly so (41.5 vs 33.5%, $\chi^2 = 1.51$). The severity of the influenza illness in the two groups was also indistinguishable, but the vulnerable group seemed more likely to be concerned about their illness and to report to the dispensary because of it. It should be emphasized that vulnerability had been defined before the influenza outbreak. Analysis showed the vulnerable group was more likely to report to the dispensary for minor medical reasons of all types, probably because of an increased concern about illness. In a later report on the same population [18], Cluff reported that there was a striking association between "depressive propensity" and the persistence of symptoms of feeling sick after smallpox vaccination. He suggested that the term *depressive propensity* may be a poor descriptor, and that these persons may simply have been more acutely aware of abnormalities associated with disease in themselves and others (i.e., they may have been prone to somatization).

When reporting for follow-up 3–6 weeks after their initial visit, 14 of the 26 persons who had been ill with influenza reported that they had completely recovered, whereas the other 12 stated they were still ill. For further analyses, the well group was called the *recovered group* by the investigators, and the still-ill group was called the *symptomatic group*.

Only 1 of the 26 patients was a woman. Average age for the recovered group was 30.6, and 38.0 for those still symptomatic. The mean duration of symptoms in the recovered group was 7.9 days, with a range of 3–14 days; the duration of symptoms exceeded 3 weeks in every patient in the chronic group, but the actual time needed for complete recovery in this group was not determined.

The symptoms presented during the acute illness by both groups were typical of those of influenza and were similar in their character in both groups. Complications of the acute illness were uncommon, and recovery from them was rapid. There were no apparent differences during the acute illness in symptoms, physical or laboratory findings, or complications in the two groups.

The most frequent persisting symptoms reported by the 12 patients in the chronically symptomatic group were tiredness or weakness (10), cough (5), insomnia (3), headache (3), anorexia (3), and feeling depressed (2). In a report on this work in 1991, Cluff characterized the illness of these patients with delayed convalescence from influenza as the chronic fatigue syndrome [18].

When the results of psychological tests administered 3–6 months before the influenza outbreak were compared for the two groups, the vulnerability scores of the chronic-symptomatic group were significantly higher for both the CMI and MMPI results (Table 3). The sections of the CMI that dealt primarily with manifestations of overt emotional disturbance were also significantly higher in the chronic-symptomatic group. The scores of the symptomatic group in the MMPI test were higher than those of the recovered group in seven of the nine scales. The MMPI indices of depressive tendencies and morale loss were also significantly higher in the symptomatic group. The depression score dominated the MMPI profiles of 9 of the 12 persons with persistent symptoms, in contrast to only 3 of the 14 recovered persons.

The authors noted that the persistent symptoms seen following influenza in this study were similar to those seen in their patients with chronic brucellosis, but they were not as severe or as prolonged. However, the MMPI scores for depression and morale loss were almost identical in the two groups (recovered or symptomatic) in subjects with either brucellosis or influenza, even though in the patients with influenza the tests were obtained *before* the acute illness, whereas in the patients with brucellosis, the psychological tests were obtained *after* the acute illness (Table 4). Analysis showed these differences in scores were not explainable in their entirety by age differences between groups, even

Table 3   Scores on Preinfluenza MMPI

Scale	Symptomatic group ($N = 12$) Mean score	Recovered group ($N = 14$) Mean score
Hypochondriasis	53.8	57.8
Depression	61.0[a]	51.5[a]
Hysteria	61.0	59.7
Psychasthenia	58.0	53.5
Morale loss (raw scores)	7.2[b]	2.7[b]

[a]Significant at $p = 0.025$ as determined by t.
[b]Significant at $p < 0.01$ as determined by t.
Source: Ref. 16.

Table 4 Comparison of MMPI Scores in Two Convalescent Studies

Groups		Mean score	
		Depression	Morale loss
Recovered	Influenza[a]	51.5	2.7
	Brucellosis[b]	51.0	2.7
Symptomatic	Influenza[a]	61.0	7.2
	Brucellosis[b]	63.7	7.4

[a]Tests administered before illness.
[b]Tests administered after illness.
Source: Ref. 16.

though the mean age of the symptomatic group (38.0 years) was higher than in the recovered group (30.6).

Imboden and colleagues speculated that their psychological data in influenza patients reflected a greater *propensity* to become depressed in vulnerable persons, rather than to actual clinical depression in the symptomatic group. Thus, as in their earlier studies with brucellosis, they postulated that clinical symptoms of depression, such as fatigue, tended to become merged with the weakness that is normally experienced following any acute infectious disease. This intermingling of symptoms obscured the endpoint of the disease from the views of both physician and patient. They also opined that most convalescent patients are likely to attribute their persistent lack of well-being to persistence of the physical disease, especially as it carried the least threat to their ego and self-esteem.

In conclusion, it seems plausible that some patients who develop CFS may do so as a result of influenza infection. However, the two convalescent groups described in this study did not represent the same extremes in recovery patterns that were manifested in the brucellosis study, in which the chronic-subjective syndrome often was severe and endured for several years.

In 1970, Middleton and associates reported studies on 26 children with acute bilateral lower-limb myositis that began in association with influenza [19]. A unique feature of their report was that the onset of myositis began during the early phase of recovery from influenza, and at a time when respiratory signs and symptoms were abating or gone. Patients had severe leg pain on walking or on awakening, often along with a bizarre gait, but without neurological changes. Muscle weakness, leg muscles tender to palpation, and elevated serum creatine phosphokinase (CPK) levels were reported. Muscle biopsies and electromyography were not done. Symptoms lasted only 1–5 days, and follow-up examination 2–3 weeks later revealed no pain or tenderness of affected muscles. The authors speculated that myositis may have been caused either by the virus or by some circulating toxic factor. They pointed out that acute myositis following influenza has often been observed in adults, especially during the 1918–1919 influenza pandemic. It is tempting to speculate that if patients such as these had gone on to develop persistent symptoms, they might have been diagnosed as having fibromyalgia or fibromyositis.

EPIDEMIC NEUROMYASTHENIA

Many outbreaks or clusters of an illness resembling CFS and seemingly having an infectious etiology have been described. Probably the first one occurred in Los Angeles, in 1934, and was reported by Gilliam [20]. By 1957, 11 similar outbreaks had been reported from the United States, 6 from England, 2 from Iceland, and 1 each from Denmark, Germany, South Africa, and Greece. They have been reported under various names and were reviewed in detail by Henderson and Shelokov [8]. Their characteristics are summarized in Figure 1. They were almost certainly *not* caused by influenza or brucella infection. Two outbreaks in the United States were reported in 1957; both were unique in that the syndrome was identified by the term epidemic neuromyasthenia instead of by the place of the outbreak [20,21]. These reports are significant both historically and scientifically; therefore, they are worthy of detailed discussion here.

In 1957, Shelokov and associates, at the National Institute of Allergy and Infectious Disease, described a sharp outbreak that began in 1953 of a disease in nurses (most of them young, adult women) working at a psychiatric hospital in suburban Maryland outside Washington, DC [21]. At first, the illness was thought to be poliomyelitis. Most of the 41 cases occurred during the first 2 weeks of July. About half the illnesses were associated with demonstrable localized muscular weakness, severe enough to be called paresis, along with myalgia, stiffness of the neck, tenderness in the back muscles, headache, depression, diarrhea, and fever up to 101°F, along with depressed morning temperatures. Other features included sore throat, pleuritic chest pain, insomnia, somnolence, cutaneous sensory disturbances, vasomotor disturbances, and abdominal pain. Muscle weakness commonly involved one or both legs or the arm and hand on the dominant side. Weakness was transient, but was confirmed in many cases by quantitative testing. Neither atrophy nor flaccidity was seen. Diagnostic studies for poliomyelitis were negative. Depression was common, and it was associated with nervousness, anxiety, unprovoked crying spells, difficulty in concentration, and irritability. Intermittent coldness or warmth of an extremity, numbness, tingling, and hyposensitivity or hypersensitivity to pain and touch unrelated to segmental nerve distribution were common. Neuromuscular signs and symptoms were a characteristic feature of this illness. After early improvement, patients entered a characteristic subacute phase that often resulted in prolonged debility that, in retrospect, closely resembles what we now call CFS. This pattern suggests (in addition to other theories) an infectious agent started the illness and then triggered a process not necessarily requiring the perpetuation of the original infection for its continuation. Clinical and laboratory tests as well as a wide variety of other diagnostic tests available then were negative or not helpful. Therapy was simply supportive. All patients reported that their health gradually improved over a period of several months, despite repeated exacerbations brought on by such things as physical exertion, menses, or cold weather. Extensive epidemiological and laboratory studies attempting to determine the etiology of the illness were negative, except for the possible implication of organisms of the Bethesda–Ballerup group of paracolon enteric bacteria. This was done both by culture of stools and by paired serum antibody tests. Fifty-five percent of the patients had positive stool cultures for these organisms, whereas only 11% of asymptomatic nurses tested positive. However, it was *not* possible to perform these tests on an appropriate sample of control nurses who had not been ill. In an attempt to implicate viruses, monolayers of monkey kidney, HeLa, human fibroblast, and human chorion–amnion cell cultures were inoculated, as well as chicken embryos by yolk-sac and allantoic routes, suckling and adult mice, and intracerebral and intramuscular inoculation of monkeys. All of these studies were negative for viruses or any other organism.

The authors concluded that the evidence for an infectious etiology of this outbreak was not clear-cut, and that a toxic etiology was also possible. The incubation period was estimated as 5–8 days. No common source exposure could be identified, although the hospital premises appeared the primary source of infection over a period of several months. They concluded that Bethesda-Ballerup organisms should be sought in stools from future outbreaks, but that they might have been present merely as "fellow travelers."

A similar outbreak in the town of Punta Gorda, on the Gulf Coast of Florida in 1956, also labeled epidemic neuromyasthenia, was reported by Poskanzer and associates [22] in the same issue of the journal in which Shelekov and his associates [21] reported the 1953 outbreak in Washington, DC.

The Punta Gorda outbreak began in late February and March 1956, and involved primarily young and middle-aged adults, most of them female. At least 150 cases occurred among 2500 residents of Punta Gorda, with prostrating symptoms similar to those reported by Shelekov in the Washington outbreak [21], and associated with severe, long-term emotional and physical sequelae. In addition, terrifying dreams, confusion, memory defects, inability to perform calculations, hyperventilation attacks, dysphagia, nausea, anorexia, vomiting, diarrhea, dizziness, vertigo, blurred vision, and diplopia were commonly noted. A temperature higher than 100°F was rare. Exacerbations occurred at irregular intervals, but especially after physical exertion or during menses. Most patients were able to carry out their normal activities by 6 months after the onset, but many were still confined to bed rest (Fig. 3). Physical findings were few compared with the frequency of symptoms, but they were similar to those seen

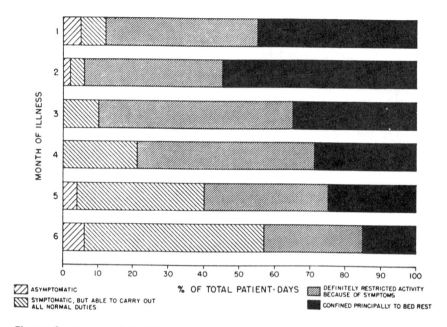

Figure 3 Degree of disability among selected patients in the Punta Gorda outbreak, according to month of illness. (From Ref. 22.)

in CFS. Notably, 9 of 21 patients examined had muscle tenderness 5 months after onset, and many of them would probably qualify also for the diagnosis of fibromyalgia/fibrositis. All clinical laboratory studies were negative, including cerebrospinal fluid examinations, electroencephalograms, and microbiological studies, including attempts to isolate viruses. Stool cultures and serum agglutinin tests for Bethesda–Ballerup organisms were done and were, in essence, negative.

A house-to-house community epidemiological survey was done in Punta Gorda; it included 1041 of the 2500 inhabitants. Fifty-one cases were found. The overall attack rate was 6.3:100 persons, which suggested there were at least 150 cases in Punta Gorda. There were no cases younger than aged 12; there were 42 cases in females and 20 in males. Attack rates for white and black females older than 10 were identical (9.5%). The disease appeared more severe in females, who accounted for 10 of 11 hospital admissions for the syndrome. In addition, 86% of 106 patients seen by physicians were female, as contrasted with 68% females in the survey population.

Although extensive epidemiological studies were conducted, and many possible routes of transmission were investigated, these studies were not fruitful.

Notably, a disproportionately high rate of illness was experienced by medical and other health care personnel during this outbreak. Of 38 such individuals surveyed, 16 (42%) reported compatible symptoms (Table 5), which was a much higher rate than was found in a comparable-aged control group in the community.

The authors cautiously drew a few inferences about the possible causes of the disease in Punta Gorda. They believed the evidence did not support the diagnosis of mass conversion reaction, poliomyelitis, trichinosis, brucellosis, leptospirosis, or infection with coxsackie virus, mumps, infectious mononucleosis, or hepatitis virus.

In 1959, Acheson [23], Henderson and Shelokov [8], and their colleagues comprehensively reviewed the literature concerning epidemic neuromyasthenia. Both papers called attention to the confusing terminology used in the literature to describe outbreaks of an illness similar to the outbreaks of epidemic neuromyasthenia they described. Henderson and Shelokov pointed out that, beginning with Iceland disease in 1954, various authors have called a similar illness by the names benign myalgic encephalomyelitis, Akureyri disease, epidemic vegetative neuritis, acute infective encephalomyelitis, encephalomyelitis, persistent myalgia following sore throat, a poliomyelitis-like disease, atypical poliomyelitis, encephalomyelitis resembling poliomyelitis, and epidemic neuromyasthenia.

Henderson and Shelokov [8] and Acheson [23] reviewed 23 such outbreaks around the world, described them in detail, called attention to their many clinical similarities (see Fig. 1), to their tendency to occur in hospital personnel between April and September, to be confused initially with poliomyelitis, to the lack in most patients of laboratory findings that were helpful in diagnosis, to the relatively good long-term prognosis, with gradual recovery punctuated by relapses over a period of years, to the *absence of fatalities* from the disease

Table 5 Epidemic Neuromyasthenialike Illness Among Medical and Associated Personnel in Punta Gorda

Age group (yr)	Males		Females	
	Totals	No. ill	Totals	No. ill
10–19	0	0	2	2
20–29	2	1	3	2
30–39	3	2	11	5
40–49	2	1	5	1
50–59	0	0	7	2
60–69	0	0	3	0
Totals	7	4	31	12

Source: Ref. 22.

reported anywhere, and to the resultant lack of pathological material and information based on autopsy experience.

The incubation periods of the illnesses were variable, but in several outbreaks were less than 1 week, or about 5–6 days, with a possible range of 4 days to 2–3 weeks. There was *no* evidence in most of the outbreaks that the disease was spread from patients to medical staff (despite that hospital staff members often developed the illness), or that it was food- or water-borne. The worldwide distribution of outbreaks, along with the marked differences in types of communities affected, were thought to preclude an insect vector or a toxic agent, although both of these had been sought in a few outbreaks without success. They concluded that it was untenable that *all* patients, or even *most* patients, in *all* the reported outbreaks were hysterical, but that a more reasonable viewpoint was that many patients may indeed have had a hysterical reaction that was based on their knowledge of patients with definite infection who had signs and symptoms of involvement of the nervous system.

Both reviews described in detail the methods used in these outbreaks to attempt to identify etiological agents. Since the clinical manifestations were dissimilar to those of any known bacterial infection, attention was focused on the isolation of viruses. Despite intensive efforts to implicate viruses in many of the outbreaks, the results before 1957 were largely nonproductive. Cerebrospinal fluid, feces, throat washings, acute-phase sera, and blood clots were inoculated by a variety of routes and by frequent blind passage into many different laboratory animals, including suckling and adult mice, guinea pigs, rats, ferrets, hamsters, rabbits, and monkeys, with and without cortisone. An illness was induced in monkeys inoculated with specimens from an Australian outbreak [24], but the agent could not be passaged, and there has been no confirmation of these results in other outbreaks. In 9 of 14 outbreaks, attempts were made to isolate poliomyelitis virus or coxsackievirus, or to implicate them serologically, without success. In addition, embryonated eggs of various ages were injected with various specimens into the chorioallantoic membrane, allantoic sac, yolk sac, and amnion, with negative results. Tissue culture systems employed with negative results include monkey testicle; monkey kidney; HeLa cells; human embryo skin, brain, liver, and spleen, and human infant kidney, fibroblast, and chorioamnion. These attempts often suffered because specimens were almost always collected many weeks after the illness had its onset, and at a time when the etiological agent might not be present in stools, blood, or other available secretions.

Complement fixation, neutralization, and agglutination tests on sera were negative, for all practical purposes, in the outbreaks studied. Heterophil antibody tests aimed at diagnosing infectious mononucleosis were positive in only 5 of 128 patients from two outbreaks, and repeat determinations usually failed to show a change in titer indicating recent infection.

Tests for antibodies for the following agents were also reported as negative (when studied) in the outbreaks reviewed by Henderson and Shelokov and by Acheson [8,23]: poliomyelitis, lymphocytic choriomeningitis, encephalomyocarditis virus; Eastern equine encephalitis, Western equine encephalitis, Port Augusta encephalitis, St. Louis encephalitis, Japanese B encephalitis, louping ill, Russian spring–summer encephalitis; influenza A, B, and C; Q fever; leptospirosis, trichinosis, toxoplasmosis; adenovirus, herpes simplex, rabies; psittacosis, lymphogranuloma venereum, brucellosis, tularemia, typhoid, paratyphoid; coxsackieviruses A and B, echoviruses; *Salmonella typhimurium,* and syphilis. Occasional serological tests for mumps were positive, but most were not.

In 1958, Likar and Dane reported an illness in Northern Ireland that resembled this syndrome and that appeared to be caused by viruses of the Russian spring–summer encephalitis–louping ill group [25], but results for this group were negative in all the other outbreaks in which it was considered.

Perhaps the most important conclusion to draw from these reports is that a CFS-like illness can occur in outbreaks, and that it is more likely that infectious agents were responsible for the syndrome than that it was caused by chemicals, toxins, or mass hysteria.

Henderson and Shelokov [8] and Acheson [23] concluded their reviews of outbreaks of epidemic neuromyasthenia with an acknowledgment that, although the etiologies and pathophysiology of these illnesses are still unknown, the outbreaks share many common features and have a distinct and unique nature. Taken together these considerations indicate a single descriptive name would be useful. Iceland disease and the closely related Akureyri disease were popular terms to describe them for a time, and had merit because some of the first clear descriptions of outbreaks of the syndrome came from those places. However, investigators in Iceland (as well as others) objected to those names. The term benign myalgic encephalomyelitis was introduced in England for a similar illness in 1956, and is still popular there. However, the reviewers [8,23] have pointed out that the illness is in no way benign, except in that it is not a fatal illness, and that there is no proof that a nervous system inflammatory process is part of the illness.

Although the appellation *chronic fatigue syndrome* (CFS) is arguably the most popular name for the illness now in the United States, other names for it are also used here, particularly the chronic fatigue immune dysfunction syndrome (CFIDS). The terms benign myalgic encephalomyelitis (or ME) and the postviral fatigue syndrome (PVFS) have caught on and persisted in the United Kingdom. In large measure, the latter's popularity stems from the studies of Behan and his associates in the United Kingdom [26], who have compiled a large body of evidence supporting their notion that the syndrome with the name benign myalgic encephalomyelitis or ME is related to infection with coxsackieviruses and other enteroviruses.

THE POSTVIRAL FATIGUE SYNDROME, BENIGN MYALGIC ENCEPHALOMYELITIS, AND THEIR RELATION TO CHRONIC ENTEROVIRAL INFECTION

The symptoms of ME and PVFS are similar to those of CFS and consist of myalgia, fatigue, emotional disturbances, chronicity, and frequent relapses; a possibly significant difference is a greater frequency of transient or fluctuating paresis and other neurological findings in ME. This presentation will focus primarily on those studies concerned with an infectious etiology of PVFS and ME; more detailed discussions of the clinical findings can be found in reports by Behan and his associates [26,27].

One of the earliest and best-studied outbreaks of ME affected the medical, nursing, and ancillary staff of the Royal Free Hospital in London in 1955 [28]. Initially, it was felt by some that it was an outbreak of poliomyelitis; others believed hysteria played an important role in the perpetuation of the outbreak. Relapses were a common feature. There were two fatalities during the outbreak, from conditions unrelated to ME; one patient died from metastatic ovarian carcinoma, and the other died from a drug overdose. Postmortem examination in the latter revealed evidence interpreted as an early stage of disseminated sclerosis, with demyelination, but no viral inclusions or primary neuronal damage. All attempts to isolate viruses or other etiological agents from specimens collected from patients in the early stages of the so-called Royal Free disease were negative when tested in numerous systems.

Behan and his associates in Glasgow, Scotland, reported their studies on 50 patients with typical signs and symptoms of PVFS/ME in 1985 [26]. Twenty-one of their 50 patients had an association with medical persons or activities. No muscle weakness was demonstrated in any muscle group tested until it was exercised, after which weakness lasting for up to 1–3 h was detected. Muscle biopsies were abnormal in all 20 patients who underwent biopsy. Widely scattered necrotic muscle fibers, without associated inflammation, were common, and histochemical stains showed an increased size and number of type II fibers in all. By electron microscopy, mitochondria were increased at the periphery of muscle fibers and occasional tubular inclusions were seen. Antibodies to smooth muscle were detected in the sera of 18 patients.

Routine electrophysiological testing was normal, but when conventional and single-fiber electromyographic (EMG) and nerve conduction studies were done, they revealed definite abnormalities, such as abnormal jitter (thought indicative of subtle primary muscle lesions compatible with a viral illness) in about 75% of patients in the peripheral part of the motor unit, and probably also in the muscle fiber [29]. Nuclear magnetic resonance (NMR) studies of muscle metabolism were done, and were said to show early intracellular acidosis that was of unknown cause during exercise, but was associated with muscle fatigue along with increased type II muscle fibers [30]. These findings in muscle metabolism were of great interest, and they directed attention to muscles as the potential target of a chronic viral infection in PVFS/ME. For further interpretation of these data see Chapter 9.

Defective immunoregulation was associated with ME in at least 35 (70%) of the 50 patients Behan et al. studied [26]. It consisted primarily of lymphocyte dysfunction during the acute and chronic stages of the illness. Patients showed a significant reduction in the number of suppressor–cytotoxic (T8) lymphocytes during the acute illness, whereas helper–inducer (T4) lymphocytes were significantly reduced in patients with chronic symptoms. Immunoglobulin concentrations were normal. Several patients had abnormal complement fractions, such as reduced CH_{50} or C_4 concentrations. Most patients had positive assays for immune complexes in serum. They indicated that these results were similar to those they had previously obtained in patients with polymyositis [26].

Test for antibodies to viruses other than coxsackieviruses were thought to be unrevealing in Behan's studies. Thirty-five of the 50 patients had antibody titers of 1:512 or greater to coxsackievirus B, using a modified micrometabolic inhibition test (this finding was stated to be expected in only 4% of random controls). In six patients, specific coxsackievirus IgM antibodies were detected by means of an enzyme-linked immunosorbent assay (ELISA) technique, but no single strain of coxsackievirus B could be implicated. Behan pointed out that previous studies of two similar outbreaks had shown a relation to coxsackievirus B [27,31].

Behan and his colleagues believed their investigation suggested a major role for coxsackieviruses in ME and PVFS, but they stated *they had no doubt that other viruses may cause a similar disease.* They believed their results suggested the syndrome is due to the interaction of viral infection and immunological processes, with the production of damage to intracellular enzymes that resulted in abnormal muscle metabolism, especially on exercise, and that further study of these mechanisms was indicated.

In 1988, Yousef and collaborators from London and the Enterovirus Reference Laboratory in Glasgow reported studies of chronic enterovirus infections in 76 patients with the postviral fatigue syndrome and 30 matched controls [32]. No patient studied had evident neurological disease, but many had cognitive defects. Complex laboratory tests not available elsewhere, that were designed to implicate enteroviruses were performed on specimens from numerous patients.

Enterovirus isolation from concentrated fecal samples was attempted using Vero cell cultures, both directly and after an acid dissociation–sucrose centrifugation procedure designed to separate virus from IgG antibodies in stools, with an estimated efficiency of 50%. Cell cultures were examined daily for a cytopathic effect for 3 weeks, during which two blind passages were done. Positive cultures were identified presumptively by a characteristic cytopathic effect (CPE) and by electron microscopy, and were confirmed by indirect immunofluorescence with a monoclonal antibody (5-D8/1) the investigators had prepared that was directed against the enteroviral group-specific protein VP1. This monoclonal antibody 5-D8/1 (produced against heat-inactivated coxsackievirus B5) reacted in a highly sensitive and reproducible way with VP1 polypeptide of all tested enteroviruses, except hepatitis A, and *only* against enteroviruses. This monoclonal antibody was also used to detect enteroviral antigens free in serum or in circulating immune complexes by using peroxidase labeled 5-D8/1 as a detector, instead of rabbit polyclonal antibody. The VP1 antigen detection tests were also done on sera from all patients with positive fecal cultures after acid centrifugation; controls were patients with PVFS who had negative fecal cultures using the same techniques.

Enteroviruses were isolated by Yousef et al. from feces of 17 (22%) of 76 PVFS patients, but from only 2 (6.7%) of controls (who were mostly neighbors of patients) [32]. In the PVFS patients, 15 of 17 viral isolations were positive only after acid centrifugation, whereas neither of the two isolates from controls required acid centrifugation ($p < 0.01$). Thus, the frequency of virus isolation from feces of patients was increased more than eightfold following acid-dissociation of virus from neutralizing antibodies that prevented infection of Vero cell cultures by viruses.

Notably, 12 of the 17 enteroviruses isolated from feces after acid centrifugation produced a visible CPE only after a second blind passage in cell culture. The isolation of virus from feces of two control patients was thought related to the fact that specimens were collected at a time of the year when enteroviral infections were to be expected in the community. Three of the four isolates obtained by direct culture were coxsackievirus B5, the fourth was echovirus 11. Two of the coxsackievirus B5 isolates were from controls. Twelve isolates obtained from PVFS patients by acid-centrifugation were coxsackieviruses (B1–5), three were echoviruses, and two were untypable at reference laboratories using antiserum pools covering all enteroviruses except types 68–71. Patients with positive stool cultures were studied again 12 months later; 5 of the 17 still yielded the same virus, whereas all 4 persons initially positive only by direct culture were culture-negative 12 months later.

Thirteen of the 17 culture-positive patients with PVFS had detectable enterovirus heterotypic IgM antibodies 12 months after isolation of virus, suggesting active infection. Patients from whom virus was isolated by direct culture in 1986 had no detectable enterovirus-specific IgM responses in 1987.

Next, a survey for the presence of IgM circulating immune complexes in sera was done by Yousef et al. on a different group of 87 patients with PVFS, [32]. Of these, 64 (74%) were positive for immune complexes, and that 44 (51%) of the 87 had detectable serum enterovirus VP1 antigen in amounts greater than three times the standard deviation (SD) above the mean of 36 normal controls.

All positive patients were retested after 4 months, and 39 (89%) were still positive. No controls had enterovirus antigen in serum, and the difference between patients and controls in frequency of detection of the VP1 antigen was highly significant ($p < 0.001$). The VP1 antigen was detected in the sera of 15 of the patients who were culture-positive only after acid centrifugation of feces, but not from either of the 2 patients who were positive on direct culture (which suggested transient carriage in the latter). An additional 7 of 16 culture-negative PVFS patients had low levels of detectable VP1 in serum. The authors ended by noting briefly that clinical monitoring of their patients showed that the correlation between clinical improvement and disappearance of both VP1 antigen and IgM complexes from the circulation was high, but they did not show data supporting this statement.

Yousef and associates further pointed out that even lytic enteroviruses can persist in various cell lines in vitro [32], and also that there are reports that demonstrate chronic (persistent) enterovirus infection in humans who have chronic muscle and cardiac diseases [33,34]. However, they also noted that attempts to culture enteroviruses from muscle biopsies obtained during outbreaks of PVFS have been negative.

Archard and co-workers reported related studies shortly thereafter that showed persistence of enteroviral RNA in muscle of patients with the postviral fatigue syndrome [35]. To do this they employed techniques analgous to those they used previously to demonstrate enteroviral RNA in affected tissues from patients with chronic inflammatory myopathies of cardiac or skeletal muscle [33,34]. Muscle specimens obtained by needle biopsy from the quadriceps of 96 patients suffering from PVFS for up to 20 years and from 4 normal controls were studied. Nucleic acids isolated from small portions of these specimens were hybridized with an enterovirus group-specific probe derived by reverse transcription and molecular cloning of the RNA genome of a coxsackievirus B2. The RNA was immobilized on nylon filters using a slot-blot apparatus along with negative controls and purified coxsackievirus B2 RNA as a positive control. Filters were probed with highly conserved virus-specific cDNA labeled with ^{32}P by random oligomeric primer extension. Filters were autoradiographed and scanned after hybridization. Signal strength generated with the viral-specific probe was compared with that of the control and was expressed as a ratio, termed the hybridization index (HI).

The signals produced by 96 specimens from PFS patients fell into two groups. In the first, 76 specimens gave low background HI values within the range of the muscles from normal controls. The remaining 20 (21%) specimens from 96 PVFS patients were positive for the presence of enterovirus-specific RNA and gave hybridization indices more than 3 SD greater than the controls or other PVFS patients. In analagous experiments, more than 50 samples of normal human muscle that they probed have been negative for enteroviral RNA.

Other studies performed on these patients included muscle NMR imaging, single fiber EMG, serum creatine kinase (CK) assay, coxsackievirus B-specific IgM and neutralizing antibody determinations, and histopathological assessment of muscle biopsies. None of these characteristics distinguished the virus probe-positive group from the remainder except the serum CK. Of 11 patients with mildly elevated CK values, 9 were positive for enterovirus RNA.

These investigators pointed out that muscle lesions of other patients with myopathies they studied have shown only focal demonstration of enterovirus RNA. Therefore, they speculated that sampling errors arising from the small amount of muscle tissue taken from these PVFS patients may have led to an underestimate of the true frequency of enteroviral RNA within their muscles. They also pointed out that it is clear enteroviruses are capable of persisting in affected tissue for many years, and that this chronic infection may negate "some non-housekeeping functions within (muscle) cells such that the cells survive but with an altered metabolism," and that this interference may explain the abnormal findings seen on NMR and EMG in some patients. They also pointed out that coxsackievirus IgM antibodies may only reflect disease of recent onset, thus explaining why only about 50% of patients with PVFS have significant neutralizing antibody titers enteroviruses. In addition, they suggested that other patients might be infected with enteroviruses not included in the available coxsackievirus B–specific neutralization test.

Since their patients had been ill for up to 20 years, and if enteroviruses are capable of triggering PVFS, the latter may be capable of persisting in affected tissues for many years, thereby accounting for the chronicity of the illness.

Gow, Behan, and their colleagues then turned to the polymerase chain reaction (PCR) as a more sensitive way than probing for RNA sequences to search for enteroviral sequences in muscle of patients with PVFS [36,37]. The PCR was believed to be more than 1000-fold more sensitive than previous hybridization protocols and, in addition, background hybridization associated with complementary DNA probes is eliminated when this technique is used.

These investigators studied 60 patients with typical severe PVFS admitted during an 18-month period to the Institute of Neurological Sciences in Glasgow. There were 27 men and 33 women in the study, with a mean age of about 35–40 years and a range of 15–58 years. The initial event in all patients was a febrile illness, with upper respiratory or gastrointestinal symptoms so severe that the patient was confined to bed for several days. Prolonged excessive somnolence with reversal of normal sleep patterns was also present, along with a fluctuating severity of all symptoms. Extensive diagnostic and laboratory studies were done, including lumbar puncture, computed tomography (CT), and serological screens for numerous viral infections, including coxsackieviruses B1–5 by neutralization. Needle muscle biopsies were carried out in all patients. Controls were 13 men and 28 women, with a mean age of about 48–56 years, which was somewhat older than the PVFS group. All controls were undergoing routine surgical procedures that permitted taking small muscle samples from the operative site. Most of the control patients had a serious disease, but none were known to have muscle disease.

Muscle samples for PCR were snap-frozen and stored in liquid nitrogen until studied. The RNA prepared from muscle was copied into complementary DNA, and PCR was performed with a mixture of sense and antisense human or viral primers in the 5'-nontranslated region, including use of Ableson tyrosine kinase gene primers to give rise to a positive control for the quality of RNA and amplification. Only samples giving a positive *ABL* gene were used for RNA analysis by enteroviral PCR, and care was taken to avoid contamination during amplification. Several different types of negative controls were included.

Routine laboratory investigations disclosed no abnormalities in these patients, and muscle biopsies showed no evidence of inflammation or necrosis. Only mild to moderate atrophy of type II fibers was detectable, which was consistent with a chronic illness. None of these patients had elevated serum creatine kinase levels.

Of the 60 patients, 12 had neutralizing titers higher than 256:1 of the coxsackieviruses B1–5; 6 of the 12 were positive for enteroviral RNA by PCR, and 6 were not; 3 were positive for Epstein–Barr virus (EBV) IgM. Of the 41 controls, 6 had titers higher than 256:1 of the coxsackieviruses B1–5 (PCR-negative in all); 1 was positive for EBV-specific IgM (PCR-negative), and 3 had high CF titers to CMV (all PCR-negative). Thus, there were significant positive serological findings in 25% of patients and 24% of controls. The investigators believed the specificity of both the primers and PCR techniques they used were good. Of the 60 patients with PVFS (only 20% of whom were seropositive for coxsackievirus infection), 32 (53%) were positive by PCR for enteroviral RNA, whereas 6 (15%) of the 41 controls were positive ($p < 0.001$). The relative odds ratio for PFS in those with enteroviral RNA was 6.7 (95% confidence interval 2.4–18.2). In this study, no healthy young adult control was positive by PCR; of the 6 controls who were PCR-positive, all had a malignant tumor. Enteroviral sequences were detected in 12 (44%) of the 27 male patients with PVFS and in 20 (61%) of the female PVFS patients. They estimated one viral genome was present per 2000 muscle cells in positive specimens. There were no correlations between duration of disease, presenting illness, or age and positivity by PCR. Only 21% of PVFS muscle biopsies were positive for enteroviral sequences, but none of the controls were positive.

As in their previous studies, it was postulated that the frequent (47%) negativity for RNA in muscle biopsies from patients with PVFS may have been related to the focality of lesions, to the use of probes that were too specific, to the lack of sensitivity of PCR, or because other etiological agents might cause infection of muscle and PVFS. The authors concluded by emphasizing that PCR is still a research tool, and that it should not yet be used for diagnosis of PVFS.

Because of the difficulty in obtaining muscle biopsies in patients with PVFS, Gow and Behan next carried out a parallel and similar PCR study on peripheral blood leukocytes from 20 patients and 20 normal controls to determine whether enteroviral RNA could be detected in patients' blood [37]. The results showed no difference between the two groups, with 16% positivity of lymphocytes in patients and controls, which was in keeping with their serological findings. Nevertheless, they believed it was of great interest that patients with PVFS were 6.7 times more likely to have the enteroviral genome in their muscles than were controls. Ultrastructural study of muscle biopsies showed evidence of mitochondrial damage in 45 of 50 cases, with clustering of injured organelles (Fig. 4). These findings were described in greater detail in a subsequent report [38], and were considered evidence that PVFS might be due to mitochondrial damage caused by a virus.

These authors also pointed out that Oldstone has shown, in animal models, that viruses may infect tissues persistently without producing any morphological effects, even though they may interfere with the normal specialized function of the host cell [39]. He also showed that viral persistence is especially likely when the agent infects long-lived cells, such as lymphocytes or cells in the nervous system. No one has yet had the opportunity to search for enteroviral RNA in cells in the nervous system of patients with PVFS, but to do so might be the definitive test of the putative enteroviral etiological hypothesis.

Recent work on a small sample of patients with PVFS suggested they have an unusual ratio of sense to antisense copies of enteroviral RNA in their tissues, which may account for its persistence [40]. It is well-known that enteroviral infections can persist in agammaglobulinemic patients [41]. Gow and his associates [36,37] speculated that enteroviruses may persist in the central nervous system in PVFS, perhaps interfering with the cellular production of neurotransmitters, and that their persistence may also be associated with depression. To this, I am compelled to add that, if enteroviruses do persist in the central nervous system in PVFS patients, they might be in a position to interfere with neuroendocrinological functions, such as the hypothalamic–pituitary–adrenal axis, which has been shown by Demitrack and his associates [42] to be abnormal in patients with CFS.

There is no general agreement or confirmation concerning the validity or meaning of the enteroviral studies reviewed in the foregoing. In a letter to *Lancet* in 1989 [43], Halpin and Wessely reported their studies on the frequency of detection of VP1 coxsackieviral antigen in sera from 47 patients with PVFS and 50 randomly selected inpatient controls on a general neurological ward. Specimens were sent by them to St. Mary's Hospital in London (where Yousef's studies on VP1 and coxsackievirus infection has likely been performed [32], along with other "routine" specimens. Results were obtained on only 73 of 97 specimens. Nine (30%) of 30 patients with PVFS were positive for VP1,

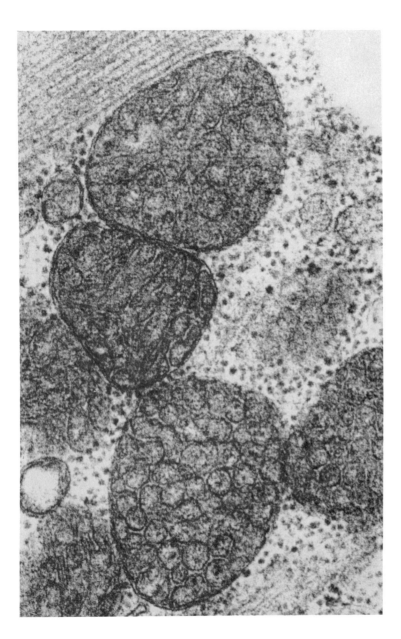

Figure 4   Ultrastructural examination of skeletal muscle biopsy from a patient with the postviral fatigue syndrome: pleomorphic mitochondria showing proliferation of cristae, with apparent formation of compartments. Numerous glycogen granules are also present (× 39,000). (From Ref. 37.)

compared with 5 (12%) of 43 controls, which was just barely significant (p = 0.05). There were no other clinical or laboratory differences between positive and negative PVFS patients. The diagnoses in the 5 positive controls were multiple sclerosis (2), glioma (1), hemichorea (1), and cerebrovascular disease (1). The writers of the letter concluded that the presence of the VP1 antigen in serum is of research interest, but that the sensitivity and specificity of the tests for it are currently unsuitable for routine clinical use.

In 1991, Miller and colleagues reported on the use of coxsackievirus B antibody tests in diagnosing the postviral fatigue syndrome [44]. They conducted a case–control study of 243 patients with PVFS of recent onset who were referred by local general practitioners over a 1-year period. Blood samples were obtained at entry and 6 months later for determination of coxsackievirus B IgM and IgG antibodies using the MU-antibody-capture ELISA test for IgM antibodies and the micrometabolic inhibition method for IgG-neutralizing antibodies, as well as for a variety of other immunological tests. The rates of positivity for coxsackievirus B IgM at entry were 23% for controls and 24% for patients; for IgG the rates were 55% for controls and 56% for patients. The pattern of symptoms of patients with PVFS was similar in those who were either coxsackievirus IgM-positive or IgM-negative. There was no predictive value of rising or falling antibody titers between entry and at 6 months; nor were there differences between categories of patients. Of the numerous other immunological tests performed, there were few significant differences. The mean value for immune complex concentrations was higher than the normal range in 35 (14%) patients and in 35 controls (no significant difference). The investigators concluded that the routine serological tests available for detecting coxsackievirus B antibodies do not help in diagnosing the postviral fatigue syndrome. In patients with acute PVFS, there was a significant reduction in mean values for circulating B lymphocytes and natural killer (NK) lymphocytes, compared with controls. The opinion of the authors was that the newer tests for chronic active enterovirus infection that are being developed promise to be more useful than currently available tests as an aid to diagnosis of PVFS.

In conclusion, these reports, taken at face value and as a whole, are suggestive that a chronic enteroviral infection of a novel and unusual nature may be responsible for a significant proportion of the illnesses we call CFS, ME, or PVFS. If the theory that CFS results from persistent or chronic overproduction of cytokines as a result in some way of an unusual infectious process is correct, then it is also conceivable that enteroviral infection may be an infection capable of initiating that process relatively frequently. It will be necessary for other investigations to confirm the key findings reported in this section before they are accepted as a significant advance. As detailed, the methods needed to do so appear complex and highly technical, and there are few laboratories both capable and willing to embark on such studies. It is nevertheless important and worthwhile for these studies to be pursued.

CHRONIC ACTIVE EPSTEIN–BARR VIRUS INFECTION

Infectious mononucleosis is usually caused by the Epstein–Barr virus (EBV), and generally, is an acute infection of short duration and without serious long-term sequelae. It is characterized by fever, malaise, myalgia, headache, the presence of atypical lymphocytosis and heterophil antibodies in peripheral blood, anorexia, sore throat, lymphadenopathy, and abdominal pain. It has long been known that patients with uncomplicated infectious mononucleosis may complain of fatigue for up to 6 months after their acute illness. However, it was not until the major cause of infectious mononucleosis was proved to be EBV, and specific IgM and IgG antibody tests for diagnosing the infection and ways to cultivate the virus in the laboratory became available that it was possible to delineate accurately its course and spectrum [45]. It was soon found that most patients infected with EBV did not develop the infectious mononucleosis syndrome; instead they developed few or no symptoms, but a long-lasting latent EBV infection that could be documented in almost all patients with infectious mononucleosis after the acute illness had resolved. Although some important long-term adverse complications were occasionally seen as a consequence of the persistent infection, latency was usually evident only by virtue of immunological test results and by detection of periodic asymptomatic activation of the infection accompanied by the presence of EBV in blood and salivia.

In 1982, Tobi and colleagues in Israel [46] called attention to a prolonged illness, characterized by fever, myalgia, weakness, malaise, and lymphadenopathy, that was not typical of infectious mononucleosis, but was associated with serological evidence of persistent and possibly active EBV infection. In the following year, Hamblin and colleagues, in England, described a disorder of T-cell regulation in patients who developed a chronic illness after infectious mononucleosis that resembled CFS [47]. T-suppressor cells were found in a greater percentage than was normal in the peripheral blood of these patients, whereas T-helper cells were found in lower than normal numbers. Complete recovery was said to occur eventually in association with a return to normal of lymphocyte subset populations. In 1985, two reports appeared in the same issue of a journal that called attention to a persisting CFS-like illness in adults along with serological evidence suggestive of chronic active EBV infection, [48,49]. It was characterized by fatigue, myalgia, nervous system symptoms, and other manifestations, similar to those seen in epidemic neuromyasthemia, chronic brucellosis, and CFS, but came to be known to many patients and clinicians as the chronic EBV syndrome.

In the first report of this pair, Jones et al. described 44 patients (26 adults and 18 children younger than 15) referred for a relapsing or persistent illness similar to CFS and characterized by pharyngitis, lymphadenopathy, fever, headache, arthralgia, fatigue, depression, dyslogia, and myalgia [48]. Epstein–

Barr virus antibody titer patterns, which were compatible with, but not diagnostic of, active EBV infection, but that persisted for at least 1 year, were found in 39 (89%) of the patients. Specifically, their antiviral capsid antigen antibody and early antigen antibody titers were significantly greater than those of age-matched controls (Fig. 5). Two general patterns of antibody responses were observed in these patients. In the first, significant positive antibody titers (usually IgG) to viral capsid antigens (VCA), early antigens (EA), and nuclear antigens (EBNA) were observed in 31 patients (70%); a second group consisting of 8 males (18%) was similar, except that antibodies to the nuclear antigen were borderline or absent. Only 10 (26%) of these 39 seropositive patients had positive heterophil antibody tests at the time of onset of symptoms suggestive of CFS, and no patient had detectable heterophil antibodies during the following year. Furthermore, the presence in peripheral blood of atypical lymphocytes was uncommon in these patients. No patient had serological or cultural evidence of recent cytomegalovirus (CMV) infection. Surprisingly, 5 of the 44 patients (11%) with the syndrome were EBV antibody-negative throughout the study period. Forty-one percent of their patients were children whose antibody patterns were similar to those of the adults. Of 33 age-matched asymptomatic control persons, 30 had antibodies to viral capsid and nuclear antigens, but only 3 (9%) had detectable anti-early antigen antibodies, and these were are at low levels. Notably, patients with the CFS-like illness differed significantly from the controls ($p < 0.001$) in their antibody patterns and titers.

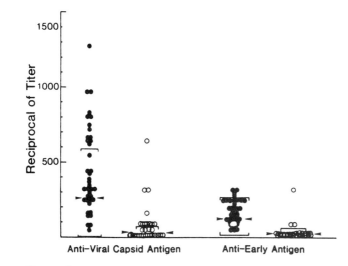

Figure 5 Geometric and arithmetic mean values of patient (solid circles) and control (open circles) EBV antibody titers. Horizontal lines represent geometric mean (1 SE) ($p < 0.001$). (From Ref. 48.)

On continued study, it was found that their patients did not easily fit into distinct clinical stages based on the absolute levels or patterns of these antibodies. The only common serological feature was that the early antigen antibody titer waxed and waned throughout the clinical course in 39 (89%) of the patients. This finding was interpreted to indicate that the persistently elevated early antigen titer suggested either a chronic lytic infection, reinfection, or reactivation of a dormant or latent process, or an immunoregulatory problem. The absence of antibodies to EBV nuclear antigen (EBNA) in eight patients was thought to suggest either an uncontrolled infection or an inherent difference in the infecting strain of the virus.

Only 1 of the 34 patients in this study, with presumed chronic active EBV infection and CFS, had detectable circulating interferon, in contrast with 7 of 7 patients with acute infectious mononucleosis. In contrast with the findings of Hamblin and co-workers [47], analysis of lymphocyte phenotypes by Jones and his associates [48], showed the ill patients did not differ significantly from the controls, and that studies of their mononuclear cell reactivity to various mitogens also were not significantly different from controls. However, Jones concluded their tests did not exclude an immune abnormality in these patients. They also noted that their observations did not prove that EBV commonly causes a prolonged viral-like illness, but that they were provocative and worthy of further prospective controlled studies.

The simultaneously reported study of Straus et al. [49] concerned 31 patients, older than 16, with a syndrome resembling CFS who were referred to the National Institutes of Health (NIH) for evaluation. No diagnosis other than chronic Epstein–Barr virus infection was established in any of them before referral. Interestingly, 8 of the 31 patients were only briefly evaluated at NIH, because when they arrived there they failed to meet the case definition; one each had Sjogren's syndrome, systemic lupus erythematosus, and lymphoma; and one had transverse myelitis and Hodgkin's disease. The other 3 patients evaluated only briefly were seronegative for EBV infection.

Thus, only 23 of the patients sent to the NIH were actually suspected by Straus et al. of having chronic EBV infection; all were studied extensively and followed for a mean of more than 2 years [49]. All were white adults, most were older than 30, and most were either in college or had a college degree. One group of 13 patients (57%) had a chronic illness resembling CFS that began within a year after a mononucleosislike disease, characterized by prolonged fever and adenopathy, 7 of them in association with a positive heterophil test. Ten of the 13 (80%) had never fully recovered from the acute mononucleosislike illness. Six other patients had a mononucleosislike illness more than 1 year *before* the onset of the symptoms that brought them to the NIH, and 4 patients (17%) did not recall having a mononucleosislike illness before thier present illness. The initial episodes of mononucleosis in these patients were relatively severe; 6 had hepatitis and 4 required hospitalization. In those patients who had recovered completely from acute mononucleosis, their acute illness lasted a mean of 3 months.

The illness of these patients when seen at the NIH was flulike, with myalgia, pharyngitis, tender adenopathy, and severe fatigue. Exacerbations had occurred one to six times in them, with more tolerable periods in between. Significantly, most of the patients had considerable psychosocial problems involving work or major conflicts with families or public agencies concerning their support. Most had consulted numerous physicians and had turned to nontraditional therapies because of anger and lack of trust in physicians. Eleven patients were evaluated by a psychiatrist at the NIH, where 6 were diagnosed as having somatization disorders, and 2 were diagnosed as having depression or an anxiety neurosis. Thus, 8 (35%) of the 23 patients studied had a diagnosis of a psychological disorder.

Despite extensive laboratory tests as well as other evaluations, few objective abnormalities were detected in these patients. Sedimentation rates were rarely abnormal. Two patients had mildly elevated abnormal liver function tests. Liver biopsy in one showed chronic persistent hepatitis that was negative on biopsy for both EBV antigens and EBV DNA. This patient was found to have chronic hepatitis C infection several years later [Straus S, personal communication]. In my experience, patients with chronic active hepatitis caused by hepatitis B or C sometimes have a clinical illness with a pattern that is similar to CFS, but it is usually considered a manifestation of the known viral infection, and, therefore, is perplexing neither to patient nor physician. Such patients might be considered to have CFS secondary to chronic active viral hepatitis. This strengthens the notion that CFS can be caused by a chronic active viral infection.

Serial Epstein–Barr virus-specific antibody titers were performed by Straus and colleagues an average of five times on these patients during their follow-up at the NIH. The geometric mean titers for IgG antibodies to EBV capsid antigen and early antigen were significantly elevated in their patients, compared with matched controls (Table 6). Five of the 23 patients had intermittently positive IgM antibody titers to early antigen; these were thought to be either false-positive results or indicative of reactivation of the infection. Fourteen of 23 patients had IgG antibody titers to viral capsid antigen of 1:640 or higher at least once during follow-up, whereas only 1 of 23 healthy controls had a titer that high. Nineteen (83%) of 23 patients had elevated antibody titers to early antigen, whereas only 6 (26%) of 23 controls were positive. Seven (30%) of 23 patients lacked detectable antibodies to EBV nuclear antigens (EBNA) at least once, and 4 never had detectable EBNA antibodies, whereas all of the EBV seropositive controls had them. It has been hypothesized that the lack of EBNA antibodies may reflect defective regulation or control of the infection by the immune system. Importantly, 3 patients with the characteristic syndrome never showed "abnormal"

Table 6 Serologic Titers for EBV on One or More Occasions for CFS Patients and Matched Controls

Antibody[a]	Titer	Patients (no.)	Controls (no.)	p value[b]
VCA-IgM	≥1:10	5	0	<0.05
VCA-IgG	≥1:320	19	3	<0.001
VCA-IgG	≥1:640	14	1	<0.001
EA-D	≥1:10	9	1	<0.005
EA-R	≥1:10	18	5	<0.005
EA (D or R)	≥1:10	19	6	<0.005
EA (D or R)	≥1:20	16	2	<0.005
EBNA	≥1:5	7	0	<0.001

[a]VCA, viral capsid antigen; EA-D, antibodies to the diffuse components of early antigen; EA-R, antibodies to the restricted components of early antigens, EBNA, antibodies to the EBV nuclear antigens.
[b]Statistics by Fisher's exact test.
Source: Ref. 49.

EBV-specific antibody titers or patterns; 2 of them had experienced typical heterophil-positive infectious mononucleosis and had never recovered from it. Although a range of antibody titers was seen in patients tested on several occasions, again, there was no clear relation between specific titers and the clinical status of the patient. In other words, high titers and atypical patterns were seen as often during remissions as during exacerbations. Therefore, the putative abnormality causing their illness was thought by Straus and his co-workers to be a persistent productive infection that was not controlled by immune factors, or not reliably reflected in antibody titers, or of unknown causation [49].

Throat washings from 5 of 11 patients ill with CFS were positive for the presence of the EB virus, which the investigators considered was about what one would expect for seropositive *well* patients late after the primary illness, but not as high a rate as would be expected during the acute illness.

Circulating lymphocytes of 10 patients were studied to quantitate the proportion transformed and capable of spontaneous outgrowth in culture, and there was no significant difference in results for the patients and 14 concurrently tested healthy seropositive controls. Although interferon can be found in sera of patients with acute mononucleosis, circulating interferon was not found in sera of 18 CFS patients tested. However, the activity of an interferon-induced enzyme, $2'$, $5'$-oligoadenylate synthetase, was increased in 5 patients studied; in 11 of 15 patients tested, moderately elevated circulating immune complex levels were also found. Persisting suppressor T-cell activity, typically found in patients recovering from acute mononucleosis, was also found in 18 of 19 patients. Epstein–Barr virus-specific antibody titers did not correlate well with clinical status, circulating immune complexes, or $2'$, $5'$-adenylate synthetase activity. However, the latter may be present in various states or induced by substances other than interferon [50].

Straus and his co-workers noted that, although many of their patients had an illness that was out of proportion to the evidence of active infection and that many of them appeared neurotic, studies also revealed a series of subtle, yet objective abnormalities in many of them [49]. The serological tests for EBV were thought to be inappropriate for persons without recent acute EBV infection, specifically the high IgG titers to viral capsid antigen and to early antigen. These results suggested persistent or reactivated EBV infection. The failure to detect antibodies to EBV nuclear antigens late after the acute infection suggested that an immune impairment was present. In addition, they noted elevated levels of circulating immune complexes, mild immunoglobulin deficiencies, and increased T-cell-mediated immune suppression despite the presence of increased numbers of T-helper cells and normal numbers of T-suppressor cells. They believed the observed suppression was apparently because of an in vitro ability of peripheral T lymphocytes from these patients to suppress immunoglobulin synthesis by mitogen or EBV-stimulated allogeneic B cells, although this abnormality was not specific for the disorder.

Tosato and colleagues then examined T-cell function in 16 of the foregoing patients with so-called chronic active EBV infection [51]. They reported that the frequency of circulating EBV-infected B cells that manifested spontaneous in vitro outgrowth in their patients was comparable with the frequency found in normal EBV-seropositive persons, and that the levels of EBV-specific suppressor activity were also normal. Upon stimulation with polyclonal activators, unseparated cells from these patients produced a relatively normal number of immunoglobulin-secreting cells. When purified T cells from these patients were mixed with normal cells in coculture, immunoglobulin production was strikingly suppressed, and the degree of T-cell suppression correlated directly with the abnormally elevated titer of antibody to the early antigen of EBV. A similar phenomenon is also seen during normal convalescence from acute EBV-induced infectious mononucleosis. Thus, Straus et al. postulated that from an immunological viewpoint, patients with so-called chronic active EBV infection were "frozen" in an unresolved state found only briefly during normal convalescence from acute EBV infection [49,51].

Straus [49] and Jones [48] and their colleagues concluded that their findings did not prove that EBV infection was responsible for their patients' illnesses, but they did indicate further investigation of that possibility was warranted. Two reports on further investigations by others appeared 2 years later and added new information concerning the role of EBV in CFS [52,53].

Buchwald et al. reported that 105 (21%) of 500 unselected patients, between the ages of 17 and 50 seeking primary care at a university medical center in

Boston, Massachusetts, because of chronic fatigue, were found to have suffered for a mean of 16 months from a syndrome clinically consistent with chronic active EBV infection [52]. Although the geometric mean antibody titers of these patients to various EBV antigens were higher in patients than those of age- and sex-matched control patients, the differences were not statistically significant (Table 7). Therefore, they concluded there was no good evidence that CFS in their practice was related to EBV infection, and that EBV serological tests from patients with CFS should be interpreted with caution. They also noted that the pattern of high titers of antibodies to EBV capsid antigen and early antigen that were reported to be typical of patients with CFS may be seen in an occasional healthy patient.

These authors also emphasized that their patients were distinct from the two unfortunate patients reported by Schooley et al. [54], who had extraordinarily high titers of EBV antibodies, particular to IgG viral capsid antigen ($\geq$ 1:5140) and early antigen ($\geq$ 1:640). These patients were suffering from a serious and sometimes fatal illness (unlike CFS) that was associated with definite, uncontrolled active EBV infection and was characterized by interstitial pneumonia, pancytopenia, and a fatal outcome unless patients were treated with acyclovir [54]. They emphasized that, although the syndrome is sometimes correctly called chronic active EBV infection, it is important that this syndrome be distinguished from the CFS associated with questionably or only moderately high antibody titers to EBV antigens. Notably, the geometric mean IgG VCA antibody titiers were 600 and 518, respectively, in the patients reported by Jones and by Straus and colleagues [47,48], whereas they were $\geq$ 1:5140 in Schooley's patients.

Patients in the study of Buchwald et al. [52] were not necessarily seeking care primarily because of fatigue, and they tended to be less sick or disabled than those in other studies on CFS. Their physical examinations were generally benign. However, it was clear that many of Buchwald's patients suffered considerable morbidity, and also that it was a surprisingly common syndrome in their practice. Sixty percent of Buchwald's patients stated that their chronic fatigue had created substantial stress both at home and in the workplace.

Holmes and colleagues reported the results of studies on a cluster of 134 patients with suspected chronic EBV syndrome in Incline Village, Nevada, in 1985 [53]. Many of their 134 patients had a relatively mild or brief illness, or had another possible explanation for their illness. These investigators focused on those 15 (11%) of the 134 patients who had the most severe, prolonged, and unexplained fatigue. Three groups of persons were studied: case patients, noncase patients, and controls (the latter a mixture of office staff members and patients with illnesses unrelated to the study) who were age, sex, and race matched to the case patients.

Analysis of the results of their study was complicated because laboratory tests were done in three different laboratories. Nonetheless, cases had higher percent-

Table 7 Comparison of EBV Serological Results in Different CFS Patient Groups and Their Matched Control

	Geometric mean titers ± SD					
	VCA-IgG		EA-Ab		EBNA-Ab	
	Patients	Controls	Patients	Controls	Patients	Controls
All patients (N = 40)	134.9 ± 3	81.2 ± 5	18.2 ± 6	10.0 ± 7	13.2 ± 2	8.5 ± 3
Patients with chief complaint of chronic fatigue (n = 12)	151.3 ± 2	38.0 ± 10	11.8 ± 7	12.3 ± 10	12.9 ± 2	6.0 ± 3
Patients with fatigue plus sore throat plus headaches plus myalgias (n = 18)	117.5 ± 2	52.5 ± 8	13.8 ± 6	6.0 ± 8	10.7 ± 2	6.0 ± 4
Patients with most severe fatigue (intermittently bedridden/homebound) (n = 16)	147.9 ± 2	102.3 ± 5	16.2 ± 6	15.9 ± 7	11.5 ± 2	9.6 ± 3
Patients with cervical adenopathy or enlarged submandibular glands (n = 12)	123.0 ± 2	50.1 ± 9	28.2 ± 3	10.5 ± 8	10.5 ± 2	7.4 ± 4
Patients with a history of mononucleosis (n = 10)	162.2 ± 2	93.3 ± 11	16.2 ± 7	6.3 ± 7	15.1 ± 2	8.1 ± 2

Source: Ref. 52.

ages than noncase patients of IgG antibody titers greater than those considered as threshold abnormal values for EA, VCA, and EBNA antibodies, and these differences were statistically significant in three instances. In the case–control study, higher percentages of cases had titers higher than thresholds than did controls for EA IgG and VCA IgG antibodies, and these differences were significant in three instances. Differences were also higher for EBNA IgG, but were not statistically significant. None of the cases or controls were positive for VCA IgM antibodies. They concluded that, although patients tended to have higher EBV antibody titers than did controls, there were no threshold titers at which patients could be "effectively" differentiated from controls.

Notably, the serological differences Holmes and his associates identified between cases and controls were not limited to EBV. Similar differences in mean elevations of antibody titers were also noted for cytomegalovirus, herpes simplex virus 1 and 2, and possibly measles virus antibody titers. Mean total serum IgG, IgA, and IgM concentrations were comparable in the two groups.

Their analysis also indicated that a high proportion of nonresident patients had referred themselves to outbreak area physicians specifically for EBV testing in 1985 (possibly because the illness had been picked up by the news media), thereby creating the impression of an outbreak of EBV infections in the Nevada area. Therefore, the existence of an epidemic could not be proved or disproved by this study. Relatively few patients in this study had been ill as long as those described in previous reports of chronic EBV infection, although 12 of the 14 case patients were still symptomatic 14 months after the investigation. Finally, lymphadenopathy and splenomegaly were more often a part of the early stages of the illness than in other reports of CFS related to chronic EBV infection.

This study also called attention to the fact that EBV serological testing is notoriously unreliably reproducible from one laboratory to another or from one time to another in the same laboratory (at least with the immunofluorescent antibody serological tests used in these studies). This study also raised the distinct possibility that a polyclonal B-lymphocytic response may be present in patients with CFS (caused by EBV infection or other agents), and that relatively high antibody titers to a wide variety of infectious agents, as well as to other antigens, may be a characteristic of CFS, and thus might confound studies designed to implicate a variety of etiological agents.

Further evidence that elevated antibody titers to various candidate etiologies of CFS may merely represent polyclonal B-cell hyperactivity was provided during the studies of Levine et al. of four clusters of the chronic fatigue syndrome in the Lake Tahoe region of Nevada and California [55], which included the Incline Village outbreak reported by Holmes et al. [53]. The geometric mean antibody titers to human herpesvirus-6 (HHV-6) was higher (132.6 mean) than that of control subjects (89 mean) in Levine's studies. The mean titers to EBV EA (6.0) were also higher than those of the controls (2.1), but the mean EBV VCA titers

(239.7) were no higher than those of controls (254.0). Once again, they found no relation between EBV antibody titer patterns and the clinical course of the illness.

In 1988, Jones and associates reported preliminary findings on antibody titers to EBV-specific DNase and DNA polymerase in patients with CFS [56]. These antibodies are expressed only during virus replication. Sera from six groups of subjects, representing various EBV-related illnesses, were studied. Only subjects with extremely elevated antibody titers to EBV viral capsid antigen (anti-VCA >10,000) had elevated levels of anti-EBV DNase and anti-EBV DNA polymerase. Three of six patients with these highly elevated anti-EBV enzyme antibody levels developed fatal lymphomas. Fourteen patients with CFS who had anti-early antigen (EA) titers of 80 or greater for more than 1 year had enzyme-neutralizing antibody titers that were normal and comparable with those of healthy EBV-seropositive medical students. Thus, their studies did *not* support the hypothesis that CFS is usually attributable to chronic active EBV infection, nor in contrast, that elevated EBV early antigen titers are reliable in diagnosing CFS related to EBV infection. However, only 14 patients with the EBV antibody titers usually associated with CFS were studied, and if there are other infectious etiologies of the syndrome as well as EBV, some of these individuals may have had an organism other than EBV responsible for initiating their illness.

In 1990, Gold and associates reported their results of a comprehensive, prospective, clinical and virological study of 26 patients with CFS [57]. Patients studied had been referred to the Viral Disease Clinic at the Harborview Medical Center in Seattle. All were at least 18 years old, and all had experienced symptoms typical of CFS for at least 9 months. All had EBV VCA IgG antibody titers of 1:80 or greater and EBV EA antibody titers of 1:20 or greater. Patients were followed at regular intervals for clinical status, changes in antibody titers, EBV cultures of blood and saliva, immunological studies (including enumeration of various T-cell subsets), and psychiatric evaluation. Controls were volunteers recruited from their medical center.

A history of clinical mononucleosis was reported in 14 (54%) of the 26 patients with CFS. No patient was human immunodeficiency virus (HIV)-positive. Subjects had previously seen a median of five health care providers for their illness, and had symptoms for a median of 3.5 years before enrollment. Thirteen were functionally impaired by their illness, and 9 were unable to work at all. All 18 control individuals worked or went to school during the day, but none slept during the day. Patients complained of a mean of 11 different symptoms typical of CFS; 20 of the 26 were depressed, but only 7 had sought counseling of psychiatric treatment, and 17 (65%) had musculoskeletal complaints. Few of them had abnormalities on general physical examination, but 5 had neurological abnormalities. The frequency of atypical lymphocytosis or antibodies to CMV or toxoplasma or antinuclear antibodies was similar in both patient and control groups.

At enrollment, the geometric mean titer of IgG antibodies to EBV VCA was 134.3 in patients, but significantly lower in controls, 39.6. The EA titers were also higher in patients (41.3) than in controls (9.2). These differences were thought to simply reflect the fact that patients were selected for study on the basis of their elevated titers, whereas controls were not. In contrast, the frequency of isolation of EBV from throat washings and lymphocytes was similar in the two groups; two patients and two controls had EBV isolated from peripheral blood lymphocytes. No patient had EBV in throat washings, whereas one control had EBV DNA in a throat washing, as demonstrated by in situ hybridization. Antibodies to HHV-6 were found in 19 of 23 patients and in all 12 controls; the geometric mean titers and their ranges were similar in both groups.

There were no significant differences between patients and controls in mean number of lymphocytes, T4/T8 ratios, or phytohemagglutinin (PHA) responses. Patients with CFS demonstrated lower in vitro interleukin (IL)-2 production by peripheral lymphocytes in response to phytohemagglutinin stimulation than did controls ($p < 0.03$), whereas in vitro natural killer (NK) lymphocyte cytotoxicity responses to K562 cells were higher in patients than in controls ($p = 0.03$).

Patients with CFS had significantly more lifetime (72%) as well as current (42%) major depressive episodes than controls (22% and 0%, respectively). Thirteen of 18 patients had one or more depressive episodes predating CFS, 2 had CFS predating depression, and 3 had the onset of CFS and depression concurrently. Patients with CFS had more somatic symptoms than controls (9.8 vs 1.1), indicating a "high degree of psychiatric distress."

Of the 26 CFS patients, 21 were followed for at least 3 months after enrollment; the mean duration was 11.3 months (range 3–21). Their symptoms (including fatigue) decreased over a relatively brief period (a mean of 11.3 months); overall, 14 patients (57%) improved or returned to normal functioning during the study, despite that no special treatment was given.

Clinical improvement in patients with CFS was not associated with any changes in EBV antibody titers or culture status. None of 21 patients developed a fourfold change in VCA IgG titer between andy two time points, and only 3 of 21 demonstrated a fourfold or greater change in EBV early antigen titer; these 3 patients improved clinically, as did 9 of 18 patients with unchanged EA titers. No changes in HHV-6 or other immunological responses were observed.

Gold and her co-workers speculated that the decreased in vitro IL-2 production by stimulated lymphocytes and the elevated NK activity they observed in their patients may have been secondary to their affective disorders [57]. Although it is not the purpose of this chapter to enumerate and evaluate various immunological abnormalities associated with CFS (see Chapter 8), a few comments here about their relation to the hypothetical etiology may be in order. Klimas and associates reported clear evidence of cellular immune dysfunction in 30 patients with CFS meeting the CDC criteria, many of whom were depressed [58].

Whereas IL-2 levels were elevated in plasma of patients with CFS in a report by Cheney and Dorman [59], IL-2 levels and levels of cytokines such as interferons and tumor necrosis factor were no different from controls in a report by Straus and colleagues [60]. Linde et al. asked whether serum levels of IL-2 and soluble cellular receptors were different in 35 patients with CFS who met CDC criteria from those of 60 patients with acute infectious mononucleosis or from 20 healthy matched control subjects [61]. Measured markers for T-lymphocyte activation (soluble IL-2 and soluble CD8) and for monocyte activation (neopterin) were elevated during acute infectious mononucleosis, but in only a few patients with CFS. The levels of IL-1α were significantly higher in patients with infectious mononucleosis and in those with CFS than in controls. They stated it is not likely that EBV activation causes the symptoms of CFS in view of their inability to detect most of the markers for lymphocyte activation that are seen in acute mononucleosis in the serum of patients with CFS. However, some of the observed differences between patients with CFS and healthy controls were considered by these authors as a strong indicator for further studies. Straus et al. noted that IL-2 and tumor necrosis factor levels in their patients with CFS did not differ significantly from controls, and that most of their CFS patients had undetectable levels of interferons [60].

One might conclude from these immunological studies that they are intriguing, but conflicting, and in any event not what one might expect in chronic active viral infection. Different ways of studying the role of cytokines in the pathogenesis of CFS might be more productive and are in order.

Gold et al. acknowledged that the CDC criteria for diagnosis of CFS [6] were established *after* patients had been enrolled in their study [57]. In retrospect, only 6 of their 26 patients fulfilled the CDC criteria; yet, it seems probable that most of their patients met the revised criteria [7]. Although the 6 who met the earlier criteria had a significantly greater number of symptoms than the other 20 (16 vs 10; $p < 0.01$), there was no significant difference between the two groups on follow-up. They also pointed out that most patients who present to medical attention with chronic fatigue after a thorough evaluation do not fulfill the formal CDC criteria developed to guide research on the syndrome, and that the data they collected on a broader cohort are still of value to physicians caring for less severely ill patients.

In summary, Gold and her co-workers could find no evidence that the unchecked replication of EBV is causative of chronic fatigue in patients with high EBV antibody titers, regardless of their pattern [57]. In addition, their finding of 50% improvement in fatigue as well as other symptoms of these patients over a short period of follow-up should be encouraging to physicians as well as to patients.

Horwitz et al. reported results of their longitudinal EBV-specific serological studies on 140 sera obtained from 88 patients, all but 4 of whom were healthy after having had infectious mononucleous caused by EBV confirmed by them 10–104 months previously [62]. Elevated levels of IgG antibody to VCA ($\geq$ 1:320) were still present in 31% of those tested at 30–38 months and in 27% at 40–104 months. Antibodies to EA-restricted component were detectable at titers of 1:10, or higher, in 44% and 39% and at $\geq$ 1:40 in 19% and 12% at 30–38 and 40–105 months, respectively; with only two exceptions, titers of antibody to EBNA ranged from 1:5 to 1:160 in all of 140 specimens. Greater reactivity and higher titers to VCA and EA were noted in both females and older patients. They interpreted their results to suggest that enhanced EBV activity may persist for as long as 30–104 months after infectious mononucleosis in healthy persons, and that caution must be exercised before accepting laboratory evidence of reactivation of EBV [i.e., the presence of antibodies to EA, restricted (R) or diffuse (D) components, and high titers of IgG antibodies to VCA] as the cause of a patient's clinical illness. They also indicated that it is still unclear whether reactivation of the EBV carrier state is capable by itself of producing clinical symptoms, even though this has been demonstrated with other viruses, such as cytomegalovirus and herpes simplex virus.

Sumaya reported similar EBV serological and virological studies on patients with a CFS-like illness and controls in 1991 [63]. There was a broad range of normal values for EBV antibody titers among different healthy groups. Although a higher mean antibody titer to the EBV early antigen complex (usually the D component) was found in CFS patients, there was no concurrently elevated IgG antibody to EBV capsid antigen. Among 29 patients in the CFS group, 5 (17%) had throat washings positive for infectious EBV, a rate comparable with that found among the healthy controls, 4 (25%) of 16. The rate of spontaneous proliferation of peripheral blood lymphocytes, a measure of the burden of EBV in the lymphocyte pool, showed a tendency, but not a statistically significant one, for a greater burden in the CFS-like group (10 positive of 37) than in normal adults (1 of 37), but less than that of patients with acute mononucleosis (9 of 17). As had been shown previously by Tosato [51], when Sumaya used a semiquantitative technique, no differences in the viral load in peripheral blood mononuclear cells were seen for CFS-like patients and healthy controls. Noting that various laboratories have reported several aberrant immune responses in patients with CFS, Sumaya concluded that patients with CFS often have an underlying dysfunction of the immune system that in some way produces mild and variable serological and virological findings detectable with EBV and other viruses, and that it is still conceivable that EBV may contribute to or exacerbate CFS.

In 1988, Straus et al. reported the results of studies on the efficacy of acyclovir (Zovirax) in CFS in a double-blind, placebo-controlled trial designed to determine whether treatment of CFS with an antiviral drug that might terminate a chronic infection with EBV was worthwhile [64]. Since they considered acyclovir to be safe as well as to inhibit synthesis of the Epstein–Barr virus in vitro and in vivo, such a trial would be not only a test of the role of activation of EBV infection in the pathogenesis of CFS, but it might provide much needed relief of the suffering of these patients. Many observers considered this trial to be the ultimate test of the EBV hypothesis.

Twenty-seven adults with the diagnosis of CFS who met the CDC criteria and who had persisting antibodies to EBV early antigens (titers $\geq$ 1:40) or undetectable levels of antibodies to EBV nuclear antigens ($<$ 1:2), or both, were enrolled into the study. Patients had had debilitating fatigue for an average of 6.8 years before the study. After an extensive initial evaluation, patients were randomly assigned to receive acylovir or placebo in a double-blinded fashion for 37 days, first intravenously, and then by mouth. After such therapy, there was a 6-week washout period during which no therapy was given. Patients then received the alternative treatment, again in a blinded fashion. There were also periods of study for 6 weeks before and after the treatment phases. Treatment consisted of an inhospital intravenous infusion of placebo or acyclovir (500 mg/m^2) over a period of 60 min in saline every 8 h for 7 days, along with vigorous oral hydration. At the end of the week, patients were discharged to take 800 mg acyclovir by mouth, four times daily, for 30 days. Patients were also permitted to take a variety of other common medications as well as antibiotics for documented infections. The patients were readmitted to the NIH Clinical Center at the end of each phase (a total of six times during the study) for reevaluation by a single physician who was blinded to treatment regimen. Various serological, immunological, and other laboratory tests, wellness scores, and self-assessments of mood, anxiety, depression, fatigue, and confusion were performed during those evaluations.

All the patients were white and of relatively high socioeconomic status and educational level. Some were capable of light or part-time work or study. Fatigue had begun insidiously in four cases, with gastroenteritis or influenzalike features in ten patients and with mononucleosislike features in seven. Patients in the two groups were well-matched.

Of 27 study participants, 3 were withdrawn from the study because of reversible renal failure during acyclovir infusions. Of the 24 patients who completed the study, 21 scored themselves as improved during one or more of the treatment phases. Perceptions of improvement typically occurred during the first week of treatment and lasted for only 2 or 3 weeks after the end of treatment. Four patients (17%) reported improvement that lasted for at least 1 year, but all 4 still had fatigue. Improvement began during placebo periods in 3 of those 4 whose improvement lasted for 1 year. Eleven patients (46%) felt better during acyclovir treatment, whereas 10 (42%) felt better during placebo. No objective evidence distinguished those who responded favorably while receiving acyclovir from those who did not. Both placebo and acyclovir were associated with mood changes; levels of anxiety, depression, and confusion were greater during acyclovir treatment than during placebo treatment, and anger was marginally greater (Table 8). During phases in which patients felt better, reduction in fatigue was impressive, and levels of vigor and sense of well-being were also higher. Acyclovir treatment did not lead to a marked change in the number of hours of rest taken by patients during the day, even when they reported improvement in well-being. Body temperature did not change significantly whether or not patients felt better, and averaged about 36.98°C (98.6°F).

Each patient's levels of EBV antibodies were remarkably stable throughout the study, with significant decreases being uncommon, and no correlation of changes in titer with treatment or clinical improvement. A variety of immunological parameters were studied, and none of them correlated with treatment or clinical status. Interestingly, interferon levels above 4 IU/ml were noted in 10 of 73 sera from patients, but from only 2 of 23 untreated age- and sex-matched controls; in addition, interferon levels in serum did not correlate with levels of 2′,5′-oligoadenylate.

Treatment with high doses of acyclovir was associated with appreciable toxicity, especially gastrointestinal symptoms, headache, and dizziness. Despite attempts to ensure hydration, three patients had reversible renal failure, with crystalluria, back pain, and elevation of serum creatinine.

Despite the known activity of acyclovir against EBV, and the use of high and

Table 8 Differences in Individual Mood States and Wellness Scores, Body Temperature, and Hours of Sleep Between Study Phases According to Whether CFS Patients Were Treated with Acyclovir or Placebo

Variable	Acyclovir vs placebo	
	Difference[a]	p value
Anxiety	2.92 ± 1.11	0.02
Depression	3.97 ± 1.59	0.02
Anger	2.30 ± 1.18	0.07
Vigor	−2.05 ± 1.26	0.12
Fatigue	1.26 ± 1.10	0.27
Confusion	1.83 ± 0.61	<0.01
Wellness score (0–100)	−1.08 ± 3.01	>0.5
Temperature (°C)	−0.02 ± 0.03	>0.5
Rest (h/day)	−0.05 ± 0.38	>0.5

[a]Plus–minus values represent mean (±SEM) paired differences in serial measurements made during the treatment phases. Positive differences indicate an increase in the level of the listed variable while receiving acyclovir, negative values a decrease.
Source: Ref. 64.

occasionally toxic doses of acylovir that were sufficient to achieve blood levels above the median inhibitory concentration, clinical improvement could not be attributed to acyclovir. Because of this result, Straus and colleagues suggested that active replication of EBV is *not* a primary determinant of the signs and symptoms of CFS. However, this does not necessarily indicate that EBV is not causative of CFS in some other way, such as by triggering a process that does not require replication of EBV for its perpetuation.

It has been reported by Andersson et al. that if acute EBV-associated infectious mononucleosis is treated with intravenous acyclovir for 7 days, virus shedding may be significantly reduced or eliminated, and that factors, such as duration of fever, tonsillar swelling, pharyngitis, and self-assessment, showed significant improvement as a group ($p < 0.01$) [65]. However, other individual symptoms and signs of illness were largely unaffected, possibly because many of the symptoms of the illness may be the result of adverse side effects of beneficial host defense mechanisms involving cytokines, antibodies, killer lymphocytes, and other mediators of that complex network of lymphocytic and mononuclear cell responses that we lump together loosely and refer to as cellular and humoral immune mechanisms. These mechanisms are almost certainly not quickly affected, either directly or indirectly, by the effects of acyclovir on viral replication in B lymphocytes or epithelial cells in the nasopharynx.

It still remains possible and, in my own view, probable that EBV is capable of causing chronic fatigue and other symptoms in some persons by initiating or triggering a chain of events, the nature of which has so far defied elucidation, that is the final common pathway leading to CFS.

If EBV is one of many different infectious agents capable of triggering this process in patients unfortunate enough to have "the CFS diathesis," then it may, at some future date, be possible to show that acyclovir may be useful in a subset of patients in whom EBV is definitely responsible for the condition, or that acyclovir may be useful as an adjunct to other forms of therapy for the disease in those patients.

Straus and his colleagues pointed out that the improvement they noted in their patients during treatment with either placebo or acyclovir must have been attributed to a placebo effect [64]. Many of their patients were surprised when they learned the study results; some were relieved to hear them, and a few dismissed the findings. Importantly, Straus said "most of the patients are now more circumspect about anecdotal reports of beneficial treatments." They also indicated their results show "that affect plays an important part in the perception of illness severity in the chronic fatigue syndrome. Significant improvement in levels of anger, depression and other mood states correlated with overall clinical improvement." With these emotional reactions and the improvement in symptomatology—which was the chicken and which was the egg?

The studies cited so far are important if for no other reason than that they indicate there are enough objective abnormalities of an immunological nature that have been detected in CFS to make it very unlikely that it is simply a psychological process, whether one wants to call it depression, somatization, psychoneuroneurosis, malingering, or whatever. I also believe that EBV is one of the infectious agents that are capable of initiating that as yet undefined process.

CANDIDIASIS AND THE "YEAST CONNECTION"

The concept that *Candida albicans* or the other *Candida* species, which commonly colonize the oral and vaginal mucosa, the skin, and the intestines of healthy human beings, might be the cause of a wide variety of human illnesses in the absence of overt evidence of yeast infection (such as thrush, vaginitis, esophagitis, or other) was first enunciated in 1978 and expanded on in 1981 by Truss, an internist in Birmingham, Alabama [66,67]. He believed the consequences of colonization with yeasts have been aggravated by the use of antibiotics, birth control pills, immunosuppressants (especially adrenal corticosteroids), repeated pregnancies, the prolonged high-carbohydrate intake characteristic of our society, and by other factors that adversely affect control of this fungus. He published six case descriptions to bolster his concept that *C. albicans* and the many antigens and toxins it produces may cause severe chronic illness. They included illnesses usually considered psychosomatic, but that he believed were, in fact, related to disturbed chemical and physiological processes in the brain, and that cleared with antiyeast therapy. He stated that virtually any organ can function improperly because of this condition, which he called chronic candidiasis or candidosis, which seemed to be especially common in women. Manifestations included depression, anxiety, hyperactivity, hyperirritability, increased susceptibility to adverse reactions to inhaled or ingested chemicals, drugs and food, interference with hormone functions, menstrual disturbances, altered libido, anorexia nervosa, decreased breast size, premenstrual tension, and impairment of memory and concentration. He indicated that these were "almost always superimposed upon the many physical manifestations originating at the sites of yeast growth or related allergic responses." In many of his patients, he claimed, such symptoms responded to treatment orally with nystatin, an antiyeast drug, and a low-carbohydrate diet.

Truss acknowledged that his patients and the details of their illnesses did not prove a cause-and-effect relation between *Candida* and these conditions, but he felt they were useful in providing ideas for further exploration. He claimed that *Candida* "lives in virtually every human being, . . . it can be cultured from the mouth, stool and vagina in most people, . . . that probably everyone has antibodies to the 70 antigens of the fungus in their blood, and that . . . they will have positive skin tests to *Candida* vaccines of assured potency." Therefore, he believed tests such as cultures and antibody or skin tests were of no value in telling when, by immunological tolerance or allergic, autoimmune, and possibly toxic mechanisms, *Candida* has caused such disturbances of body functions. He went on to state that the loss of normal suppressor lymphocyte cellular functions induced by *C. albicans* allowed immune responses to normal cells to occur, which resulted in autoimmune or hypersensitivity processes.

Curiously, Truss also described five patients with multiple sclerosis, in 1981 [67], who responded to treatment with nystatin. He reported that some of them had abnormally low levels of natural killer lymphocytes and that these levels improved with nystatin therapy.

Truss concluded by stressing the importance of the emergence of a picture of a universally present organism (*Candida*) of great complexity and variety, with its own physiology and growth characteristics influenced strongly by many factors in our lives. "Simple . . . complex . . . poorly understood . . . constantly changing . . . quantitatively and qualitatively . . . and represented by abnormal function in many organs, which result in the candidiasis syndrome" [67].

All in all, his was and still is a very difficult hypothesis, or series of connected hypotheses, to prove or disprove. On the other hand, so far the *existence* of this syndrome has not been supported, even partially, by any properly conducted scientific studies.

In 1983, both Truss [68] and Crook [69] authored books elaborating on chronic candidiasis, or the so-called yeast connection, as it had come to be known. Aimed at lay readers, these books and their theories were eagerly and uncritically adopted by patients with a wide variety of illnesses, including chronic fatigue syndrome. Patients used these ideas for self-diagnosis, to support the notions that their illnesses were not psychological in origin, and that treatment with dietary manipulations and other therapies would result in a cure of their illness if only one could find a sympathetic and knowledgeable physician who was willing and able to help them.

In 1986, a commentary on this issue was published by a food scientist, E. R. Blonz [70], who discussed the question: "Is there an epidemic of chronic candidiasis in our midst?" He indicated that there is a growing segment within the medical community that actively treats patients with the complaint of "candida" and also a wide variety of nonspecific symptoms with dietary instructions and antifungal drugs. He noted that the American Academy of Allergy and Immunology has taken the position that this concept of candidiasis is speculative and unproved, and he expressed caution concerning the potential side effects (including hepatitis) of oral antifungal agents. He stated that it is inappropriate to believe there is an epidemic of the nature and proportions stated, and he stressed that the wide range of symptoms and the lack of reliable diagnostic tests would make it difficult for *any* sick person to be certain they were *not* suffering from this ailment. He said there is the further danger that in the search for a cure for the yeast syndrome, the ensuing ineffective treatment might obscure or delay the diagnosis of more serious illnesses. He also pointed out that there is a need for scientific study of the many theories on which the candidiasis syndrome is based, and that until these questions are answered, patients will be both in a position of vulnerability to entrepreneurial adventurism (and exploitation) and, in many cases, subject to needless suffering.

Renfro et al. subsequently compared eight patients with chronic fatigue, who believed they had a candida-related illness, with 92 patients with chronic fatigue who did not, and were unable to find any differences between them [71]. They were also unable to identify any findings (including skin test reactivity to candidal antigens) specific for the yeast connection. Furthermore, in seven of the eight patients who believed they had the yeast connection, a psychiatric illness was believed to underly their fatigue; of the remaining 92 patients with CFS, 59 had underlying psychiatric diagnoses. The patients who believed they had chronic candidiasis were more likely to have seen a nonmedical caretaker and were likely to be taking large quantities of vitamins. Three patients who believed they had oral or vaginal candidal infections had negative fungal cultures from those sites and elsewhere. Interestingly, these authors noted that some patients were more accepting of a diagnosis of major depression or anxiety disorder if it was presented to them as an imbalance of brain chemistry. Since it is undoubtedly true that psychiatric disease is associated with alterations in the activities of neurotransmitters and other biochemical functions found in the brain, theirs is not a surprising observation. The surprising thing is that it has taken so long for us to recognize the importance of their observation.

In 1990, Dismukes and his colleagues reported the results of the first randomized, double-blind study of any sort on this entity, which they called the candidiasis hypersensitivity syndrome [72]. It was a carefully designed, executed, and analyzed study. Enrollment was limited to 42 women from 21 to 40 years of age who had a history of candidal vaginitis accompanied by burning, itching, or discharge that had previously responded to antifungal therapy. They were also required to have three of five clinical features that are commonly seen with the syndrome, such as gastrointestinal symptoms of unknown cause, upper or lower respiratory symptoms, symptoms of premenstrual distress, moderate to severe depression, and difficulty with short-term memory, concentration, or lethargy. Patients who were pregnant, or were taking various medications, or who had diseases, such as diabetes mellitus, that were thought to enhance the risk of developing the syndrome were excluded from the study.

During the 32 weeks of the study, each patient serially received four different double-blind treatment regimens consisting of all the possible combinations of oral nystatin, vaginal nystatin, or placebo. Nystatin is a potent inhibitor of the growth and metabolism of *Candida* species. The objective was to determine whether nystatin given orally, vaginally, or by both routes was superior to placebo. Patients followed each regimen for an 8-week period. Patients doubled the dose of oral capsules twice during each treatment block, at the end of 2 and of 4 weeks. By the end of the study, each patient had received all of the four possible regimens. Patient responses were determined periodically by having them fill out questionnaires evaluating symptoms and their severity, and by physical examinations and fungal cultures.

The results (Fig. 6) showed that the three active drug treatment regimens and the placebo regimen reduced vaginal symptoms significantly ($p < 0.001$). There was also a suggestion that the benefit of nystatin on vaginal symptoms persisted after patients were switched to placebo. By contrast, no statistically significant treatment differences or carryover effects were detected for changes in the systemic (nonvaginal) symptoms of the candidiasis syndrome. All four treatment regimens, including the double-placebo regimen, reduced systemic symptoms significantly ($p < 0.001$), but the active regimens were no more effective than placebo. The mean rate of improvement for the active drug regimens was 25%, whereas it was 23% for the placebo. All four regimens had a positive effect on overall symptoms, mostly because of effects on vaginal symptoms. The three active treatment regimens and the placebo regimen had significant beneficial effects on psychological symptoms and indexes of "distress" measured in the study, except for obsessive–compulsive symptoms in patients receiving oral placebo and vaginal nystatin. There were no significant differences among the treatment regimens.

Dismukes and his colleagues appropriately concluded that their data did not support any significant overall effect of nystatin therapy on the systemic symptoms of the candidasis hypersensitivity syndrome. The oral plus vaginal nystatin regimen was of appreciable benefit for vaginal symptoms and for only

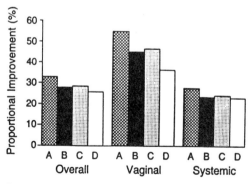

Figure 6 Proportional improvement in overall, vaginal, and systemic candidiasis symptom scores from baseline to the end of the 32-week study period. A, oral nystatin plus vaginal nystatin; B, oral nystatin plus vaginal placebo; C, oral placebo plus vaginal nystatin; D, oral placebo plus vaginal placebo. (From Ref. 72.)

4 of 15 systemic symptoms (abdominal pain or cramping, constipation, menstrual irregularity, and sneezing). There were no significant differences among any of the treatments in cognitive or psychological symptoms or physical findings. A positive placebo effect was most evident during the first 2 weeks of treatment, regardless of regimen. The double-drug (nystatin) regimen appeared to have a beneficial effect on systemic symptoms during the last 16 weeks of the study, but not the first 16 weeks, although this was not statistically significant ($p <$ 0.06). Finally, in this study, there was no relation between positive cultures for candida and systemic symptoms.

This study was criticized by Crook, Truss, and others because of study design and analysis, and especially because it did not also study the potential effects of multimodal therapy, such as avoidance of foods containing yeasts or molds, or the reduction of dietary carbohydrates, or candidal immunotherapy [73]. According to the authors, these were not included in the study design because of the increase in its complexity they would have necessitated. The authors acknowledged that further controlled studies may be needed to address these issues. However, their findings provide objective evidence that *the candidiasis syndrome is not a verifiable entity*, and that the use of empirical long-term nystatin treatment for it is not justified. It should also be stressed that the patients they studied would almost certainly *not* qualify for the diagnosis of the chronic fatigue syndrome according to CDC criteria [6,7]. Their symptoms were distinctly different from those of that condition, even though several of the symptoms of CFS were common to both.

HUMAN HERPESVIRUS TYPE 6

Brief reference has already been made to the reports of Holmes et al. [53] and Levine et al. [55] concerning the possible role of EBV infection in outbreaks of CFS in the Lake Tahoe region of Nevada and California. In patients in these studies, there was evidence of a polyclonal B-cell hyperreactivity to several viral agents, including human herpesvirus type 6 (HHV-6), a newly recognized lymphotropic and gliotropic virus believed to be the cause of exanthem subitum (roseola infantum). Relatively high serum antibody titers to HHV-6 were found in many patients from the Lake Tahoe outbreak, when compared with controls, but an etiological role for HHV-6 in CFS was not substantiated by those reports [55].

In 1989, Dale and her associates reported that antibodies to HHV-6 were detected more frequently in a group of 16 (69%) patients at NIH with CFS than they were in 14 (12.5%) age- and sex-matched laboratory controls [74]. In 1991, Josephs et al. reported on three of seven of their patients who met the CDC criteria for the diagnosis of CFS and who had positive mononuclear cell cultures for HHV-6 as well as elevated IgG antibody titers to HHV-6 late capsid antigens

[74]. They postulated that their findings represented reactivation of HHV-6 in CFS patients. The patients whose peripheral blood mononuclear cells contained both HHV-6 antigen and DNA were very lethargic and had severe adenopathy and cerebral dysfunction, exemplified by cognitive or memory difficulties. The authors suggested that short-term culture assays may prove to be a reliable test for reactivation of HHV-6 in future outbreaks. Although the results of these four reports [53,55,74,75] were intriguing and suggested HHV-6 may be the cause of a CFS-like illness, they were not conclusive.

The results of a more comprehensive and detailed study of the Lake Tahoe outbreak and its relation to HHV-6 and other agents was reported by Buchwald and her associates in 1992 [76]. These authors studied 259 patients with a viral-like illness of abrupt onset that was followed by months or years of disabling chronic fatigue and impaired cognition that shared many features with "the postinfectious fatigue syndrome, myalgic encephalomyelitis, primary fibro-myalgia, chronic mononucleosis, and the chronic fatigue syndrome."

The outbreak began in 1984 in Incline Village, Nevada, on the north shore of Lake Tahoe, and by 1985 it had assumed epidemic proportions. Formal study of the outbreak began in early 1986, a year after most of the events had unfolded, and the outbreak appeared to end in 1987. One hundred and eighty-three patients were from the Lake Tahoe area; 76 additional patients came from outside this area and were largely from urban areas of California and Nevada. About 50% of patients stated that a close contact was similarly affected. The mean age of patients was about 39 years, and about two-thirds were female.

Criteria for entry into the Buchwald study in 1986 [76] were very similar to, but not identical with, the CDC criteria for the diagnosis of CFS that were not stated until 1988 [9]. Myalgia was noted in 86% of patients, joint pain in 75%, and diarrhea in 38%. Diarrhea is an uncommon symptom in CFS, and some of these patients probably came from a nearby town where there was an outbreak of giardiasis [55]. About 25% of patients were bedridden or unable to carry out light housework or family responsibilities.

Physical examinations and routine laboratory tests were not remarkable in these patients. A few patients developed transient encephalitis, characterized by confusion, ataxia, paresis, and primary seizure disorders. Several other unusual features of the illness were revealed by immunological testing, magnetic resonance imaging (MRI), and virological studies.

Foci of high-signal intensity were seen on T2-weighted MRIs of the brain; typically they were punctate and occasionally consisted of larger patchy areas (Fig. 7). They were seen in 78% of 144 CFS patients, but also in 21% of healthy, matched controls (who were from Wisconsin, not California or Nevada). Such signals are often referred to as unidentified bright objects (UBOs), and they may be confused with the lesions of multiple sclerosis. The subcortical white matter was affected most often, but similar lesions were also seen elsewhere in the

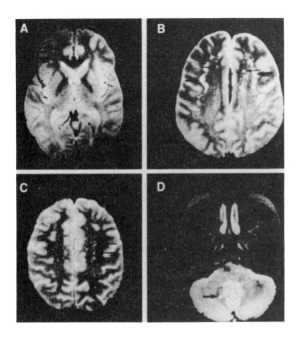

Figure 7   Magnetic resonance images of brain. (A) Transaxial section in a 44-year-old woman with cognitive impairment. Two punctate areas of high-signal intensity (arrows) are seen in the deep, right frontal white matter on a T2-weighted image. These areas probably represent white matter abnormalities. (B) Transaxial section from a 50-year-old woman with disorientation and paresis. Taken at the level of the centrum semiovale, the image shows multiple patchy areas (large arrows) of high-signal intensity in the subcortical white matter (an uncommon finding in this patient group) and smaller punctate lesions (small arrows) in the subcortical and deep white matter (a common finding in these patients). (C) Transaxial section from a 32-year-old woman with cognitive impairment. Taken at the level of high convexity, the image shows multiple punctuate areas of high-signal intensity (arrows) in the subcortical white matter. These findings were most typical of their patient group and may correspond to prominent or enlarged perivascular spaces. (D) Posterior fossa cut from a 34-year-old patient with recurrent ataxia and disorientation. The image shows an isolated high-signal lesion (arrow) in the cerebellar white matter, an unusual location for high signal in their patient group. The patient also had the more typical punctate areas of high-signal intensity in the subcortical white matter (not shown). (From Ref. 76.)

central nervous system. A relation between the site of the lesion and the clinical presentation was observed in nine patients, and serial scans showed that lesions persisted despite resolution of symptoms. Their significance is still uncertain, and great caution should be used in interpreting them.

No significant differences were seen in total T-cell or B-cell numbers in peripheral blood of patients and controls. Studies of lymphocyte phenotypes showed higher CD4/CD8 ratios in patients, both because of higher numbers of CD4-positive cells and also because of lower numbers of CD8-positive cells.

Bioassays for the presence of HHV-6 in peripheral blood mononuclear cells (lymphocytes) were positive in 70% of 113 patients, but in only 20% of 40 controls (a difference that was highly statistically significant). Most of the HHV-6 assays in 27 of the 34 (79%) patients who had serial testing indicated "active replication of HHV-6." A variety of confirmatory assays using either three specific monoclonal antibodies or PCR for HHV-6-specific DNA were done with positive cultures and were in agreement with the bioassay results.

Sixty-eight (81%) of 84 patients who were studied for HHV-6 replication underwent MRI study, and 81% of them had abnormalities, which was similar to the rate that was observed for all patients who had MRI studies (79%). However, patients with MRI abnormalities were *not* more likely to have evidence of actively replicating HHV-6 than those without abnormal MRIs.

When serological test results were analyzed, median optical density values for HHV-6 IgG ELISA antibodies in patients and controls were 1905 and 1288 respectively ($p = 0.08$). Also, 93% of patients were seropositive for EBV infection, but only two patients had serological evidence of acute primary EBV infection. The reciprocal geometric mean titers for patient groups were significantly higher than for control groups for EBV viral capsid IgG antibodies ($p < 0.0001$), but there were no statistically significant differences for VCA IgM, EA, and EBNA antibodies. Relative to human retroviruses studies (to be discussed later), antibodies to human T-cell lymphotropic virus (HTLV)-I and to HIV were not found in sera from any of the patients tested, and 14 culture supernatants tested by two assays were negative for reverse transcriptase activity.

The intriguing MRI abnormalities seen in these patients were nonspecific and are seen in a variety of other diseases [76]. They are also seen in normal persons, in whom they seem to increase with age and with the presence of cerebrovascular risk factors, although spatial distributions may help distinguish them from vascular abnormalities. Viral infections, such as HIV or HTLV-1, can also produce similar MRI changes. Characterization of them in this study was severely compromised by the absence of histopathological studies on brain tissues. The lesions seen in the subcortical white matter correspond anatomically to the cerebrospinal fluid-filled perivascular (Virchow–Robin) spaces. Enlarged Virchow–Robin spaces, such as those seen, may either be a normal variant or represent ischemia or inflammation. Buchwald and her colleagues believed that the weight of evidence suggested that MRI findings in their patients represented a genuine, but as yet undefined, pathological process, and that the value of MRI tests in CFS needs to be assessed and validated in other populations before general adoption as an aid in the diagnosis of CFS. They also believed that the immunological studies (lymphocytic phenotyping) they and others have done on patients with CFS seem to indicate the presence of an immune system that is chronically responding to a perceived antigenic challenge. They believed that both EBV and HHV-6 may have been actively replicating more often in their patients than in control subjects.

The apparent active replication of HHV-6 in their patients was thought to represent reactivation of latent infection, because most persons acquire HHV-6 infection early in life. None of the reports associating HHV-6 with CFS have related the onset of CFS to contact with an infant with roseola infantum, the primary and most easily recognizable clinical manifestation of HHV-6 infection in infants.

Buchwald et al. were of the opinion that the reactivation of HHV-6 in their patients might have been either merely an epiphenomenon, secondary to immune dysfunction or transactivation by another virus, or an unrelated event such as might result from a coincidental outbreak of HHV-6 in the community in the recent past [76]. In favor of HHV-6 being responsible for CFS in their patients is that HHV-6 is tropic for T and B cells, and for glial, neuroblastoma, and intestinal cell lines. They concluded their report by stating that their study did not directly address whether HHV-6 plays a role in producing the symptoms or the immunological and neurological dysfunction seen in their patients, and that whether their findings based on study of a relatively small geographic area will be generalizable to patients elsewhere remains to be seen.

The evidence suggests HHV-6 is one of the infectious agents that can trigger CFS, but it is not the sole cause of the syndrome. These studies are also of interest in that they add further to the evidence of objective abnormalities that are found in patients with CFS.

RETROVIRUSES

Two major groups have been investigated for their possible role in CFS: an HTLV-II-like agent and the spumaviruses. Although patients infected with HIV-1 or HIV-2 (both are retroviruses) may develop an illness (acquired immunodeficiency syndrome; AIDS) that resembles some aspects of a very severe form of CFS, their symptoms can be attributable to either the HIV infection, or to one of the many opportunistic infections to which these patients are highly susceptible. Thus, their fatigue is neither idiopathic nor cryptogenic. It is possible that the fatigue and other symptoms seen in patients with HIV infection or AIDS may be caused by mechanisms similar to those that will ultimately be found important in the pathogenesis of CFS. However, there is *no* reason for patients with so-called idiopathic or cryptogenic CFS (a diagnosis of exclusion) to worry that they will develop AIDS from an as yet undiscovered virus.

On September 4, 1990, DeFreitas and her colleagues reported (at a scientific meeting) their preliminary findings suggesting an HTLV-II-like retrovirus infection might be the cause of CFS in patients and their contacts. Their published report in 1991 [77] using molecular assays to detect specific segments of the retroviral genome suggested there was a human T-lymphotropic virus type 2 (HTLV-II) *gag* gene sequence in lymphocytes from 10 of 12 adults with CFS, from 13 of 18 ill children from an outbreak of CFS, and from 7 of 20 contacts of these patients, but from none of 20 nonexposure controls. Sequences for several other retroviral genetic regions, such as the HTLV-I *gag* gene and the HTLV-II *tax* gene, were not detectable in patients or controls. They also reported detecting antibodies to HTLV-I in 6 of 12 adults and 11 of 18 children with CFS. These data were interpreted as evidence for an HTLV-II-like virus infection in some patients with CFS that might be causative either of CFS or of a benign secondary infection.

Several groups of investigators subsequently attempted to confirm these results without success. Buchwald et al. failed to detect antibodies to either HTLV-I or HIV in a sample of their patients with CFS in the Lake Tahoe cluster [76], and mononuclear cells from 14 of their patients were negative when tested for reverse transcriptase (an enzyme characteristic of retroviruses) activity by two assays. Levy and his associates found similar negative results for a role for retroviruses in their patients from the Lake Tahoe area [78].

Khan and co-workers [79], from the CDC in Atlanta, investigated the prevalence of the HTLV-II gene marker in 21 persons from Atlanta who met published criteria for the diagnosis of CFS [6,7]. Patients were compared with two control groups: one a group of healthy CDC employees matched for age, race, and gender, and the other a matched group of healthy neighborhood controls selected primarily for analysis of risk factors.

Most of their patients had the onset of CFS between 1986 and 1990; their mean age at onset was 33 years, with a range of 16–51 years; and the median interval from onset to study was 4.5 years. Eighteen of the 21 patients were women and all were white, non-Hispanic United States citizens.

Samples from preparations of peripheral blood lymphocytes and leukocytes obtained from all 21 patients and from 21 controls failed to amplify with HTLV-II *gag* gene-specific primers, and thus were judged negative. In addition, serum samples from nine patients and nine controls tested negative for HTLV-I and HTLV-II antibodies by Western blot and synthetic peptide ELISA tests.

Risk factor analyses in patients and matched neighborhood controls showed a few significant differences. Interestingly, patients (most of whom were women) with CFS were less likely to be living with children than were controls; patients also had a smaller mean household size, and despite these facts, women patients were more likely to be multiparous. Patients were also more likely to have a household member or first-degree relative ill with a chronic fatiguing illness, and to have a history of allergies, primarily to respiratory irritants. They were not more likely to have risk factors for retroviral infection (including risky sexual behavior), to have drunk raw milk, or to have a pet with a prolonged or unexplained illness.

Khan et al. [79] speculated that the associations reported by DeFreitas et al. [77] may have resulted from false-positive results produced by inadvertent contamination of specimens or other technical problems, such as low-stringency conditions, nonspecific binding, long exposure times, and insufficient blinding. Khan concluded by stating that retroviral markers should not be used as a diagnostic test for CFS, and also that physicians should not indicate to patients that the evidence convincingly associates CFS with an HLTV-like retrovirus.

Flugel et al. reported their studies attempting to associate a human spuma-retrovirus (HSRV, spumavirus, or human foamy virus), with CFS in 1992 [80]. HSRV has not yet been definitely associated with any human disease, but its genome has some similarities to pathogenic human retroviruses, including oncoviruses and lentiviruses [77]. They evaluated the presence of antibodies to HSRV in 41 fatigued patients, 9 of whom met the CDC case definition of CFS [8], along with 20 matched controls (healthy human blood donors). Sera from patients with CFS were diluted 1:250 before testing. They used an ELISA test specific for the central domain of the HSRV envelope protein. No patient or control subject had serum antibody reactivity to HSRV. They believed the sensitivity of their test was such that their results indicate that a human spumavirus is unlikely to play an important role in CFS.

In 1992, Gow et al. reported similar negative results in their studies concerning the retroviral etiology of CFS [81]. Blood samples from 30 patients and muscle biopsies from 15 patients were examined for retroviral sequences by DNA extraction, PCR, and Southern blotting hybridization. Sera were examined for human foamy virus (spumaretrovirus) by Western immunoblotting and im-munofluorescent techniques. No differences between patient and control populations were found for any of the PCR primer sets used (*gag, pol, env,* and *tax* regions of HTLV-I/II). An endogenous *gag* band was observed in both patient and control groups. All sera were negative for antibody to human foamy virus. Thus, their results provide no evidence for retroviral involvement in CFS.

From the preliminary reports in 1991 [77] suggesting that infection with a human T-lymphotropic virus type 2 (HTLV-II-like) or a spumavirus might be associated with CFS, several research and commercial laboratories developed assays for use in testing patients with CFS for infection with these agents. Consequently, although the association between CFS and these agents had not yet been confirmed, tests for them had begun to be used routinely to evaluate patients in some areas. Gunn and associates conducted a controlled, blinded study in 1992 to determine whether three such tests (PCR assay, PCR modified assay, and culture of cells looking for a foamy cytopathic effect) could distinguish between patients with CFS and healthy controls matched for age, race, sex, and geographic area [82]. Blood samples obtained from 68 CFS patients, from four study populations and from three states, whose illnesses met the CDC definition [7,8], were tested in a blinded fashion in two of the laboratories that had developed retroviral tests for routine use. Previous tests done at these two laboratories had been positive on most of the patients who subsequently participated in this study. The results of this double-blind, controlled study were that *none* of the three assays and *neither* laboratory could differentiate between case patients and controls in either the entire study population or in any of its regional subgroups. In one laboratory, 59% of patients and controls were positive by the original polymerase chain reaction, whereas only 3 and 1%, respectively, were positive subsequently using a modified PCR. In the other laboratory, 46% of patients and 49% of controls were positive on culture for a foamy cell cytopathic effect. Gunn and associates concluded that no scientific basis exists for use of such retroviral tests to confirm the diagnosis of CFS [81]. It was also concluded that, as in the past, diagnostic tests should be performed on CFS patients solely to *exclude* other diagnoses. Taken together, all these results cast serious doubt on an etiological association of retroviruses with CFS.

LYME DISEASE, *Borrelia burgdorferii,* CHRONIC FATIGUE SYNDROME, AND FIBROMYALGIA

Lyme disease is a multisystem inflammatory disease with protean manifestations and is caused by a tick-borne spirochete, *Borrelia burgdorferi* [83]. The illness usually, but not always, begins with a characteristic skin lesion, erythema migrans (which tends to become chronic), which is often followed by spirochetal involvement of the nervous system, heart, and joints, weeks or months later. Serological tests for borrelia infection may be negative in the early weeks of the infection when erythema migrans first calls attention to the diagnosis, and the serological response may, in fact, be completely abrogated by early antimicrobial treatment of erythema migrans. Most untreated patients later develop positive antibody tests. A small percentage of patients remain antibody-negative by the usual tests, but may have positive Western blots or cellular immune responses to borrelia antigens [83]. Diagnostic errors are facilitated because some healthy persons with positive tests have no past history of the disease, and because some ill persons diagnosed with Lyme disease actually have false-positive serological tests, which are common because of the variability and unreliability of the tests in many laboratories [84]. In addition, some tests used to confirm questionable results are expensive or are not readily available; therefore, they are not done. Increasing media coverage has increased awareness and anxiety about this disease on the part of both patients and their physicians.

Because of its chronic course, protean nature, diagnostic vagaries, and, especially, because treatment of Lyme disease is not always curative, it would be surprising if Lyme disease were not considered an antecedent to CFS in some patients. In addition, Montgomery and associates reported [85] that unopsonized *B. burgdorferi* entered macrophages readily and, occasionally, persisted intracellularly in a lysosomal glycoprotein-positive compartment. Although most spirochetes within macrophages were dead, the investigators, nonetheless, were able to culture spirochetes from them. Persistence of spirochetes within macrophages provides a possible mechanism for chronic or recurrent Lyme disease and for CFS secondary to continued cytokine production or other immune responses. Finally, since Lyme disease is often associated with pain in joints, muscles, and tendons, it is not surprising that it might initiate or be confused with the fibromyalgia syndrome.

This discussion on the relation between Lyme disease, CFS, and fibromyalgia will concentrate on reports by Steere [84], Sigal [86], Dinerman [87], and their associates.

Sigal analyzed the first 100 patients referred for suspect Lyme disease to his institution in New Jersey in 1990 [86]. Overall, in only 37 of the 100 patients was Lyme disease actually judged by him to be responsible for their symptoms; and only 8 (13%) of 60 patients with possible late manifestations of the infection were thought to have Lyme disease. Nine of the 37 patients had persistent but nonspecific symptoms following appropriately treated Lyme disease; these included fatigue, malaise, difficulty with concentration or memory, or musculoskeletal complaints. They did not have any evidence of active inflammation or other diseases when seen, and some of them seemed to qualify for the diagnosis of CFS. In three of those nine patients, nonspecific symptoms slowly resolved over a 3- to 7-month period. In contrast to the fact that only 8 of 60 patients with possible late manifestations of Lyme disease actually had that diagnosis, 25 of the 100 patients referred because of suspect Lyme disease had classic fibromyalgia by generally accepted criteria [88], and 17 of the 25 (76%) were thought to have fibromyalgia following and possibly caused by documented Lyme disease. In fact, 17 (46%) of the 37 patients with good evidence of borrelia infection had fibromyalgia. Thus, there appears to be a strong association between Lyme disease and fibromyalgia. Although 9 of their 100 patients possibly had CFS in association with Lyme disease, 25 were thought to have fibromyalgia in association with Lyme disease. Fibromyalgia is now recognized as being closely related in manifestations and pathogenesis to CFS, and some persons believe they are actually two ends of the spectrum of the same disease.

Fibromyalgia (also known as fibrositis, fibromyositis, and psychogenic rheumatism) is a chronic pain syndrome characterized by diffuse muscle and joint pain, headache, paresthesia, sleep disturbance, and marked fatigue (see Chapter 12). Many investigators believe the fatigue is secondary to a nonrestorative sleep disturbance characterized by an alpha EEG nonrapid eye movement anomaly [89,90]. Symmetric tender points are usually found in multiple characteristic locations over the neck, back, and extremities (Fig. 8). Women

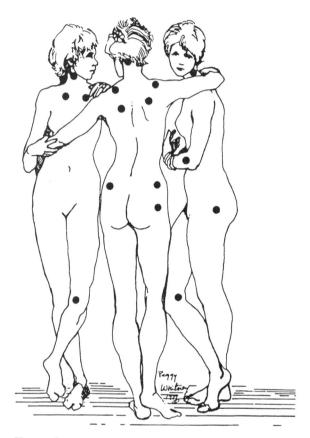

Figure 8 Eighteen tender points required by the 1990 American College of Rheumatology criteria for the classification of fibromyalgia. (From Ref. 88.)

are affected more often than men. The cause of the syndrome is not known, as is true with CFS, and there are no specific histopathological or laboratory abnormalities that confirm the diagnosis. It is nevertheless thought to be a consistent syndrome, and well-defined and tested diagnostic criteria for it have been identified [88,91]. Various infections, thyroid disease, emotional stress, and head trauma have been considered important triggers of the syndrome. Treatment is difficult, but amitriptyline, anaerobic training, and analgesics have been used and are often successful.

Sigal strongly associated fibromyalgia with Lyme disease [86]. 25 of 100 patients referred to his center for suspected Lyme disease had fibromyalgia by generally accepted criteria [88,91]. All 25 had at least 3 months of musculoskeletal complaints and multiple trigger points, but without evidence of synovitis or a systemic disease that would account for their illness (except for 3 patients who also had active Lyme disease). All 25 reported difficulty falling asleep, frequent awakening in the middle of the night (nonrestorative sleep), generalized fatigue, or neck pain. Most patients also complained of headache, which was often their major complaint. Subjective swelling of the extremities, especially the hands, was reported by many patients, but none reported Raynaud's phenomenon or irritable bowel symptoms. None of them had laboratory evidence of an occult inflammatory process.

Of the 25 patients with fibromyalgia in Sigal's report [86], 17 were thought to have it because of B. burgdorferi infection. Nine had developed erythema chronicum migrans an average of about 1 year before onset of their musculoskeletal complaints. Three patients had fibromyalgia associated with active Lyme disease at the time of evaluation. Although 9 of the 25 patients with fibromyalgia had a history of erythema migrans, 17 were IgG-positive but IgM-antibody negative for borrelia infection, and they also had an illness at the onset of fibromyalgia that was compatible with active Lyme disease. Three children with fibromyalgia had the new onset of sleep disturbances during the course of Lyme disease, and in all three the sleep disorder resolved with antibiotic therapy. Sleep disorder has been reported to be a common part of primary Lyme disease in children as well as adults, and may represent a mild, previously unsuspected encephalopathy [92]. Seven of the 25 patients had fibromyalgia unrelated to Lyme disease. All but 1 of the fibromyalgia patients had received antibiotic therapy before referral; most often it had been given to treat Lyme disease or its late complications. There was no clinical response to treatment with antibiotics in any of the fibromyalgia patients. Therapy initiated at the Lyme disease center (antibiotics, amitriptyline, and graded exercise to tolerance) was associated with resolution of fibromyalgia within 4–6 months in most patients.

Fibromyalgia is frequent in a general rheumatological clinic population, and secondary myalgia occurs in 5–10% of rheumatological disorders [93]. In a review by Goldenberg [94], 10% of fibromyalgia patients had a "viral syndrome" just before the onset of their musculoskeletal complaints, which suggested to him that fibromyalgia may be a common reaction to a variety of infectious and noninfectious disorders.

In a study similar to Sigal's [86], Dinermen and Steere [87] evaluated 679 patients at their Lyme disease clinic; 22 of them (8%) met both the CDC case definition for Lyme disease [83] and the 1990 American College of Rheumatology criteria for fibromyalgia [88]. In their patients, fibromyalgia developed either soon after the treatment of early disseminated borrelia infection or along with the onset of Lyme arthritis. For the diagnosis of fibromyalgia, patients were required to have widespread pain in combination with tenderness in 11 or more of 18 specific tender points (see Fig. 8). Fifteen of their 22 patients with both confirmed Lyme disease and fibromyalgia participated in a long-term observational study; 10 were women and 5 were men. The mean age at onset was 41 (range 23 to 60 years). Of the 15 patients, 10 had experienced erythema migrans; the other 5 had fever, headache, myalgias, and arthralgia at the onset. All 15 had signs of dissemination of the borrelia infection to multiple organ systems, including such things as gingivitis, facial palsy, carditis, or attacks of asymmetric oligoarticular arthritis. All but 1 (who had classic erythema migrans) had serological evidence of infection with *B. burgdorferi*. Fourteen of the 15 patients were treated with oral or intravenous antibiotics, and all but 1 had resolution of the signs and symptoms of Lyme disease. Nine patients developed fibromyalgia a mean of 1.7 months (range, 0–5) after antibiotic treatment for early Lyme disease; the other 6 developed symptoms during the course of Lyme arthritis, but before its treatment. None had fibromyalgia before the onset of Lyme disease. Other symptoms in their patients with fibromyalgia were fatigue, headache, memory deficit, dysesthesias, poor concentration, and restless sleep with morning somnolence. Although symptoms waxed and waned, these patients never felt well and continued to have symptoms for a mean of 4 years, and for as long as 10 years, during which their neurological and joint examinations were usually normal.

Only 11 of their 15 patients with confirmed Lyme disease *and* fibromyalgia were initially seropositive for *B. burgdorferi* infection. All 11 still had positive IgG (ELISA) antibody responses, usually in low titer, at the time of the observational study. Three of the four patients with negative antibody tests had received early antibiotic therapy for erythema migrans, but had positive cellular immune responses; the other had a positive Western blot. Three with negative antibody tests had received early antibiotic therapy for erythema migrans, but still had positive cellular immune responses to borrelia antigens. None of the 15 patients had an elevated erythrocyte sedimentation rate. Eleven with neurological symptoms underwent lumbar puncture, electromyography, magnetic resonance imaging of the brain, and neuropsychological testing. Two had evidence of an intrathecal antibody response to the *Borrelia* spirochete; one had an elevated protein level, and one had slight pleocytosis. One 34-year-old woman had areas of increased T2 signal intensity on MRI brain scan. Four of these five patients had evidence of memory impairment or depression; two had both. None had abnormal electrophysiological tests. Except for serological tests, few significant findings were found by tests and procedures.

All but 1 of the 15 patients with Lyme disease and fibromyalgia were retreated with antibiotics, usually ceftriaxone or penicillin, given intravenously for 2–4 weeks. Symptoms worsened during retreatment in 2 patients (without fever, which might be seen with a Jarisch–Herxheimer reaction), but 10 patients had subjective improvement in some of their symptoms that lasted as long as several months, even though tender points persisted. The remaining 4 patients had no improvement with antibiotic therapy. By 6 months after treatment, all 14 patients who had been treated with antibiotics had resumption of signs and symptoms of fibromyalgia.

Only 2 of 11 initially borrelia-seropositive patients showed a significant decline in antibody titers after treatment, and the 3 seronegative patients also developed negative spirochetal cellular immune responses after treatment.

The 14 patients who were still symptomatic despite antibiotic therapy were then treated with various combinations of low-dose amitriptyline, analgesic doses of nonsteroidal anti-inflammatory medications, and an exercise program. This therapy provided improvement of symptoms in only 6 of the 14 patients and only 1 patient was asymptomatic and off therapy a mean of 2.5 years later.

Fibromyalgia was thought to differ from classic Lyme arthritis in these patients because Lyme arthritis is typically associated with asymmetric pain and tenderness in only one or a few joints, and is associated with a greater degree of memory impairment and less anxiety and depression than is fibromyalgia. The authors stressed the difficulty of distinguishing the neuropathy of the two disorders on clinical grounds alone, and that it is usually necessary to demonstrate cerebrospinal fluid or electromyographic abnormalities to make a diagnosis of chronic neuroborreliosis. Signs of central nervous system inflammation are suggestive of active neuroborreliosis, rather than fibromyalgia. In their experience, the symptoms of chronic neuroborreliosis usually do not improve until several months after antibiotic therapy is given, and its worsening is usually associated with worsening cerebrospinal fluid abnormalities.

Dinerman and Steere concluded by noting that the pathogenesis of fibromyalgia is not known; that recent investigations by them and others have concentrated on the theory that, as with CFS, immune abnormalities are involved, and that they result in production or stimulation of cytokines and neuropeptides, which are believed to cause the symptoms [87]. They also noted that fibromyalgia has come to be considered a variant of CFS, which is believed to have a similar pathogenesis. Patients with fibromyalgia, as a group, have more tender points, more morning stiffness, and a more gradual onset than patients with CFS, who also have more fever, fatigue, painful adenopathy, and headache. Patients with depression tend to have more guilt, feelings of worthlessness, and suicidal ideations than those with CFS [95].

Because the combination of adequately treated Lyme disease followed by fibromyalgia is often different from classic CFS, it has been proposed that it should be considered a separate and unique syndrome for research purposes, if for no other [7]. In addition, it seems likely that some patients with both Lyme disease and CFS may not have fibromyalgia if strict diagnostic criteria are employed.

Dinerman and Steele believed *B. burgdorferi* infection can trigger fibromyalgia in a small percentage of patients with Lyme disease (8% in their study), and they also believed such patients should be evaluated for the presence of active spirochetal infection in the central nervous system or elsewhere [87]. If the evidence suggests active infection, they suggested patients should receive oral or intravenous antibiotic therapy for borrelia infection for 10–30 days. They emphasized that most patients referred to their clinic with a diagnosis of "chronic Lyme borreliosis" and in whom they diagnosed fibromyalgia did not meet the CDC clinical or serological criteria for Lyme disease. They also noted that fibromyalgia does not seem to respond well to the antibiotic therapy that is usually effective in Lyme disease. They recommended judicious use of amitriptyline, analgesics, exercise, and reassurance of patients that fibromyalgia is neither a crippling rheumatic disease nor a degenerative neurological disease.

In a more recent paper focused on the notorious frequency of overdiagnosis of Lyme disease, Steere and his associates analyzed the diagnoses, serological tests, and treatment results of 788 patients referred to a Lyme disease clinic in a university hospital [83]. It was found that only 180 (23%) of the 788 patients actually had active Lyme disease. Another 156 patients (20% of the total) had a prior history of Lyme disease, but seemed to have another illness at the time of referral, most commonly CFS or fibromyalgia. In 49 of the 156 patients (or 15% of those with borrelia infection), these symptoms began soon after recognition of the objective manifestations of Lyme disease; thus, CFS seemed to be triggered by Lyme disease in these patients. The remaining 452 patients did not have evidence of borrelia infection, but had positive serological test results in another laboratory that were not confirmed in Steere's laboratory. Finally, 79% of these patients with an incorrect diagnosis had been treated with antibiotics elsewhere without responding. Most of these 452 patients referred with an incorrect diagnosis had either CFS (142; 31%) or fibromyalgia (84; 19% of the total). Thus, Steere's results indicate that both CFS and fibromyalgia are often correctly and incorrectly associated with Lyme disease. In sum, only 49 (about 25%) of 191 of their patients diagnosed with CFS actually developed CFS in association with proved Lyme disease. Although CFS was associated in this report with the onset of Lyme disease, the latter was clearly not implicated in the onset of CFS in most patients with that diagnosis.

It seems likely that Lyme disease is not *the* cause of either fibromyalgia or the chronic fatigue syndrome, but that it can be a trigger for either one of them. Fibromyalgia arguably seems more likely than classic CFS to occur after Lyme disease. Since there is much overlap in the symptoms and other features of fibromyalgia and CFS, they may occur simultaneously in some unfortunate persons. Aggressive antibiotic therapy of fibromyalgia or CFS following Lyme disease is *not* likely to have sustained benefits, and if not, nonantibiotic treatment regimens are preferred (amitryptiline, analgesics, graded exercise, reassurance, and psychotherapy), especially if there are significant emotional problems.

Buchwald and her co-workers determined Epstein–Barr virus antibody profiles in 50 patients with primary fibromyalgia and compared them with the profiles of age- and sex-matched healthy and unhealthy control subjects and found no significant differences between them [96]. Fye and his co-workers reported a similar study that involved 19 patients with the fibrositis (fibromyalgia) syndrome, 21 with CFS, and groups of 20 persons with either osteoarthritis, rheumatoid arthritis, or no disease [97]. They found no relation between EBV and fibromyalgia, and antibody titers to EBV VCA were significantly higher in CFS patients than in patients with fibromyalgia.

Buskila and colleagues investigated a possible relation between HIV infection and fibromyalgia [98], and found that 15 (29%) of 51 patients with HIV met the criteria for fibromyalgia (10 tender of 14 possible "fibrositic" points). About the same frequency of fibromyalgia was found in patients with psoriatic arthritis, but a higher rate (57%) was seen in patients with rheumatoid arthritis. There was no association of fibromyalgia with duration or stage of HIV infection, or with zidovudine therapy. The results suggested to them that a chronic viral infection may cause fibromyalgia, but its low rate in HIV infection suggests HIV may not have been directly causative in their patients. They stressed the importance of diagnosing and treating fibromyalgia in HIV patients, and of reassuring patients about its nature.

Leventhal and associates reported three patients who developed fibromyalgia after episodes of documented acute parvovirus B19 infection, as documented by positive IgM and IgG antibody titers [99]. Two of them had sleep abnormalities, with profound alpha-wave intrusion throughout non–rapid eye movement sleep. All three were women, and two were nurses who may have contracted the infection in the course of their hospital duties. There was no indication in this report, or in others in the literature, that parvovirus infection is followed by CFS in children or adults.

Nash and his colleagues followed an elderly woman with a syndrome mimicking primary fibromyalgia [100], who had evidence of a chronic (persistent) coxsackievirus B2 infection over a 4-year period. Muscle biopsy showed nonspecific abnormalities, and in situ hybridization with coxsackievirus B1–5 RNA probes were negative; she later became seropositive for rheumatoid factor. This patient's illness suggests those enteroviral studies that were used to define a possible etiological relation with CFS might be of interest in patients with fibromyalgia.

Wallace and colleagues evaluated the immunological status of 16 patients with fibrositis and 55 healthy controls [101]. They also determined serum levels of six cytokines. They found that patients with chronic fibrositis did not differ from controls in cytokine levels, IgG subclasses, EBV titers, lymphocyte subsets, mitogen stimulation, or circulating immune complexes.

MISCELLANEOUS INFECTIONS

Poliomyelitis

Poliomyelitis is now rare in developed countries, and there is no evidence in recent times that implicates it in CFS. However, many of the early clusters of epidemic neurasthenia developed during the poliomyelitis season, and the illness was often misdiagnosed as poliomyelitis [21]. It is of interest to consider whether the postpolio syndrome (PPS) might represent CFS occurring in persons who previously suffered from classic poliomyelitis and who later recovered much or most of their muscular function. The answer appears to be negative. An excellent discussion of this syndrome can be found in a recent editorial by Yarnell, from a postpolio clinic in San Francisco [102]. Most of the symptoms of PPS appear to be caused by neural or musculoskeletal wear and tear, and there is no evidence indicating persistence of the virus in the spinal cord or elsewhere in PPS. Electromyographic findings differ from those found in CFS and show evidence of defective neuromuscular transmission in aging reinnervated motor units, with the result that some of the muscle fibers fail to fire and do not contribute to the force of contraction. Recent evidence suggests the defect in some patients may be due to anticholinesterase-responsive defects in neuromuscular junction transmission that may improve with treatment with edrophonium [103]. Thus, PPS does not seem related to CFS.

Chlamydia pneumoniae

Komaroff and colleagues recently published the results of their studies that showed a lack of any association of CFS with a chronic infection caused by *C. pneumoniae*, a recently recognized organism that causes, among other things, acute and chronic infections of the respiratory tracts of children and adults [104].

Viral Hepatitis

It is abundantly clear to physicians caring for patients with chronic active or chronic persistent viral hepatitis B or C that many of them have symptoms similar to those of CFS, and that these symptoms may wax and wane according to the degree of activity of the liver infection, as measured by enzymatic or other liver function tests [Fekety R, unpublished observations]. Studies designed to elucidate the pathogenesis of CFS might be worth performing in these patients, as they could provide a way to test hypotheses concerning the factors and mechanisms responsible for CFS in patients who are definitely ill with a chronic viral infection. Interesting findings could than be looked for in patients with idiopathic or cryptogenic chronic fatigue syndromes. It should be emphasized that there is no evidence that chronic viral hepatitis plays any role in production of the illness in the vast majority of patients with CFS in developed countries. In fact, Dale and her associates specifically examined this issue and found that only 1 of 36 patients with typical CFS had evidence of hepatitis C virus (HCV) infection, as determined by reliable antibody tests of infection [49,105].

Borna Disease Virus

Borna disease virus (BDV) is a poorly characterized, currently unclassified virus that has an affinity for the CNS and especially for the limbic system, an area of the brain where many investigators suspect infectious agents responsible for CFS may lurk or cause damage. Because BDV can cause infection of humans, and may cause chronic progressive diseases of the brain and immune system, Bode and associates looked for serological evidence of BDV infection in 50 adult patients with CFS, using an indirect immunofluorescent test for BDV [106]. No evidence of BDV antibodies were found, and the investigators concluded that BDV is unlikely to be an important etiology of CFS.

Inoue–Melnick Virus

Dale and her associates reported the results of a serological study designed to ascertain whether a prior infection with Inoue–Melnick virus (IMV) was a prominent feature of their patients with CFS [74]. This virus is not well defined, but it resembles the herpesviruses in many ways, including its DNA content, and it has been recovered from patients with subacute myeloopticoneuropathy, a disease with some similarities to CFS. Forty coded serum samples from patients with CFS, adults with various infections caused by herpesviruses, chronic neurological disorders associated with fatigue, and age- and sex-matched healthy controls were studied. Neutralizing antibodies to IMV were sought, as well as antibodies to various herpesviruses. Among patients with CFS, 25% were IMV seropositive, as were 36% of the controls. In contrast, antibodies to HHV-6 were found more often in CFS patients (69%) than in controls (12.5%). Seropositivity to other herpesviruses were detected with equal frequency in patients and controls. Thus, there was no indication IMV was causative of CFS.

Rubella Immunization

In 1988, Allen postulated that immunization of females with the live attenuated rubella virus strain RA27/3, a more potent stain of the virus that was introduced for vaccination in 1979, was responsible for an alleged increase in the frequency of CFS since 1979, or for the elevated antibody levels to various viruses that have been reported in patients with CFS, since the rubella virus is lymphotropic as well as arthrotropic [107]. The Institute of Medicine of the U. S. National Academy of Sciences issued a committee report that examined the relation between vaccination with the RA27/3 strain and chronic arthritis in 1992 [108]. It indicated the evidence is limited in scope, but does not prove a causal relation between this vaccine strain and chronic arthritis in adult women. Arthralgias, carpal tunnel syndrome, and paresthesias have also been reported in these patients. Chronic fatigue syndrome or fibromyalgia has not been common or troublesome in patients with chronic arthritis following rubella vaccination. In addition, CFS in its many guises existed long before rubella vaccine was introduced, and men who have not been vaccinated have developed CFS. There seems to be no reason at present to suspect rubella vaccination is a cause of CFS.

Future "New" Infectious Diseases

It now seems almost inevitable that newly discovered infectious agents will be considered potential causative agents of CFS. This is particularly true when the newly discovered illnesses they cause are protean, frightening, or difficult to diagnose or rule out with certainty on the basis of laboratory tests. This pattern will probably continue in the future. Therefore, one prophecy may be in order.

In 1942, Houghton and Jones reported a small epidemic of what *may* have been the CFS/fibromyalgia syndrome following a putative streptoccocal sore throat [109]. Seven nurses were affected with muscle pains, headache, fever, and other symptoms that became chronic. In their publication, these authors noted a resemblance between their patients' illnesses and those of soldiers with trench fever diagnosed during World War I. Trench fever was eventually found to be caused by an unusual gram-negative bacterium known as *Rochalimaea quintana*. A close relative, *R. henselae*, has recently been found to cause a variety of cutaneous and systemic infectious diseases in healthy as well as im-munocompromised adults, including cat scratch disease, bacteremia, and fever of unknown origin [110]. It would be surprising if investigators did not attempt soon to determine whether patients with CFS have an unusual form of rochalimaeal infection. Fishing expeditions like this in the past have created a lot of interest, especially in the lay press, but few useful approaches to diagnosis and treatment of CFS.

SUMMARY AND CONCLUDING REMARKS

More than ten different infectious agents that have been suspected of playing an etiological role in the pathogenesis of CFS have been reviewed in this chapter. It is apparent that none qualifies as the sole cause of that illness. Nevertheless, it is also clear that several of these agents are strongly implicated in development of the syndrome in a proportion of patients. The list of probably important etiological agents include *Brucella*, enteroviruses (including coxsackieviruses), the Epstein–Barr virus, human herpesvirus-6, and *Borrelia burgdorferi*. Perhaps the influenza virus should also be added to the list. It is likely that other old or newly recognized agents will be added in the future. Hepatitis B and hepatitis C viruses, *Mycobacterium tuberculosis*, and HIV should be added to a separate category of agents that definitely can cause a syndrome resembling CFS. But in the latter situations, CFS is secondary to an infection known to cause symptoms like those of CFS. In contrast, other patients who develop CFS soon after contracting acute infections, such as influenza, brucellosis, or Lyme disease, or other agents causing persistent latent infection (such as EBV and HHV-6) might, for practical reasons, be considered to have *idiopathic or cryptogenic CFS*. This emphasizes the fact that the pathogenesis of their illness is less easily understood than that of patients who have CFS secondary to a chronic active infectious process in which fatigue and other symptoms of CFS are characteristic, expected, understood, and accepted.

If, as seems likely, more than one infectious agent is capable of inducing the syndrome called CFS, then it is necessary to involve, in addition to those infecting agents, one or more cofactors that are also pathogenetically important, presumably along a final common pathway; that is, additional factors that trigger one or more as yet unidentified key processes need to be considered. Some might argue that the putative cofactor is simply a psychiatric illness, such as depression or psychoneurosis, the symptoms of which are magnified by the infection, and then appropriated and used by the patient as an acceptable cause of their symptoms long after the infection has resolved. However, many objective abnormalities characteristic of CFS that are clearly not part of classic psychiatric diseases have been detailed in this and other chapters in this book. They suggest that psychological factors, however important, are not sufficient by themselves to explain the development of CFS.

It is my strong belief that emotional factors and symptoms are inextricably linked to CFS in many, if not most, patients, but that CFS is not simply a psychiatric disorder. Consider that Demitrack and his colleagues [42] have recently reported studies indicating that patients with CFS have a subtle neuroendocrine abnormality, involving the hypothalamic–pituitary–adrenal (HPA) axis, that results in adrenal corticoid hyporesponsiveness, in contrast with the adrenal hyperresponsiveness that is seen in classic depression. Furthermore, Zubieta and colleagues have also reported that rapid eye movement (REM) sleep is normal in their patients with CFS, whereas their depressed patients were very different and showed reduced REM latency and increased REM density and activity [111]. In addition, CFS patients showed a substantial and significant increase in percentage of stage 4 sleep, compared with depressed patients or controls, along with a striking increase in time spent in delta sleep. Their data associate a specific sleep disturbance with CFS, which is in contrast with the findings seen in depressed inpatients or outpatients. The sleep abnormalities in CFS might be explainable by persistent, unretrained immune activation and cytokine release, perhaps secondary to a reduction in the normal counterregulatory restraint of the HPA axis, or possibly by a chronic active infection of the nervous system, particularly in the limbic region.

Currently popular theories attempting to understand the multifactorial causation of CFS usually invoke an unusual reaction to various infectious agents, possibly because of an immune dysfunction that results in chronically or intermittently active disease, along with an exaggerated or prolonged response to it by mononuclear cells. These cellular defenders produce cytokines, such as interleukin-1, tumor necrosis factor, and interferons. Perhaps a novel cytokine or a complex cytokine network that has not yet been discovered or delineated is involved. Cytokines participate in normal host defenses against invading organisms and other inflammatory processes. When produced in response to a variety of infections, cytokines appear responsible for many of the manifestations of infection, such as fever, malaise, fatigue, myalgia, sleep disorders, confusion, delerium, and cognitive defects. Some of these symptoms, such as the desire to rest or sleep and loss of appetite, may be beneficial to the infected host. Appropriately, much scientific effort is now being expended to validate and define the nature and details of the cytokine network in CFS, and in infectious diseases in general.

It is my working hypothesis that CFS is a Pavlovian-conditioned cytokine response to the repetitive simultaneous occurrence of infection and stress, especially of a psychological nature. In time, psychological stress by itself becomes capable of initiating those cytokine responses characteristic of infection. Infectious diseases that are relatively prolonged and that result in the cytokine responses similar to those of CFS would be most likely to be associated with CFS, but other infections occurring at times of emotional stress might also strengthen the conditioned response. This theory is in no way contradictory to, or incompatible with, an important role for various immunological abnormalities, neuroendocrine responses, or novel sleep disorders in the pathogenesis of CFS. Furthermore, persons with mild or atypical depression or psychoneurosis might have the illness accentuated by the effects of the cytokines produced in response to a variety of infectious agents.

Invoking such a conditioned response in CFS has important therapeutic implications. First, reduction in psychologically stressful events would tend to be deconditioning and therapeutically beneficial, as might pharmacological therapy of depression. Second, either prevention of infections or early successful treatment of them would also tend to break the conditioned response. There might be other novel ways to decondition patients. More work in this area is needed.

Although there is a considerable body of circumstantial scientific evidence that could be cited in support of the hypothesis invoking conditioned cytokine responses following "stress" in the pathogenesis of CFS, it is not possible to develop it in detail here. The theory is mentioned in the hope that it will whet the reader's appetite, and also because it provides one mechanism to explain how so many different infections, immunological diseases, inflammatory processes, and psychological factors can be tied together to explain the complex, fascinating, and controversial illness known as chronic fatigue syndrome.

REFERENCES

1. Tumulty PA, Nichols E, Singewald M, Lidz T. An investigation of the effects of recurrent malaria. Medicine 1946; 25:17–75.
2. Frank JD. Emotional reactions of American soldiers to an unfamiliar disease. Am J Psychiatry 1946; 102:631–40.
3. Greenfield NS, Roessler R, Crosby AP. Ego strength and length of recovery from infectious mononucleosis. J Ner Mental Dis 1959; 129:125–8.
4. Graham NMH, Douglas RM, Ryan P. Stress and acute respiratory infection. Am J Epidemol 1986; 124:389–401.
5. Cohen S, Tyrrell DAJ, Smith AP. Psychological stress and susceptibility to the common cold. N Eng J Med 1991; 325:606–12.
6. Holmes GP, Kaplan JE, Gantz NM, et al. Chronic fatigue syndrome: a working case definition. Ann Intern Med 1988; 108:387–9.
7. Schluederberg A, Straus SE, Peterson P, et al. Chronic fatigue syndrome research: definition and medical outcome assessment. Ann Intern Med 1992; 117:325–31.
8. Henderson DA, Shelokov A. Epidemic neuromyasthenia—clinical syndrome? N Engl J Med 1959; 260:757–64; 814–18.
9. Evans AS. Chronic fatigue syndrome: thoughts on pathogenesis. Rev Infect Dis 1991; 13(suppl 1):S56–9.
10. Evans AC. Chronic brucellosis. JAMA 1934; 103:665–7.
11. Spink WW. What is chronic brucellosis? Ann Intern Med 1951; 35:358–74.
12. Apter NS, Halstead WC, Eisele CW, McCullough NB. Impaired cerebral functions in chronic brucellosis. Am J Psychiatry 1948; 105:361–6.
13. Trever RW, Cluff LE, Peeler RN, Bennett IL. Brucellosis. I. Laboratory-acquired acute infection. Arch Intern Med 1959; 103:381–97.
14. Cluff LE, Trever RN, Imboden JB, Canter A. Brucellosis. II. Medical aspects of delayed convalescence. Arch Intern Med 1959; 103:398–405.
15. Imboden JB, Canter A, Cluff LE, Trever RW. Brucellosis. III. Psychological aspects of delayed convalescence. Arch Intern Med 1959; 103:406–14.
16. Imboden JB, Canter A, Cluff LE. Convalescence from influenza. A study of the psychological and clinical determinants. Arch Intern Med 1961; 108:393–99.
17. Cluff LE, Canter A, Imboden JB. Asian influenza. Infection, disease, and psychological factors. Arch Intern Med 1966; 117:159–63.
18. Cluff LE. Medical aspects of delayed convalescence. Rev Infect Dis 1991; 13 (suppl 1):S138–40.
19. Middleton PJ, Alexander RM, Syzmanski MT. Severe myositis during recovery from influenza. Lancet 1970; 2:533–35.
20. Gilliam AG. Epidemiologic study of an epidemic diagnosed as poliomyelitis occurring among the personnel of the Los Angeles County General Hospital during the summer of 1934. Public Health Bulletin, U.S. Treasury Department. No. 240, 1938.
21. Shelokov A, Habel K, Verder E, Welsh W. Epidemic neuromyasthenia. An outbreak of poliomyelitis-like illness in student nurses. N Engl J Med 1957; 257:345–55.
22. Poskanzer DC, Henderson DA, Kunkle EC, Kalter SS, Clement WB, Bond JO. Epidemic neuromyasthenia. An outbreak in Punta Gorda, Florida. N Engl J Med 1957; 257:356–64.

23. Acheson ED. The clinical syndrome variously called benign myalgic encephalomyelitis, Iceland disease and epidemic neuromyasthenia. Am J Med 1959; 26:569–95.

24. Pellew RAA, Miles JAR. Further investigations on a disease resembling poliomyelitis seen in Adelaide. Med J Aus 1955; 2:480–2.

25. Likar M, Dane DS. An illness resembling acute poliomyelitis caused by the virus of Russian spring/summer encephalitis louping ill group in Northern Ireland. Lancet 1958; 1:456.

26. Behan PO, Behan WMH, Bell EJ. The postviral fatigue syndrome—an analysis of the findings in 50 cases. J Infect 1985; 10:211–22.

27. Fegan KG, Behan PO, Bell EJ. Myalgic encephalomyelitis: report of an epidemic. J R Coll Gen Pract 1983; 33:335–37.

28. Medical Staff of the Royal Free Hospital. An outbreak of encephalomyelitis in the Royal Free Hospital Group, London, in 1955. Br Med J 1957; 2:895–904.

29. Jamal GA, Jausen S. Electrophysiologic studies in the postviral fatigue syndrome. J Neurol Neurosurg Pschiatry 1985; 48:691–94.

30. Arnold DL, Bore PJ, Radda GK, Styles P, Taylor DJ. Excessive intracellular acidosis of skeletal muscle on exercise in a patient with a post-viral exhaustion fatigue syndrome. Lancet 1984; 1:1367–9.

31. Calder BD, Warnock PJ. Coxsackie B infection in a Scottish general practice. J R Coll Gen Pract 1984; 34:15–9.

32. Yousef GE, Bell EJ, Mann GF, Murugesan V, Smith DG, McCarney RA, Mowbray JF. Chronic enterovirus infection in patients with postviral fatigue syndrome. Lancet 1988; 1:146–50.

33. Bowles NE, Richardson PJ, Olsen EGJ, Archard LC. Detection of Coxsackie-B-virus-specific RNA sequences in myocardial biopsy samples from patients with myocarditis and dilated cardiomyopathy. Lancet 1986; 1:1120–23.

34. Bowles NE, Dubowitz V, Sewry CA, Archard LC. Dermatomyositis, polymyositis, and Coxsackie-B-virus infections. Lancet 1987; 1:1104–07.

35. Archard LC, Bowles NE, Behan PO, Bell EJ, Doyle D. Postviral fatigue syndrome: persistence of enterovirus RNA in muscle and elevated creatine kinase. J R Soc Med 1988; 81:326–29.

36. Gow JW, Behan WMH, Clements GB, Woodall C, Riding M, Behan PO. Enteroviral RNA sequences detected by polymerase chain reaction in muscle of patients with postviral fatigue syndrome. Br Med J 1991; 302:692–96.

37. Gow JW, Behan WMH. Amplification and identification of enteroviral sequences in the postviral fatigue syndrome. Br Med Bull 1991; 47:872–85.

38. Behan WMH, More IAR, Behan PO. Mitochondrial abnormalities in the postviral fatigue syndrome. Acta Neuropathol 1991; 83:61–5.

39. Oldstone MBA. Viruses can cause disease in the absence of morphological evidence of cell injury: implications for uncovering new disease in the future. J Infect Dis 1989; 159:384–9.

40. Cunningham L, Bowles NE, Lane RJM, Dubowitz V, Archard LC. Persistence of enteroviral RNA in chronic fatigue syndrome is associated with the abnormal production of equal amounts of positive and negative strands of enteroviral RNA. J Gen Virol 1990; 71:1399–402.

41. Wilfert CM, Buckley RH, Mohana Rumar T, et al. Persistent and fatal central

nervous system ECHOvirus infections in patients with agammaglobulinemia. N Engl J Med 1977; 296:1485–9.

42. Demitrack MA, Dale JK, Straus SE, Laue L, Listwak SJ, Krusei MJP, Chrousos GP, Gold PW. Evidence for impaired activation of the hypothalamic–pituitary–adrenal axis in patients with chronic fatigue syndrome. J Clin Endocrinol Metab 1991; 73:1224–34.

43. Halpin D, Wessely S. VP-1 antigen in chronic postviral fatigue syndrome. Lancet 1989; 1:1028–29.

44. Miller NA, Carmichael HA, Calder BD, Behan PO, Bell EJ, McCartney RA, Hall FC. Antibody to Coxsackie B virus in diagnosing postviral fatigue syndrome. Br Med J 1991; 302:140–3.

45. Henle W, Henle G, Horwitz CA. Epstein–Barr virus specific diagnostic tests in infectious mononucleosis. Hum Pathol 1974; 5:551–65.

46. Tobi M, Morag A, Ravid Z, Chowers I, Feldman-Weiss I, Michaeli Y, Ben-Chetrit E, Shalit M, Knobler H. Prolonged atypical illness associated with serological evidence of persistent Epstein–Barr virus infection. Lancet 1982; 1:61–4.

47. Hamblin TJ, Hussain J, Akbar AN, Tang YC, Smith JL, Jones DB. Immunological reason for ill health after infectious mononucleosis. Br Med J 1983; 287:85–8.

48. Jones JF, Ray CG, Minnich LL, Hicks MJ, Kibler R, Lucas DO. Evidence for active Epstein–Barr virus infection in patients with persistent unexplained illnesses: elevated anti-early antigen antibodies. Ann Intern Med 1985; 102:1–7.

49. Straus SE, Tosato G, Armstrong G, Lawley T, Preble OT, Henle W, Davey R, Pearson G, Epstein J, Brus I, Blaese MR. Persisting illness and fatigue in adults with evidence of Epstein–Barr virus infection. Ann Intern Med 1985; 102:7–16.

50. Brewster FE, Sullivan JL. Epstein–Barr virus-infected B lymphoblastoid cell lines: dynamics of interferon and 2′,5′ oligoadenylate synthetase activity. Antiviral Res 1983, 3:195–209.

51. Tosato G, Straus S, Henle W, Pike SE, Blease M. Characteristic T cell dysfunction in patients with chronic active Epstein–Barr virus infection (chronic infectious mononucleosis). J Immunol 1985; 134:3082–88.

52. Buchwald D, Sullivan JL, Komaroff AL. Frequency of "chronic active Epstein–Barr" virus infection in a general medical practice. JAMA 1987; 257:2303–7.

53. Holmes GP, Kaplan JE, Stewart JA, Hunt B, Pinsky PF, Schonberger LB. A cluster of patients with a chronic mononucleosis-like syndrome. JAMA 1987; 257:2297–302.

54. Schooley RT, Carey RW, Miller G, Henle W, Eastman R, Mark EJ, Kenyon K, Wheeler EO, Rubin RH. Chronic Epstein–Barr virus infection associated with fever and interstitial pneumonitis: clinical and serologic features and response to antiviral chemotherapy. Ann Intern Med 1986; 104:636–43.

55. Levine PH, Jacobson S, Pocinki AG, Cheney P, Peterson D, Connelly RR, Weil R, Robinson SM, Ablashi DV, Salahuddin SZ, Pearson GR, Hoover R. Viral, epidemiologic and virologic studies in four clusters of the chronic fatigue syndrome. Arch Intern Med 1992; 152:1611–6.

56. Jones JF, Williams M, Schooley RT, Robinson C, Glaser R. Antibodies to Epstein–Barr virus-specific DNase and DNA polymerase in the chronic fatigue syndrome. Arch Intern Med 1988; 148:1957–60.

57. Gold D, Bowden R, Sixbey J, Riggs R, Katon WJ, Ashley R, Obrigewitch RM, Corey L. Chronic fatigue: a prospective clinical and virologic study. JAMA 1990; 264:48–53.

58. Klimas NG, Salvato F, Morgan R, Fletcher MA. Immunologic abnormalities in chronic fatigue syndrome. J Clin Microbiol 1990; 28:1403–10.

59. Cheney PR, Dorman SE. Interleukin-2 and the chronic fatigue syndrome. Ann Intern Med 1989; 110:321.

60. Straus SE, Dale JK, Peter JB, Dinarello CA. Circulating lymphokine levels in the chronic fatigue syndrome. J Infect Dis 1989; 160:1085–6.

61. Linde A, Andersson B, Svenson SB, Ahrne H, Carlsson M, Forsberg P, Hugo H, Karstarp A, Lenkei R, Lundwall A, Loftenius A, Sall C, Andersson J. Serum levels of lymphokines and soluble receptors in primary Epstein–Barr virus infection and in patients with chronic fatigue syndrome. J Infect Dis 1992; 165:994–1000.

62. Horwitz CA, Henle W, Henle G, Rudnick H, Latts E. Long-term serological follow-up of patients for Epstein–Barr virus after recovery from infectious mononucleosis. J Infect Dis 1985; 151:1150–3.

63. Sumaya CV. Serologic and virologic epidemiology of Epstein–Barr virus. Relevance to chronic fatigue syndrome. Rev Infect Dis 1991; 13(suppl 1):S19–25.

64. Straus SE, Dale JK, Tobi M, Lawley T, Preble O, Blaese MR, Hallahan C, Henle W. Acyclovir treatment of the chronic fatigue syndrome: lack of efficacy in a placebo-controlled trial. N Engl J Med 1988; 319:1692–8.

65. Andersson J, Britton S, Ernberg I, Andersson U, Henle W, Skoldenberg B, Tissel A. Effect of acyclovir on infectious mononucleosis: a double-blind, placebo-controlled study. J Infect Dis 1986; 153:283–90.

66. Truss CO. Tissue injury induced by *Candida albicans*: mental and neurological manifestations. Orthomol Psychiatry 1978; 7:17–37.

67. Truss CO. The role of *Candida albicans* in human illness. Orthomol Psychiatry 1981; 10:228–38.

68. Truss CO. The Missing Diagnosis. Birmingham: CO Truss, 1983.

69. Crook WG. *The Yeast Connection*. Jackson, TN: Professional Books, 1983.

70. Blonz ER. Is there an epidemic of chronic candidiasis in our midst? JAMA 1956; 256:3138–9.

71. Renfro L, Feder HM, Lane TJ, Manu P, Matthews DA. Yeast connection among 100 patients with chronic fatigue. Am J Med 1989; 86:165–8.

72. Dismukes WE, Wade JS, Lee JY, Dockery BK Hain JD. A randomized, double-blind trial of nystatin therapy of the candidiasis hypersensitivity syndrome. N Engl J Med 1990; 323:1717–23.

73. Crook WG, Truss CO, Truss CV, Cutter RB, Llabre MM, Ledger WJ, Witkin SS, Campbell M, Dismukes WE, Lee JY. A controlled trial of nystatin for the candidiasis hypersensitivity syndrome [letters to the editor and authors' reply]. N Engl J Med 1991; 324:1592–94.

74. Dale JK, Straus SE, Ablashi DV, Salahuddin ZS, Gallo RC, Nishibi Y, Inoue YK. The Inoue–Melnicke virus, human herpesvirus type 6, and the chronic fatigue syndrome. Ann Intern Med 1989; 110:92–3.

75. Josephs SF, Henry B, Balachandran N, Strayer D, Peterson D, Komaroff AL, Ablashi DV. HHV-6 reactivation in chronic fatigue syndrome. Lancet 1991; 337:1346–7.

76. Buchwald D, Cheney PR, Peterson DL, Henry B, Wormsley SB, Geiger A, Ablashi DV, Salahuddin SZ, Saxinger C, Biddle R, Kikinis R, Jolesz FA, Folks T, Balachandran N, Peter JB, Gallo RC, Komaroff T. A chronic illness characterized by fatigue, neurologic and immunologic disorders, and active human herpesvirus type 6 infection. Ann Intern Med 1992; 116:103–13.

77. DeFreitas E, Hilliard B, Cheney PR, Bell DS, Kiggundn E, Sankey D, Wroblewska Z, Palladino M, Woodward JP, Koprowski H. Retroviral sequence related to human T-lymphotropic virus type II in patients with chronic fatigue immunodysfunction syndrome. Proc Natl Acad Sci USA 1991; 88:2922–6.

78. Levy JA, Ferro F, Greenspan D, Lennette ET. Frequent isolation of HHV-6 from saliva and high seroprevalence of the virus in the population. Lancet 1990; 335:1047–50.

79. Khan AS, Heneine WM, Chapman LE, Gray HE, Woods TC, Folks TM, Schomberger LB. Assessment of a retroviral sequence and other possible risk factors for a chronic fatigue syndrome in adults. Ann Intern Med 1993; 188:241–5.

80. Flugel RM, Mahnke C, Geiger A, Komoroff AL. Absence of antibody to human spumaretrovirus in patients with chronic fatigue syndrome. Clin Infect Dis 1992; 14:623–4.

81. Gow J, Simpson K, Schliephake A, Behan WM, Morrison LJ, Cavanaugh H, Rethwilm A, Behan PO. Search for retrovirus in the chronic fatigue syndrome. J Clin Pathol 1992; 45:1056–61.

82. Centers for Disease Control. Inability of retroviral tests to identify persons with chronic fatigue syndrome. MMWR 1993; 42:183–90.

83. Centers for Disease Control. Lyme disease surveillance: United States. MMWR 1991; 40:417–20.

84. Steere AC, Taylor E, McHugh GL, Logigian EL. The overdiagnosis of Lyme disease. JAMA 1993; 269:1812–16.

85. Montgomery RR, Nathanson MH, Malawista SE. The fate of *Borrelia burgdorferi*, the agent for Lyme disease, in mouse macrophages. Destruction, survival, recovery. J Immunol 1993; 15:909–15.

86. Sigal LR. Summary of the first 100 patients seen at a Lyme disease referral center. Am J Med 1990; 88:577–81.

87. Dinerman H, Steere AC. Lyme disease associated with fibromyalgia. Ann Intern Med 1992; 117:281–5.

88. Wolfe F, Smythe HA, Yunus MB, et al. The American College of Rheumatology 1990 criteria for the classification of fibromyalgia: report of the multicenter criteria committee. Arthritis Rheum 1990; 33:160–72.

89. Modolfsky H, Saskin P, Lue FP. Sleep and symptoms in fibrositis syndrome after a febrile illness. J Rheumatol 1988; 15:1701–4.

90. Moldofsky H. Nonrestorative sleep and symptoms after a febrile illness in patients fibrositis and chronic fatigue syndrome. J Rheumatol 1989; 16 (suppl 19):150–3.

91. Wolfe F, Hawley DJ, Cathey MA, Caro X, Russell IJ. Fibrositis: symptom frequency and criteria for diagnosis: an evaluation of 291 rheumatic disease patients and 58 normal individuals. J Rheumatol 1985; 12:1159–63.

92. Belman AL, Romero J, Volkman D, Dattwyler R. Neurologic manifestations of Lyme disease in children. Pediatr Res 1989; 25:353A.

93. Goldenberg DL. Fibromyalgia: an emerging but controversial condition. JAMA 1987; 257:2782–7.

94. Goldenberg DC. Fibromyalgia and other chronic fatigue syndromes: is there evidence for chronic viral disease? Semin Arthritis Rheum 1988; 18:111–20.

95. Calabrese L, Danao T, Camara E, Wilke W. Chronic fatigue syndrome. Am Fam Physician 1992; 45:1205–13.

96. Buchwald D, Goldenberg DL, Sullivan JL, Komaroff A. The "chronic active Epstein–Barr virus infection" syndrome and primary fibromyalgia. Arthritis Rheum 1987; 30:1132–6.

97. Fye KH, Whiting-O'Keefe QE, Lennette ET, Jessop C. Absence of abnormal Epstein–Barr virus serologic findings in patients with fibrositis. Arthritis Rheum 1988; 31:1455–6.

98. Buskila D, Gladman DD, Langevitz P, Urovitz S, Smythe HA. Fibromyalgia in human immunodeficiency virus infections. J Rheumatol 1990; 17:1202–6.

99. Leventhal LJ, Naides SJ, Freundlich B. Fibromyalgia and parvovirus infection Arthritis Rheum 1991; 34:1319–24.

100. Nash P, Chard M, Hazleman B. Chronic Coxsackie B infection mimicking primary fibromyalgia. J Rheumatol 1989; 16:1506–8.

101. Wallace DJ, Bowman RL, Wormsley SB, Peter JB. Cytokines and immune regulation in patients with fibrositis. Arthritis Rheum 1989; 32:1334–5.

102. Yarnell SK. Poliomyelitis: the battle continues. JAMA 1989; 261:3294–5.

103. Trojan DA, Gendron D, Cashman NR. Anticholinesterase-responsive neuromuscular transmission defects in post-poliomyelitis fatigue. J Neurol Sci 1993; 114:170–77.

104. Komaroff AL, Wang SP, Lee J, Grayston JT. No association of chronic *Chlamydia pneumoniae* infection with the chronic fatigue syndrome. J Infect Dis 1992; 165:184.

105. Dale JK, DiBisceglie, Joofnagle JH, Straus SE. Chronic fatigue syndrome: lack of association with hepatitis C infection. J Med Virol 1991; 34:119–21.

106. Bode L, Komaroff AL, Ludwig H. No serologic evidence of Borna disease virus in patients with chronic fatigue syndrome. Clin Infect Dis 1992; 15:1049.

107. Allen AD. Is RA27/3 rubella immunization a cause of chronic fatigue? Med Hypotheses 1988; 27:217–20.

108. Howson CP, Katz M, Johnston RB, Fineberg HV. Chronic arthritis after rubella vaccination. Clin Infect Dis 1992; 15:307–12.

109. Houghton LE, Jones EI. Persistent myalgia following sore throat. Lancet 1942; 1:196–8.

110. Dolan MJ, Wong MT, Regnery RL, Jorgensen JH, Garcia M, Peters J, Drehner D. Syndrome of *Rochalimaea henselae* adenitis suggesting cat scratch disease. Ann Intern Med 1993; 118:331–6.
111. Zubieta JK, Demitrack MA, Shipley JE, Engleberg NC, Eiser A, Douglass A. Sleep EEG in chronic fatigue syndrome: comparison with major depression. Biol Psychiatry 1993; 33:74A (abst. 136).

6

Human Herpesviruses and Chronic Fatigue Syndrome

John Hay
*School of Medicine, State University of New York at Buffalo,
Buffalo, New York*

Frank J. Jenkins
*Uniformed Services University of the Health Sciences,
Bethesda, Maryland*

Not to put too fine a point on it, chronic fatigue syndrome (CFS) is a confusing entity both clinically and biologically. It is still unclear exactly what constitutes the illness, or whether it is a group of related processes, despite the detailed case definition generated by the Centers for Disease Control (CDC) [1]. Obviously, if the clinical picture is still rather vague, this uncertainty is passed on to attempts to define the cause or causes of the syndrome. This is one reason why a variety of potential pathogenetic pathways to CFS have been put forward, many of which presume a viral component.

An underlying theme in many proposed mechanisms for CFS is the interplay between the immune system and a virus (or viruses), in which one feeds on the other in a cyclic fashion, leading to an altered state of equilibrium in which the patient has to deal with both the effects of an altered immune system and the problems of viral infection. Another reason to propose a role for viruses is that a feature of the very early stages of the clinical course of the syndrome is an acute flulike illness, reminiscent of viral infection.

Although a variety of viruses have been linked with CFS, those already known to interact with the immune system directly have often been favored candidates, since they might reasonably fit into a hypothetical pathogenesis scheme along the lines of that just outlined. Among these viruses are the human herpesviruses, particularly Epstein–Barr virus (EBV) and human herpesvirus-6 (HHV-6), which infect B and T lymphocytes. These viruses are also considered as attractive candidates for involvement in CFS, in that they are responsible for disease symptoms similar to those seen in CFS, including fever, malaise, lymphadenopathy, and central nervous system (CNS) involvement, as well as having the ability to cause recurring or chronic disease with several CFS-like features. However, if we are to consider the human herpesviruses as possible "CFS viruses," we also need to remember that these infectious agents are ubiquitous and are harbored in a latent or persistent state by virtually the entire population. These facts require that any scheme for the development of CFS caused by EBV or HHV-6 must accommodate factors or cofactors that set the CFS patient aside from the rest of the (normal) infected population.

EPSTEIN–BARR VIRUS

Primary infection with EBV can be symptomatic (e.g., infectious mononucleosis), but is generally clinically inapparent. Following primary infection, which usually takes place early in life, the virus persists, presumably for the remainder of the individual's life, in a latent state for which the features are just now beginning to be fully delineated. Reactivation of EBV from latency occurs frequently, leading to shedding of virus in saliva, increases in early antigen-specific antibodies, and, in the compromised host, clinical symptoms. It is unclear which factors are responsible for this reactivation, but it is known that immunodeficiency or immunosuppressive drug treatments will facilitate virus recrudescence [2]. Clinical features of EBV infection include infectious mononucleosis, which can be fatal in immunosuppressed individuals [3], and chronic active EBV infection, which can present with features of CFS, but is distinguished by clinically apparent immunological, hematological, neurological, and pulmonary problems, among others. Other EBV-associated illnesses include aplastic anemia and a variety of tumors, including Burkitt's lymphoma, nasopharyngeal carcinoma, and various B-cell and rare T-cell lymphomas.

The human herpesviruses are capable of interaction with human cells to produce lytic infection or latent infection. In lytic infection, the virus proceeds through its entire replicative cycle, and progeny virus particles are produced. In contrast, only part of the viral genome is expressed during latent infection, and no progeny virus particles are made; the latent state may be maintained for the life of the host cell.

The molecular events that characterize EBV lytic infection are known in some detail and appear, in general terms, to follow the pattern worked out for other herpesviruses [4], with a well-ordered temporal and sequential expression of genes. The first set of genes code for immediate early proteins, including the Epstein–Barr nuclear antigen (EBNA) proteins, latent membrane proteins (LMPs), and Z and R proteins, which seem to have roles in controlling viral (and cellular) gene expression, largely through regulation of transcription. The next set of proteins is expressed from early genes and includes some additional regulatory polypeptides, as well as the machinery required to allow viral DNA synthesis to occur; this includes a DNA polymerase activity and a deoxyribonuclease activity (DNase). Evidence for synthesis of these early enzymes in the infected host has been taken as a sign of active (lytic) replication of EBV (as opposed to latent infection), since these are nonstructural antigens that would not be expected to be seen unless EBV was actively growing [5]. The third, or late, set of EBV proteins expressed contains many of the structural proteins of the virus and includes several glycoproteins that are targets for neutralizing antibodies and cytotoxic T-cell responses.

The usual outcome of infection of B lymphocytes with EBV, however, is persistent latent infection and transformation of cells. Transformation frequently confers "immortality" on cells and is often a step on the pathway to tumor development. These events are controlled by both cellular and viral factors, although the processes remain to be completely understood. At least nine EBV genes seem to be important for latency or transformation; these include the EBNAs, EBNA leader protein (EBNA-LP), the LMPs, and the Epstein–Barr encoded RNAs (EBERs) [4].

If EBV is a factor in CFS, we will need to understand its latency or transforming properties as well as the lytic virus cycle to assess its potential importance in pathogenesis. In the context of potential viral involvement in CFS, EBV is arguably the most closely studied of all the candidate viruses. The reasons for this include that EBV is responsible for a chronic mononucleosis syndrome that has some features in common with CFS. Indeed, a report in 1948 (before EBV per se had been recognized) describes such a chronic postinfectious mononucleosis syndrome [6]. The early studies describing a relation between EBV and CFS relied on serological assays and were based on the assessments known to be diagnostic for infectious mononucleosis. Acute infection with EBV can be diagnosed immunologically through measurements of the levels of IgM and IgG antibodies to the viral capsid antigen (VCA), of antibodies to early antigen (EA), and to nuclear antigen (EBNA). Individuals who have recovered from EBV infection have IgG VCA and anti-EBNA antibodies, whereas those suffering from chronic infectious mononucleosis have persisting anti-EA antibodies as well as high titers of IgG VCA [7]. The earliest investigations on CFS raised the possibility that it might represent a chronic or reactivated form of infection with EBV. In 1982, elevated levels of antibody to EBV EA in the absence of the usually detected antibodies to EBNA were reported in a study of two family members with chronic fatigue [8]. A report from Israel in the same year [9] described seven patients with fatigue and many of the other clinical signs now identified with the syndrome. All showed what were then considered to be abnormal EBV serological responses, with sustained IgM and high IgG titers to VCA, high titers to the D (diffuse) component of EA, and a high EBNA titer at the start of the study. These profiles were taken by the authors to suggest reactivated EBV infection; however, no controls were included in the study.

High titers of antibodies to EBV proteins were also reported by DuBois et al. [10], but in sharp contrast to the earlier data, VCA IgM could not be detected. Nevertheless, there were elevations in titer to VCA IgG and Ea, compared with a control population, although it was not clear how well this had been matched with the patient cohort. The authors pointed out that similar findings could be seen in other disorders, such as some malignancies, autoimmune disease, immunosuppression, and such. Jones et al. reported on an even larger cohort of chronically fatigued adults and children, in an age-matched, controlled study, and found serological differences in the patient group analogous to those described by DuBois [10], including a failure to find evidence for elevated VCA IgM [11]. Although suggestions were made by the authors that the serological findings might be consistent with active EBV replication, no actual studies of EBV shedding rates were carried out. When this was done in a more broadly based study by Straus and colleagues [12], no significant differences could be discerned between the CFS and control populations in terms of infectious EBV present in throat washes or in EBV-transformed lymphocytes in the blood (Tables 1 and 2). However, higher than expected levels of VCA IgG and anti-EA, absent VCA IgM, and the occasional absence of anti-EBNA were seen in this controlled study, much as before. This group also reported a variety of immunological disturbances in some patients, including high circulating immune complexes, evidence for interferon (IFN)-induction enzymes, and increased T-suppressor cell activity. They concluded that, at this stage of analysis, it could not be said that EBV caused CFS or was necessarily involved in it.

Similar reservations were expressed by Niederman [13], who pointed out that although rises in antiviral antibody titers, for example to EA, are reasonable prognosticators for relapse in nasopharyngeal carcinoma (NPC) or Burkitt's lymphoma (BL) (and, therefore, might be relevant to a possible EBV "relapse" leading to CFS), elevated anti-EA titers are seen in healthy normal persons and in some immunosuppressed individuals. Indeed, Horwitz et al. noted that EBV

Table 1 Prevalence of Infectious (Transforming) EBV in Throat Washings

Group	No. +ve/ No. tested	%
Acute infectious mononucleosis	14/20	70[a]
Healthy adult	4/16	25[a]
Immunosuppressed/deficient	61/92	66[a]
CFS-like	5/29	17[a]
CFS	7/21	33[b]

[a]Data from Ref. 17.
[b]Data from Ref. 11.

Table 2 Semiquantitative Values of EBV-Infected Cells in the Peripheral Blood

Group	No. tested	Value
Acute infectious mononucleosis	19	2.4 ± 5.2[a]
Healthy adult	17	< 0.05[a]
Immunosuppressed/deficient	85	1.06 ± 3.7[a]
CFS-like	31	< 0.05[a]
Healthy adult		3.9 ± 1.5[b]
CFS		2.3 ± 1.3[b]

[a]Data from Ref. 17, expressed as number of EBV-infected cells/10^5 cells.
[b]Data from Ref. 11, expressed as number of EBV infected cells/10^6 lymphocytes; $p > 0.20$ (two-tailed test) for these two values.

serological findings analogous to those seen in CFS patients (e.g., persistence of anti-EA antibodies) could also be seen in healthy control patients for up to 4 years after infectious mononucleosis [14].

Buchwald and colleagues assessed CFS patients and matched controls and found no statistically different EBV titers in the two groups [15]. Hellinger et al., in 1988, compared fatigued patients with high and absent levels of anti-EA antibodies and showed that there was no difference in the disease outcome between the two groups [16]; they also demonstrated that a significant number of blood donors had elevated EBV EA antibodies, yet were clinically normal (Table 3). In a prospective study in 1990, Gold et al. followed CFS patients every 3 months for about a year while examining a wide range of clinical and laboratory variables [17]. Interestingly, approximately half of the patient group improved substantially in terms of their symptoms during the study period. Titers to VCA and EA were elevated at the start of the study, but were not significantly altered during the course of follow-up, and were not correlated with recovery.

Table 3 Results of Testing for Antibody to EBV Early Antigen

Anti-EA titer	Asymptomatic blood donors[a]	CFS patients[a]
<10	161	317[b]
>10 and <160	33	406
>160	3	46[c]

[a]These numbers represent the number of patients in each group having the listed anti-EA titer. The difference between these two populations is statistically significant at $p < 0.05$. However symptom comparisons between the [b] and [c] groups showed no significant differences.
Source: Data from Ref 15.

Similarly, there was no link between symptoms and evidence (both by viral growth and DNA hybridization assays) for EBV reactivation. It could be argued that this study dealt with an unusual CFS population, since so many patients recovered in a relatively short time.

Clearly, one of the problems with the experimental approaches outlined above is that patient cohorts have tended to be heterogeneous among studies. In addition, serological testing has been problematic because of the variability between laboratories in types of EBV-specific tests used and in assay variability in responses of control populations [18]. One specific difficulty with EBV serological testing has been the relative crudity of the antigens used, and there are good reasons to consider using more-defined proteins in assays. Examples of tests that have been employed are ratios of EBNA-1 to EBNA-2, which have been reported to be lower in CFS [19], and the absence of antibodies to K antigen [20]. More strikingly, however, at least two groups have reported that antibodies against two EBV enzymes, DNA polymerase and DNase, are present in CFS patients [21,22]. Such antibodies do suggest active virus replication, although tests for actual virus shedding in patients have not been particularly informative. Jones, in a review of this issue published in 1991, reflected on several different studies and concluded that, in general, patients with CFS, as well as those with severe disease caused by EBV, had higher titers to EBV antigens than healthy controls [23]. Again, however, he cautioned that this did not prove a causal relation between the virus and the syndrome. A more recent study from Jones and his colleagues took a more refined approach to seeking evidence for EBV in CFS patients, being carefully codified, with both open and case-controlled parameters [22]. His basic hypothesis assumed that, if EBV were involved in CFS, then patients should show patterns of behavior similar to those seen in individuals with known active EBV infection (e.g., infectious mononucleosis). Three hypotheses were tested: that peripheral blood lymphocytes from CFS patients will undergo spontaneous transformation more frequently than those from healthy individuals; that antibody responses to EBV in CFS resemble those in proved EBV disease; and that CFS-associated strains of EBV will differ from those of asymptomatic controls. The first two hypotheses were supported by the experimental data, suggesting that reactivation of lytic EBV infection may have occurred in these patients. It should be recalled, however, that in the study by Straus et al. mentioned earlier [12], there was no sign of an increase in transformed lymphocytes in CFS patients, as opposed to controls.

Finally, if a herpesvirus is involved in the ongoing disease process in CFS, treatment with an antiherpesvirus agent should have some effect on the syndrome. However, work from the Straus group [24] indicates that acyclovir treatment is not effective in CFS and that, although there are changes in viral serological markers brought about by the treatment, there is no correlation with clinical improvement.

It is difficult to reconcile all of the available information on the possible role of EBV in CFS into a discrete hypothesis, but some aspects now appear more clear. An excess of CFS patients do have abnormal EBV diagnostic signs, reminiscent of an active EBV infection. The relevance of this to CFS is uncertain because only some patients have these EBV markers, thus EBV cannot be the answer to CFS, and there must be other routes to the syndrome; alternatively, EBV activity cycles unpredictably throughout the disease. The former possibility seems the more likely.

HUMAN HERPESVIRUS-6

Human herpesvirus-6 (HHV-6) is a recently discovered member of the human herpesvirus family. Originally called human B-cell lymphotropic virus (HBLV), HHV-6 was first isolated from the peripheral blood lymphocytes (PBLs) of a patient with acquired immunodeficiency syndrome (AIDS), in 1985 [25]. Since this initial report, it has been isolated from a variety of patients, including those with AIDS, lymphoproliferative disorders, and normal healthy adults [26–31] (Table 4). The primary target cell for HHV-6 replication in vivo appears to be $CD4^+$ T lymphocytes [32], although recent studies, as discussed later, also reported the ability of HHV-6 to infect $CD8^+$ T cells [33] and macrophage–monocyte populations [34].

Although there is no cross-hybridization between the genome of HHV-6 and those of the other members of the human herpesvirus family [35], the locations of conserved HHV-6 genes based on DNA sequencing indicates that HHV-6 has a close genetic relationship to human cytomegalovirus (HCMV) [36–39]. In addition, the host range and tissue tropism of HHV-6, namely T cells and monocytes, also resembles that of HCMV.

The HHV-6–infected cells are characterized morphologically as enlarged, giant cells, with nuclear inclusion bodies and evidence for the margination of the chromatin [40,41], all of which are common characteristics for cells infected

Table 4 Detection of Infectious HHV-6 in Saliva

Subjects	Number	Virus detection[a]	
		No. positive	% positive
HIV$^+$	25	20	80
HIV$^-$	45	41	92
Total	70	61	87

[a]Virus was detected by growing saliva filtrates in cord blood lymphocytes.
Source: Ref. 31.

by members of the human herpesvirus family. At the molecular level, HHV-6 infection induces host cell protein synthesis, a feature shared with HCMV, but not with herpes simplex virus (HSV) and varicella–zoster virus (VZV) infections [42]. Infection of peripheral blood mononuclear cells (PBMCs) by HHV-6 leads to the induction of cytokines, including interleukin-1β (IL-1β), tumor necrosis factor-α (TNFα), and interferon-α (IFN-α), but not interleukin-6 [43–46] (Table 5). The induction of IFN-α in the course of HHV-6 infection of bone marrow mononuclear cells has been suggested as a cause for the recognized suppression of bone marrow cell differentiation and proliferation that can follow bone marrow transplants [45]. In so doing, these studies implicate HHV-6 as a cofactor in cases of bone marrow transplant failures. Infection with HHV-6 also is capable of transactivating the HIV LTR promoter, a potentially significant finding, given that both HHV-6 and HIV are capable of infecting the same cells [47–50]. In two studies, Lusso and coworkers [32,51] reported that HHV-6 and HIV-1 could productively coinfect $CD4^+$ cells, and that the coinfection accelerates the virally induced cytopathic effect. They showed, in a later study [33], that HHV-6 could infect human $CD8^+$ cells. The induction of CD4 in the HHV-6 infected $CD8^+$ cells permits subsequent infection by HIV-1. Furthermore, HHV-6 infection of either $CD4^+$ or $CD8^+$ cells results in down-regulation of the cell surface marker CD3 [52], the result of which would likely be impairment of T-cell function. However, these data contrast with those of Carrigan and colleagues and Levy and his colleagues [53,54], in which HHV-6 infection of $CD4^+$ cells or PBMCs led to suppression of HIV replication. However this issue may resolve, it is clearly based on current understanding that HHV-6 infection of susceptible immune cells can affect the competence of lymphocytes and, therefore, may serve as a cofactor in the pathogenesis of diseases in which an immune disturbance is a suspected element.

    Human herpesvirus-6 is a cause of roseola infantum (or exanthem subitum), a benign childhood disease characterized classically by high fever for 2–3 days, followed by a lacy, transient rash [28]. Although most roseola cases are

Table 5   Effects of HHV-6 Infection on Cytokine[a] Production in Peripheral Blood Mononuclear Cells

Sample	IL-1β	IL-6	TNF-α
Uninfected cells	960 + 101	3100 + 180	165 + 20
HHV-6–infected cells	3250 + 364	2600 + 168	1765 + 234
PAA + HHV-6	3100 + 333	5100 + 401	1300 + 146
UV-inactivated HHV-6	4250 + 637	6500 + 701	1500 + 206
Heat-inactivated HHV-6	700 + 130	3200 + 299	140 + 19

[a]IL, interleukin; TNF, tumor necrosis factor.
Source: Data from Ref. 44.

self-limited, convulsions are reported and, in some instances, encephalitis may evolve following the high fever and convulsions [28,55,56]. Several studies of children with roseola have demonstrated that seroconversion to HHV-6 accompanies the course of pathogenesis of the disease [28,57–60]. Takahashi and colleagues have documented that levels of IFN-α and natural killer (NK) cell activities rise during the acute phase of HHV-6–associated roseola infection [46].

Studies on the DNA genomes of HHV-6 isolates demonstrated that most of the isolates could be divided into two groups, based on their restriction enzyme digestion profiles [61–64]. Further analyses showed that, in addition to their restriction digest patterns, the two groups of viral strains differed from each other in their abilities to replicate in continuous cell lines and to react with certain HHV-6–specific monoclonal antibodies [reviewed in 65]. One group is typified by the Z29 isolate [27], whereas the other is characterized by the U1102 strain [66]. Even more striking was the finding that HHV-6 isolates from roseola patients always belong to the Z29-like group, whereas the isolates from patients with immunodeficiency disorders always belong to the U1102 group. This led some investigators to suggest that the classification of HHV-6 be reconsidered [65] and that the roseola virus be considered HHV-6B, while the U1102-like viruses be renamed HHV-6A. It remains to be seen whether the HHV-6 viruses apparently associated with some CFS patients will fall into one or other (or both) of these categories. Given the knowledge that the HHV-6 isolates obtained from patients with immune dysfunctions have belonged to the U1102-like group, it can be speculated that HHV-6 isolates from CFS patients will belong to this group of HHV-6.

Seroepidemiological studies have demonstrated that HHV-6 is ubiquitous. Enders and co-workers have shown that maternal antibodies in newborns to HHV-6 decrease from birth to 6 months, and that the rate of prevalence is 79.5% between the ages of 7 months and 5 years, 81.3% between the ages of 6 and 10 years, and 66% between the ages of 10 and 40 years [67]. Similarly, Yoshikawa and colleagues [68] and Gopal and co-workers [69] reported seroprevalence rates of 80–83%, respectively, in normal healthy adults. Although the prevalence of HHV-6 antibodies is accepted as being high in the general population, the ability to detect HHV-6 in cultured PBLs, however, is controversial, with reports placing levels at between zero and 50% [69,70]. The prevalence of virus in blood cells most likely reflects the level of HHV-6 latency in these cells. The high seroconversion rates along with the lower prevalence rates of HHV-6 virus in the blood raises the question of mode of transmission. Since most seroconversions occur during the first few years of life, several laboratories have assessed the orpharynx and saliva for the presence of infectious HHV-6. Infectious HHV-6 has been isolated from saliva and the mouths of normal adults at fairly high rates, ranging from 3 to 22% in one study [70] to 63% and higher than 85% in two other studies [31,69]. Cells expressing HHV-6 antigens have also been found in biopsy samples of salivary glands [71]. These results suggest that oral shedding is likely to be a major vehicle for HHV-6 transmission.

The only human disease clearly identified with HHV-6 infection is roseola infantum. However, considerable effort is being expended toward identifying other diseases, in both children and adults, in which HHV-6 infection may be involved. Toward this end, several disorders have been reported as either having been caused by HHV-6, or as presenting with an active HHV-6 infection during the course of the disease. In one study, Kurata and co-workers reported HHV-6 infection in 5 of 17 biopsied lymph nodes from patients with necrotizing lymphadenitis [41]. Other studies have implicated the reactivation of HHV-6 in patients undergoing immunosuppression for transplant surgeries [72,73]. Carrigan and colleagues [74] reported two cases of interstitial pneumonitis associated with HHV-6 following bone marrow transplants, and HHV-6 has been implicated in fulminant hepatitis in children and adults [75–77]. The underlying theme in these diverse disorders (and the relation to HHV-6 infection) appears to be that of an immune system under attack or of specific immunosuppression. The exact role of HHV-6 in these different disorders is unclear, but a virus that is both able to infect immune cells rapidly and that may establish reversible latency within them remains an attractive candidate for direct involvement in disease pathogenesis.

In that context, HHV-6 is currently one of the key viral suspects being pursued as an etiological factor in CFS. Early work, however, from Gold et al. [17] and Komaroff and Goldenberg [78] seemed to discount a role for HHV-6 in CFS, based on serological studies. More recently, Steeper and colleagues reported a 30% incidence of active HHV-6 infection in patients with a mononucleosislike illness that was not caused by either Epstein–Barr virus or cytomegalovirus [79]. In this study, active replication was determined by either a fourfold increase in HHV-6-specific IgG antibody titer or by the presence of HHV-6 IgM antibody. In a small pediatric population (eight patients), however, Marshall et al. could find no serological evidence for a link between HHV-6 and CFS [80]. However, in a larger study, Buchwald and associates reported a 70% prevalence of "active" HHV-6 infection (defined through an assay for infectious virus in peripheral blood mononuclear cells) among patients suffering from CFS ($n = 113$) compared with a 20% incidence rate among matched controls ($n = 40$) [81]. In this study, HHV-6 replication was detected in primary cell cultures of the patient's lymphocytes. However, it is possible that latent HHV-6 was reactivated by the process of isolation and culture of lymphocytes. These results were augmented using immunofluorescence assays with HHV-6 monoclonal antibodies and polymerase chain reaction (PCR) analysis of lymphocyte DNA using HHV-6-specific DNA primers. In subsequent studies, Iyengar and his colleagues report the generation of monoclonal antibodies to late and early antigens of HHV-6 and show that African Burkitt's lymphoma and Hodgkin's disease patients specifically have antibody responses to the early antigen (p41/38) [82]. There are some indications that CFS patients also specifically make antibodies to these early antigens (Ablashi D, personal communication), suggesting that active virus replication is taking place in these patients (58%), but not in controls (14%). Despite this impressive volume of data, direct evidence for a role of HHV-6 in chronic fatigue syndrome is still lacking (as many authors, including those with "positive" data, take pains to point out). As we have discussed earlier for EBV, differing views on the possible connection between HHV-6 and CFS existing in the literature may well be due, at least in part, to differences in assays used for HHV-6 antibodies, antigens, or virus. However, it is important to consider that a significant portion of CFS patients apparently demonstrate active HHV-6 replication and, that even though HHV-6 may not be the cause of CFS, it could certainly contribute to the symptoms. For example, increased circulating IFN-α levels have been reported in some studies of CFS patients [83,84], and HHV-6 infection increases IFN-α levels. Recent studies on HHV-6 in bone marrow transplant patients indicated that increased IFN levels could be a cause of increased bone marrow graft rejections.

Additional studies on the effects of HHV-6 replication on the immune system and on its role as an opportunistic virus are required to fully understand its potential in human pathogenesis. It will also be of interest to determine if a difference in adult pathogenicity and immune distress exists between the two proposed groups of HHV-6 (HHV-6A and HHV-6B).

OTHER HERPESVIRUSES

Other human herpesviruses have been examined in the context of CFS, notably herpes simplex virus (HSV), cytomegalovirus (CMV), and the so-called Inoue–Melnick virus (IMV) [85]. This last virus has only been suggested to be a herpesvirus, based on physicochemical properties. The evidence for HSV involvement in CFS is based on sparse data that suggest some reactivation, but this has not been pursued; the current wisdom would suggest no obvious role for HSV. In contrast, CMV titers have been raised in several studies of CFS patients [9,10,12] and, although there have been reports of patients in whom CFS was clearly triggered by a primary CMV infection, no consistent pattern of association of this virus with disease has been shown.

One consistent hypothesis in CFS is that an immune imbalance triggers latent viruses to reactivate. If this is indeed taking place, one might expect to see similar patterns of reactivation among many such viruses. In the case of the two major players in the CFS–herpes axis, evidence is accumulating that this is so. In that context, Levy (personal communication) recently demonstrated that, in a wide survey of CFS candidate viruses (including retroviruses and enteroviruses), serological evidence for only EBV and HHV-6 could be detected as different from controls. He suggested that a "hit-and-run" mechanism for CFS, stemming from the initial (viral?; influenza?) insult might be tenable; this "hit" would trigger an altered immune response that, in turn, would lead to activation of a variety of viruses. These viruses might then also play a role in further alterations of the host's immunity and in possible disease. If this mechanism were accurate, it would be predicted that a wider range of latent viruses would be activated in CFS patients than has currently been described. That this is not so either suggests that the theory is flawed, or that the presence of other viruses has not been effectively examined.

One important set of future experiments that may shed some light on this enigmatic syndrome is to test one cohort of patients, with appropriately matched controls, for the presence of the variety of viral agents with literature claims on CFS, using correlations with disease severity. These viruses include EBV, CMV, Inoue–Melnick virus, HHV-6, an HTLV-II-like virus, a human spumavirus, rubella virus, and enteroviruses. The possibility exists that CFS represents a range of syndromes, each triggered by a different virus infection, with additional possible geographic variations.

ACKNOWLEDGMENT

We gratefully acknowledge support from USPHS grant no. A1 32247.

REFERENCES

1. Holmes GP, Kaplan JE, Gantz NM, Komaroff AL, Schonberger LB, Straus SE, Jones JF, DuBois RE, Cunningham-Rundles C, Pahwa S, Tosato G, Zegans LS, Purtilo DT, Brown N, Schooley RT, Brus I. Chronic fatigue syndrome: a working case definition. Ann Intern Med 1988; 108:387–9.
2. Srtauch B, Siegel N, Andrews L, Miller G. Oropharyngeal excretion of EBV by renal transplant recipients and other patients treated with immunosuppressive drugs. Lancet 1987; 1:234–7.
3. Robinson J, Brown N, Andiman W, et al. Diffuse polyclonal B cell lymphoma during primary infection with EBV. N Engl J Med 1979; 302:1293–7.
4. Kieff E, Liebowitz D. EBV and its replication. In: Fields BN et al, eds. Virology. 2nd ed. New York: Raven Press, 1990:1889–920.
5. Jones JF, Williams M, Schooley RT, Robinson C, Glaser R. Antibodies to EBV-specific DNase and DNA polymerase in the chronic fatigue syndrome. Arch Intern Med 1988; 148:1957–60.
6. Isaacs R. Chronic infectious mononucleosis. Blood 1948; 3:858–61.
7. Kroenke K. Chronic fatigue syndrome: is it real? Postgrad Med 1991; 89:44–55.
8. Ballow M, Seeley J, Purtilo DT, St Onge S, Sakamoto K, Rickles FR. Familial chronic mononucleosis. Ann Intern Med 1982; 97:821–5.
9. Tobi M, Morag A, Ravid Z, Chowers I, Feldman-Weiss V, Michaeli Y, Ben-Chetrit

E, Shalit M, Knobler H. Prolonged atypical illness associated with serological evidence of persistent EBV infection. Lancet 1982; 1:61–4.

10. Dubois RE, Seeley J, Brus I, Sakamoto K, Ballow M, Harada S, Bchtold TA, Pearson G, Purtilo DT. Chronic mononucleosis syndrome. South Med J 1984; 77:1376–82.

11. Jones JF, Streib J, Baker S, Hergerger M. Chronic fatigue syndrome: 1. EBV immune response and molecular epidemiology. J Med Virol 1991; 33:151–8.

12. Straus SE, Tostao G, Armstrong G, Lawley T, Prebble OT, Henle W, Davey R, Pearson G, Epstein J, Brus I, Blaese M. Persisting illness and fatigue in adults with evidence of EBV infection. Ann Intern Med 1985; 102:7–16.

13. Niederman JC. Chronicity of Epstein Barr virus infection. Ann Intern Med 1985; 102:119–21.

14. Horwitz CA, Henle W, Henle G, Rudnick H, Latts E. Long term serologic follow-up of patients for Epstein–Barr virus after recovery from infectious mononucleosis. J Infect Dis 1985; 151:1150–3.

15. Buchwald D, Komaroff A. Review of laboratory findings for patients with chronic fatigue syndrome. Rev Infect Dis 1991; 13:S12–8.

16. Hellinger WC, Smith TF, Van Scoy RE, Spitzer PG, Forgas P, Edson RS. Chronic fatigue syndrome and the diagnostic utility of antibody to Epstein Barr virus early antigen. JAMA 1988; 260:971–3.

17. Gold D, Bowden R, Sixbey J, Riggs R, Katon WJ, Ashley R, Obrigewitch RM, Corey L. Chronic fatigue: a prospective clinical and virologic study. JAMA 1990; 264:48–53.

18. Sumaya CV. Serologic and virologic epidemiology of Epstein–Barr virus: relevance to chronic fatigue syndrome. Rev Infect Dis 1991; 13:S19–25.

19. Henle W, Henle G, Anderson J, Ernberg I, Klein G, Horwitz CA, Marklund G, Rymo L, Wellinder C, Straus SE. Antibody responses to Epstein–Barr virus-deter-mined nuclear antigen (EBNA)-1 and EBNA-2 in acute and chronic Epstein–Barr virus infection. Proc Natl Acad Sci USA 1987; 84:570–4.

20. Miller G, Grogan E, Rowe D, Rooney C, Heston L, Eastman R, Andiman W, Niederman J, Lenoir G, Henle W, Sullivan J, Schooley R, Vossen J, Strauss S, Issekutz T. Selective lack of antibody to a component of EB nuclear antigen in patients with chronic active Epstein–Barr virus infection. J Infect Dis 1987; 156:26–35.

21. Natelson BH, Ye N, Moul DE, Jenkins FJ, Oren DA, Tapp WN, Cheng Y-C. Antibodies to Epstein–Barr virus replicating enzymes: a biomedical marker for severe fatiguing illness. (submitted).

22. Jones JF, Streib J, Baker S, Herberger M. Chronic fatigue syndrome: 1. Epstein–Barr virus immune response and molecular epidemiology. J Med Virol 1991; 33:151–8.

23. Jones JE. Serological and immune responses in chronic fatigue syndrome with emphasis on the Epstein–Barr virus. Rev Infect Dis 1991; 13:S26–31.

24. Straus SE, Dale JK, Tobi M, Lawley T, Preble O, Blaese RM, Hallahan C, Henle W. Acyclovir treatment of the chronic fatigue syndrome: lack of efficacy in a placebo-controlled trial. N Engl J Med 1988; 319:1692–8.

25. Salahuddin SZ, Ablashi DV, Markham PD, Josephs SF, Sturzennegger S, Kaplan M, Halligan G, Biberfeld P, Wong-Staal F, Kramarsky B, Gallo RC. Isolation of

a new virus, HBLV, in patients with lymphoproliferative disorders. Science 1986; 234:596–601.

26. Agut H, Guetard D, Collandre H, Dauguet C, Montagnier L, Miclea JM, Baurmann H, Gessain A. Concomitant infection by human herpesvirus 6, HTLV-1 and HIV-2. Lancet 1988; 1:712.

27. Lopez C, Pellet P, Stewart J, Goldsmith C, Sanderlin K, Black J, Warfield D, Feorino P. Characterization of human herpes virus 6. J Infect Dis 1988; 157:1271–3.

28. Yamanishi K, Okono T, Shiraki K, Takahashi M, Kondo T, Asano Y, Kurata K. Identification of human herpes 6 a causal agent for exanthem subitum. Lancet 1988; 1:1065–7.

29. Pietroboni GR, Harnett GB, Bucens MR, Honess RW. Antibody to human herpesvirus 6 in saliva. Lancet 1988; 1:1059.

30. Harnett GB, Farr TJ, Pietroboni GR, Bucens MR. Frequent shedding of human herpesvirus 6 in saliva. J Med Virol 1990; 30:128–30.

31. Levy JA, Ferro F, Greenspan D, Lennette ET. Frequent isolation of HHV-6 from saliva and high seroprevalence of the virus in the population. Lancet 1990; 1:1047–50.

32. Lusso P, Markham PD, Tschachler E, Veronese FM, Salahuddin SZ, Abalshi DV, Pahwa S, Krohn K, Gallo RC. In vitro cellular tropism of human B-lymphotropic virus (human herpesvirus-6). J Exp Med 1988; 167:1659–70.

33. Lusso P, Maria AD, Malnati M, Lori F, DeRocco SE, Baseler M, Gallo RC. Induction of CD4 and susceptibility to HIV-1 infection in human CD8[+] T lymphocytes by human herpesvirus 6. Nature 1991; 349:533–5.

34. Kondo K, Kondo T, Okuno T, Takahashi M, Yamanishi K. Latent human herpesvirus 6 infection of human monocytes/macrophages. J Gen Virol 1991; 72:1401–08.

35. Josephs SF, Ablashi DV, Salahuddin SZ, Kramrsky B, Franza BR, Pellet P, Buchbinder A, Memon S, Wong-Staal F, Gallo RC. Molecular studies of HHV-6. J Virol Methods 1988; 21:179–90.

36. Efstathiou S, Gompels UA, Craxton MA, Honess RW, Ward K. DNA homology between a novel human herpesvirus (HHV-6) and human cytomegalovirus. Lancet 1988; 1:63–4.

37. Lawrence GL, Chee M, Craxton MA, Gompels UA, Honess RW, Barrell BG. Human herpesvirus 6 is closely related to human cytomegalovirus. J Virol 1990; 64:287–99.

38. Martin MED, Thomson BJ, Honess RW, Craxton MA, Gompels UA, Liu M-Y, Littler E, Arrand JR, Teo I, Jones MD. The genome of human herpesvirus 6: maps of unit-length and concatemeric genomes for nine restriction endonucleases. J Gen Virol 1991; 72:157–68.

39. Neipel F, Ellinger K, Fleckenstein B. The unique region of the human herpesvirus 6 genome is essentially colinear with the U^L segment of human cytomegalovirus. J Gen Virol 1991; 72:2293–97.

40. Nii S, Yoshida M, Uno F, Kurata T, Ikuta K, Yamanishi K. Replication of human herpesvirus 6 (HHV-6): morphological aspects. In: Lopez C, eds. Immunobiology and prophylaxis of human herpesvirus infections. New York: Plenum Press, 1990:19–28.

41. Kurata T, Iwasaki T, Sata T, Wakabayashi T, Yamaguchi K, Okuno T, Yamanishi K, Takei Y. Viral pathology of human herpesvirus 6 infection. In: Lopez C, ed. Immunobiology and prophylaxis of human herpesvirus infections. New York: Plenum Press, 1990:39–47.

42. Black JB, Lopez C, Pellet PE. Induction of host cell protein synthesis by human herpesvirus 6. Virus Res 1991; 22:13–23.

43. Flamand L, Gosselin J, D'addario M, Hiscott J, Ablashi DV, Gallo RC, Menezes J. Human herpesvirus 6 induces interleukin-1β and tumor necrosis factor alpha, but not interleukin-6 in peripheral blood mononuclear cell cultures. J Virol 1991; 65:5105–10.

44. Gosselin J, Flamand L, D'addario M, Hiscott J, Stefanescu I, Ablashi DV, Gallo RC, Menezes J. Modulatory effects of Epstein–Barr, herpes simplex, and human herpes-6 viral infections and coinfection on cytokine synthesis. A comparative study. J Immunol 1992; 149:181–7.

45. Knox KK, Carrigan DR. In vitro suppression of bone marrow progenitor cell differentiation by human herpesvirus 6 infection. J Infect Dis 1992; 165:925–9.

46. Takahashi K, Segal E, Kondo T, Mukai T, Moriyama M, Takahashi M, Yamanishi K. Interferon and natural killer cell activity in patients with exanthem subitum. Pediatr Infect Dis J 1992; 11:369–73.

47. Ensoli B, Lusso P, Schachter F, Josephs SF, Rappaport J, Negro F, Gallo RC, Wong-Staal F. Human herpes virus-6 increases HIV-1 expression in co-infected T cells via nuclear factors binding to the HIV-1 enhancer. EMBO J 1989; 8:3019–27.

48. Horvat RT, Wood C, Joshephs SF, Balachandran N. Transactivation of the human immunodeficiency virus promoter by human herpesvirus 6 (HHV-6) strains GS and Z-29 in primary human T lymphocytes and identification of transactivating HHV-6(GS) gene fragments. J. Virol 1991; 65:2895–902.

49. Campbell MEM, McCorkindale S, Everett RD, Onions DE. Activation of gene expression by human herpesvirus 6 is reporter gene-dependent. J Gen Virol 1991; 72:1123–30.

50. Geng Y, Chandran B, Josephs SF, Wood C. Identification and characterization of a human herpesvirus 6 gene segment that *trans* activates the human immunodeficiency virus type 1 promoter. J Virol 1992; 66:1564–70.

51. Lusso P, Ensoli B, Markham PD, Abalshi DV, Salahuddin SZ, Tschachler E, Wong-Staal F, Gallo RC. Productive dual infection of human CD4$^+$ T-lymphocytes by HIV-1 and HHV-6. Nature 1989; 337:370–3.

52. Lusso P, Malnati M, DeMaria A, Balotta C, DeRocco SE, Markham PD, Gallo RC. Productive infection of CD4$^+$ and CD8$^+$ mature human T cell populations and clones by human herpesvirus 6. J Immunol 1991; 147:685–91.

53. Carrigan DR, Knox KK, Tapper MA. Suppression of human immunodeficiency virus type 1 replication by human herpesvirus-6. J Infect Dis 1990; 162:844–51.

54. Levy JA, Landay A, Lennette ET. Human herpesvirus 6 inhibits human immunodeficiency virus type 1 replication in cell culture. J Clin Microbiol 1990; 28:2362–4.

55. Moore WF. Roseola infantum. Hawaii Med J 1963; 22:431–5.

56. Ishiguro N, Yamada S, Takahashi T, Takahashi Y, Togashi T, Okuno T, Yamanishi

K. Meningo-encephalitis associated with HHV-6 related exanthem subitum. Acta Paediatr Scand 1990; 79:987–9.

57. Knowles WA, Gardner SD. High prevalence of antibody to human herpesvirus-6 and seroconversion associated with rash in two infants. Lancet 1988; 2:912–3.

58. Asano Y, Suga S, Yoshikawa T, Urisu A, Yazaki T. Human herpesvirus type 6 infection (exanthem subitum) without fever. J Pediatr 1989; 115:264–5.

59. Suga S, Yoshikawa T, Asano Y, Yazaki T, Hirata S. Human herpesvirus-6 infection (exanthem subitum) without rash. Pediatrics 1989; 83:1003–6.

60. Yoshiyama H, Suzuki E, Yoshida T, Kajii T, Yamamoto N. Role of human herpesvirus 6 infection in infants with exanthema subitum. Pediatr Infect Dis J 1990; 9:71–74.

61. Jarrett RF, Gallagher A, Gledhill S, Jones MD, Teo I, Griffin BE. Variation in restriction map of HHV-6 genome. Lancet 1989; 1:448–9.

62. Kikuta H, Lu H, Matsumoto S, Josephs SF, Gallo RC. Polymorphism of human herpesvirus 6 DNA from five Japanese patients with exanthem subitum. J Infect Dis 1989; 160:550–1.

63. Pellet PE, Lindquester GJ, Feorino P, Lopez C. Genomic heterogeneity of human herpesvirus 6 isolates. In: Lopez C, ed. Immunobiology and prophylaxis of human herpesvirus infections. New York: Plenum Press, 1990:9–18.

64. Aubin J-T, Collandre H, Candotti D, Ingrand D, Rouzioux C, Burgard M, Richard S, Huraux J-M, Agut H. Several groups among human herpesvirus 6 strains can be distinguished by Southern blotting and polymerase chain reaction. J Clin Microbiol 1991; 29:367–72.

65. Schirmer EC, Wyatt LS, Yamanishi K, Rodriguez WJ, Frenkel N. Differentiation between two distinct classes of viruses now classified as human herpesvirus 6. Proc Natl Acad Sci USA 1991; 88:5922–26.

66. Downing RG, Sewankambo N, Serwadda D, Honess R, Crawford D, Jarrett R, Griffin BE. Isolation of human lymphotropic herpesviruses from Uganda. Lancet 1987; 2:390–1.

67. Enders G, Biber M, Meyer G, Helftenbein E. Prevalence of antibodies to human herpesvirus 6 in different age groups, in children with exanthema subitum, other acute exanthematous childhood diseases, Kawasaki syndrome, and acute infections with other herpesviruses and HIV. Infection 1990; 18:12–5.

68. Yoshikawa T, Suga S, Asano Y, Yazaki T, Ozaki T. Neutralizing antibodies to human herpesvirus-6 in healthy individuals. Pediatr Infect Dis J 1990; 9:589–90.

69. Gopal MR, Thomson BJ, Fox J, Tedder RS, Honess RW. Detection by PCR of HHV-6 and EBV DNA in blood and oropharynx of healthy adults and HIV-sero-positives. Lancet 1990; 335:1598–9.

70. Kido S, Kondo K, Kondo T, Morishima T, Takahashi M, Yamanishi K. Detection of human herpesvirus 6 DNA in throat swabs by polymerase chain reaction. J Med Virol 1990; 32:139–42.

71. Fox JD, Briggs M, Ward PA, Tedder RS. Human herpesvirus 6 in salivary glands. Lancet 1990; 336:590–3.

72. Kikuta H, Itami N, Matsumoto S, Chikaraishi T, Togashi M. Frequent detection

of human herpesvirus 6 DNA in peripheral blood mononuclear cells from kidney transplant patients. J Infect Dis 1991; 163:925.

73. Asano Y, Yoshikawa T, Suga S, Yazaki T, Hirabayashi S, Ono Y, Tsuzuki K, Oshima S. Human herpesvirus 6 harbouring in kidney. Lancet 1989; 2:1391.

74. Carrigan DR, Drobyski WR, Russler SK, Tapper MA, Knox KK, Ash RC. Interstitial pneumonitis associated with human herpesvirus-6 infection after marrow transplantation. Lancet 1991; 338:147–9.

75. Sobue R, Miyazaki H, Okamoto M, Hirano M, Yoshikawa T, Suga S, Asano Y. Fulminant hepatitis in primary human herpesvirus-6 infection. N Engl J Med 1991; 862.

76. Asano Y, Yoshikawa T, Suga S, Yazaki T, Kondo K, Yamanishi K. Fatal fulminant hepatitis in an infant with human herpesvirus-6 infection. Lancet 1990; 335:862–3.

77. Dubedat S, Kappagoda N. Hepatitis due to human herpesvirus-6. Lancet 1989; 2:1463–4.

78. Komaroff AL, Goldenberg D. The chronic fatigue syndrome: definition, current studies and lessons for fibromyalgia research. J Rheumatol Suppl 1989; 19:23–7.

79. Steeper TA, Horwitz CA, Ablashi DV, Salahuddin SZ, Saxinger C, Saltzman R, Schwartz B. The spectrum of clinical and laboratory findings resulting from human herpesvirus-6 (HHV-6) in patients with mononucleosis-like illnesses not resulting from Epstein–Barr or cytomegalovirus. Am J Clin Pathol 1990; 93:776–83.

80. Marshall GS, Gesser RM, Yamanishi K, Starr SE. Chronic fatigue in children: clinical features, Epstein–Barr virus and human herpesvirus 6 serology and long term follow-up. Pediatr Infect Dis J 1991; 10:287–90.

81. Buchwald D, Cheney PR, Peterson DL, Henry B, Wormsley SB, Geiger A, Ablashi DV, Salahuddin SZ, Saxinger C, Biddle R, Kikinis R, Jolesz FA, Folks T, Balachandran N, Peter JB, Gallo RC, Komaroff AL. A chronic illness characterized by fatigue, neurologic and immunologic disorders, and active human herpesvirus type 6 infection. Ann Intern Med 1992; 116:103–13.

82. Iyengar S, Levine PH, Ablashi D, Neequaye J, Pearson GR. Sero-epidemiological investigations on human herpesvirus 6 (HHV-6) infections using a newly developed early antigen assay. Int J Cancer 1991; 49:551–7.

83. Morrison LJA, Behan WHM, Behan PO. Changes in natural killer cell phenotype in patients with post-viral fatigue syndrome. Clin Exp Immunol 1991; 83:441–6.

84. Lloyd A, Hickie I, Brockman A, Dwyer J, Wakefield D. Cytokine levels in serum and cerebrospinal fluid in patients with chronic fatigue syndrome and control subjects. J Infect Dis 1991; 164:1023–4.

85. Dale JK, Straus SE, Ablashi DV, Salahuddin SZ, Gallo RC, Nishibe Y, Inoye YK. The Inoye–Melnick virus, human herpesvirus type 6, and the chronic fatigue syndrome. Ann Intern Med 1989; 110:92–3.

7

Retroviruses and Chronic Fatigue Syndrome

Walid Heneine and Thomas M. Folks
National Center for Infectious Diseases, Centers for Disease Control and Prevention, Atlanta, Georgia

During the past several years, much attention has been given to an illness called chronic fatigue syndrome (CFS). CFS is a disease of unknown cause(s) characterized by severe debilitating fatigue and associated nonspecific symptoms and signs, including fevers, pharangitis, headaches, myalgias, neurocognitive difficulties, sleep disturbances, and depression [1]. Criteria for a CFS research case definition were developed in 1988 [1], although a historical review suggests that CFS may be an old clinical problem [2]. It appears to affect young adults most commonly and has been reported more frequently in females than in males. The cause of CFS remains obscure, despite reports suggesting immunological abnormalities, neuroendocrinological dysfunction, psychological dysfunction, and involvement of infectious agents, particularly viruses. A viral etiology has been suspected because the onset of CFS often is reported to resemble an acute viral illness [2], and because chronic postinfectious fatigue has been described as a sequelae of several viral infections. In fact, CFS has been reported to be associated with multiple viral agents, such as Epstein–Barr virus (EBV), cytomegalovirus (CMV), enteroviruses, and human herpesvirus-6 (HHV-6), but such associations have not been firmly established or widely accepted [2].

This chapter was written by Walid Heneine and Thomas M. Folks in their private capacities. No official support or endorsement by the Centers for Disease Control and Prevention is intended or should be inferred.

Table 1 Characteristics of Representative Retroviruses

Subfamily	Disease	Natural host
Oncoviruses		
Human T-cell lymphotropic virus type I	T-cell lymphoma, neurological disorders	Man
HTLV-II	Unknown pathogenicity	Man
Bovine leukemia virus (BLV)	B-cell lymphoma	Cattle
Moloney murine leukemia virus	T-cell lymphoma	Mouse
Feline leukemia virus	T-cell lymphoma, immunodeficiency, and other diseases	Cat
Simian type D viruses	Immunodeficiencies	Monkey
Mouse mammary tumor virus	Mammary carcinoma, T-cell lymphoma	Mouse
Lentiviruses		
Human immunodeficiency viruses (HIV-1 and HIV-2)	AIDS	Man
Simian immunodeficiency virus	AIDS	Monkey
Visna/Maedi virus	Pneumonia, meningoencephalitis	Sheep, goats
Caprine arthritis–encephalitis virus	Arthritis, pneumonia, encephalitis	Goats, sheep
Equine infectious anemia virus	Fever, anemia	Horses
Spumaviruses		
Human spuma virus	Apparently benign	Man
Simian spuma viruses	Apparently benign	Monkey

Because of the involvement of retroviruses in other chronic diseases, multiple attempts were recently made to identify a possible role for retroviruses in CFS. These viruses are the focus of intense research because they are important human and animal pathogens, and also because their unique replication cycle makes them novel and interesting subjects of study [3]. Retroviruses are a large family of RNA viruses that replicate by a double-stranded DNA intermediate, synthesized from the virion by an RNA-dependent DNA polymerase (reverse transcriptase). This intermediate, known as the provirus, is integrated into the host cell DNA and acts as a template for the production of viral genomic and mRNA by using the host cell replicative machinery [3]. Primarily on the basis of pathogenicity, rather than genome relationships, the retrovirus family is divided into three subfamilies: the oncoviruses, lentiviruses, and spumaviruses. Retroviruses are associated with many diseases, including ones with rapid- to long-latency malignancies, wasting diseases, neurologic disorders, and immunodeficiencies, as well as lifelong viremia in the absence of any obvious disease. Well-characterized representative retroviruses from these three subfamilies are listed in Table 1.

An increasing number of reports indicate that retroviruses may be involved in several chronic diseases of humans (Fig. 1). Examples include claims concerning the isolation of a putative retrovirus from multiple sclerosis [4], the detection of intracisternal A type particles in Sjögren's syndrome [5], the presence of human T-lymphotropic virus type I (HTLV-I) gene fragments in mycosis fungoides [6], and the identification of human spuma retrovirus sequences in Graves disease [7]. In chickens, the presence of an avian leukosis virus (*ev22*) has been linked to the development of autoimmune thyroiditis [8]. In addition, some animal models of chronic diseases of unknown etiology have been associated with the expression of various retroviral genes. For instance, transgenic mice expressing the *tax* gene of HTLV-I develop an inflammatory arthropathy resembling rheumatoid arthritis [9], whereas those expressing the human spuma *bel* gene develop a progressive encephalopathy and myopathy [10].

These diverse reports encourage searches for retroviruses in an ever-broadening variety of illnesses. It is in this light that several attempts have been made to discern a role for retroviruses in CFS by employing several laboratory techniques. These investigations primarily have used serological or molecular tests for specific known retroviruses, or general tests for reverse transcriptase activity in cells cultured from CFS patients to detect novel retroviruses. Serological test results for human immunodeficiency virus (HIV) types 1 and 2

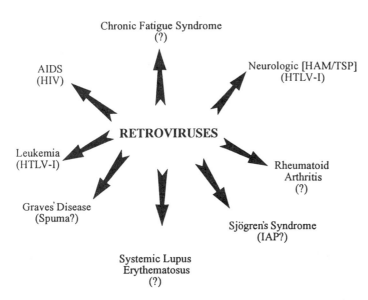

Figure 1 Human diseases in which retroviruses have been implicated or suspected HAM/TSP, HTLV-I-associated myelopathy/tropical spastic paraparesis; IAP, intracisternal A particles. Disorders for which an association is suspected but unconfirmed are followed by a question mark.

have been consistently negative in CFS patients [11,12]. Similarly, efforts to detect evidence of prior human spuma retrovirus infection in CFS patients by serological studies [13,14] or by the polymerase chain reaction (PCR) [15] have proved to be negative. These published findings, in contrast to the unpublished report on the isolation of such a virus from cell cultures of patients with CFS [16], do not support a role for human spuma retrovirus in CFS. A recent controlled and blinded study further confirmed the inability of the putative spuma retrovirus culture assay to distinguish between case-patients and controls [17].

The possibility of oncovirus involvement in CFS has been evaluated more extensively. Several groups sought serological or molecular evidence of HTLV-I and HTLV-II infection in CFS patients [11–13,15,18–21]. With the exception of a report by DeFreitas et al. [18], no evidence of HTLV-I or HTLV-II has been found. By using PCR to screen for HTLV-I and HTLV-II proviral sequences in the peripheral blood mononuclear cells (PBMCs), DeFreitas et al. reported the detection of an HTLV-II *gag* sequence in 10 of 12 adults with CFS, 13 of 18 children with CFS, and in 7 of 20 contacts of these patients, but in none of noncontact controls. No other HTLV-I *gag* or HTLV-II *tax* sequences were detected. In addition, most patients in that study were positive for HTLV-I/II antibodies by Western blotting and for the HTLV-II *gag* RNA transcript sequence by in situ hybridization. These data were interpreted by the authors as evidence of an association between an HTLV-II-like virus and CFS. However, subsequent investigations aimed at assessing and confirming this retroviral association with CFS found no evidence of either the HTLV-II *gag* sequence or of the HTLV-I/II antibodies in CFS patients and matched controls [13,15,20,21]. A representative PCR result from a study of patients and controls in Atlanta, Georgia, is shown in Figure 2 [20].

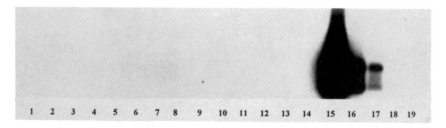

Figure 2   A representative polymerase chain reaction analysis of the human T-lymphotropic virus type II (HTLV-II) *gag* gene sequence in patients with the chronic fatigue syndrome and healthy controls from Atlanta, Georgia. Autoradiograph is shown for eight patients (lanes 1, 2, 4, 5, 7, 8, 10, and 11); four health controls (lane 3, 6, 9, and 12); 2 µg of carrier DNA containing 20, 2, 0.2, 0.02 ng of DNA from HTLV-II–infected cell line (Mo-T) (lanes, 15, 16, 17, and 18, respectively); noninfected Hut-78 (lane 13); molecular size marker (lane 14); and reagent cocktail control (lane 19). (Adapted from Ref. 20.)

These negative results could not be attributed to differences in methodologies; for instance, the PCR technique used in one such study [20] had a sensitivity and specificity comparable with that of DeFreitas et al. [21]. It is possible that inadvertent contamination of specimens and other technical problems might explain the previously reported positive PCR results. For example, the internal HTLV-II *gag* probe used in the assays had an 85% GC content, which results in an unusually high melting temperature (80.4°C). Use of this probe at 37°C in the hybridization and washing steps, as was done in the original report [18], constituted low-stringency conditions. These conditions may have permitted nonspecific binding of the probe to endogenously amplified material, which is normally generated with this particular HTLV-II primer pair, and is close in size to the authentic HTLV-II product [13,15]. The combination of the nonspecific amplification and hybridization, along with unconventionally long exposure times (5–7 days), may have resulted in false-positive results that were incorrectly interpreted by the investigators, who were incompletely blinded to subject identity. The importance of blinding is further emphasized by the experiences in a second study. In this fully blinded study, other HTLV-II *gag*-based PCR tests failed to distinguish between CFS patients and controls [17]. Moreover, Khan et al. evaluated possible risk factors for CFS, particularly those associated with retroviral transmission in well-characterized CFS patients and matched neighborhood controls from Atlanta. Their data did not reveal epidemiological evidence recognized to facilitate transmission of known retroviruses among CFS patients (e.g., history of intravenous drug use, blood transfusion, or homosexual behavior) or hypothesized to facilitate the transmission of unidentified retroviruses (Table 2) [20]. Taken together, these data do not support a role for HTLV-II nor for an HTLV-II-like agent in CFS. No additional data have yet been provided by DeFreitas et al. or by other groups to confirm the original findings, or to support them by isolating an HTLV-II-like agent, or by better characterizing the putative molecular and serological HTLV-II marker.

Because of reports that humans can be infected with animal retroviruses [22,23], one group evaluated CFS patients for evidence of infection by several animal retroviruses, including the simian T-lymphotropic virus type I, the simian retroviruses types 1, 2, and 3 (SRV-1,-2,-3), the bovine leukemia virus (BLV), the feline leukemia virus, and the gibbon ape leukemia virus (GALV) [15]. These retroviruses were selected for three reasons: they grow in human cells in vitro [22,24,25]; they may infect humans (e.g., GALV, SRV-1, -2, and -3) [22,24]; and some of them (e.g., BLV, GALV) are easily missed by routine retroviral screening of cell cultures because of poor reverse transcriptase activity. No proviral sequences of any of these retroviruses were detected by PCR in patients or controls, yielding no support to the involvement of these prototypic animal viruses in CFS.

One study of 14 CFS patients attempted to look generically for retroviruses

Table 2 Prevalence of Potential Risk Factors and Sexual Behaviors Before Illness
Onset for the Chronic Fatigue Syndrome in Patients and Controls from Atlanta, Georgia

Variable	Patients	Controls	p value
	n/n(%)		
Blood transfusion	2/21 (10)	3/42 (7)	1.0
Exposure to human blood	3/21 (14)	8/42 (19)	0.9
Blood animal blood	2/21 (10)	4/42 (10)	1.0
Tatoo	0/21 (0)	0/42 (0)	
Acupuncture	2/21 (10)	0/42 (0)	0.2
Breastfed	6/16 (38)	18/37 (49)	1.0
Mother traveled outside US before participant was born	2/20 (10)	8/42 (19)	0.6
Father traveled outside US before participant was born	9/20 (45)	19/42 (45)	1.0
Personal travel outside the US	15/21 (71)	24/42 (57)	0.3
Intravenous drug use	0/21 (0)	0/42 (0)	
Median number of sex partners	3	3	0.9^a
Sex outside US with a native of a foreign country	2/15 (13)	4/23 (17)	1.0
Sex partner with an ill-defined fatiguing illness	1/20 (5)	1/42 (2)	1.0
Bisexual or homosexual behavior	3/21 (14)	3/42 (7)	0.6
Sex partner who used intravenous drugs	1/19 (5)	3/33 (9)	1.0
Sex partner who was a prostitute or traded sex for drugs	2/21 (10)	4/42 (10)	1.0
Sex partner who had hemophilia	0/14 (0)	0/31 (0)	
History of sexually transmitted disease	5/21 (24)	14/42 (33)	0.6
History of pelvic inflammatory disease (women)	2/17 (12)	1/34 (3)	0.4

[a]Stratified exact Wilcoxon rank-sum test.
Source: Adapted from Ref. 20.

by culturing PBMCs and monitoring the culture supernatants for reverse
transcriptase activity [12]. Despite the use of an optimized assay that was capable
of detecting retroviruses with poor reverse transcriptase activity (e.g., HTLV-I,
HTLV-II), all supernatants from cell cultures tested negative. These data cast
additional doubt on the possible involvement of known or novel retroviruses in
these CFS patients.

Despite the use of sensitive molecular, serological, and biological assays in
the search for retroviruses in CFS, no convincing evidence as yet exists that
associates this disease with a retrovirus acting as a causal agent or even as a
cofactor in the disease. However, this conclusion needs to be interpreted
cautiously because of several limitations, not the least of which is that a negative
result is not as compelling as a positive one. Specifically, the patient populations
that were assessed in the various studies were neither clinically nor epidemio-

logically homogeneous. They represented sporadic as well as cluster-associated cases of CFS from different geographic areas. It is possible that retroviral involvement in CFS could be limited to some, but not all, patient groups. Second, not all of these patient groups were comparably and extensively evaluated for known and novel retroviruses. The presence of a retrovirus in a subset of these patients could have been missed because of insufficient laboratory evaluation. Third, even when the laboratory testing was extensive, a novel retrovirus or variant of a known one could have been missed, particularly if the agent is present only transiently in the peripheral blood leukocytes or if it resides primarily in other tissues.

As new laboratory technologies are developed and new epidemiological information is accumulated, the final chapter may be written concerning the potential role of retroviruses in this debilitating syndrome. In the meantime, health care providers should not indicate to their patients that convincing evidence associates CFS with a retroviral infection.

ACKNOWLEDGMENTS

We thank Drs. Keiji Fukuda and Jonathan E. Kaplan for their critical review of the chapter and for their helpful comments.

REFERENCES

1. Holmes GP, Kaplan JE, Gantz NM, et al. Chronic fatigue syndrome: a working case definition. Ann Intern Med 1988; 108:387–9.
2. Shafran SD. The chronic fatigue syndrome. Am J Med 1991; 90:730–9.
3. Coffin J. Retroviridae and their replication. In: Fields BN, Knipe DM, et al, eds. Virology. 2nd ed. New York: Raven Press, 1990:1435–500.
4. Perron H, Gratacap B, Lalande B, et al. In vitro transmission and antigenicity of a retrovirus isolated from a multiple sclerosis patient. Res Virol 1992; 143:337–50.
5. Garry RF, Fermin CS, Hart DJ, et al. Detection of a human intracisternal A-type retroviral particle antigenically related to HIV. Science 1990; 250:1127–9.
6. Hall WW, Liu CR, Schneewind O, et al. Deleted HTLV-I provirus in blood and cutaneous lesions of patients with mycosis fungoides. Science 1991; 253:317–20.
7. LaGaye S, Vexiau P, Morozov V, et al. Human spumaretrovirus-related sequences in the DNA of leukocytes from patients with Graves disease. Proc Natl Acad Sci USA 1992; 89:10070–4.
8. Ziemiecki A, Krömer G, Mueller RG, et al. *ev22*, a new endogenous avian leukosis virus locus found in chickens with spontaneous autoimmune thyroiditis. Arch Virol 1988; 100:267–71.
9. Iwakura Y, Tosu M, Yoshida E, et al. Induction of inflammatory arthropathy resembling rheumatoid arthritis in mice transgenic for HTLV-I. Science 1991; 253:1026–8.

10. Bothe K, Aguzzi A, Lassmann H, et al. Progressive encephalopathy and myopathy in transgenic mice expressing human foamy virus genes. Science 1991; 253:555–7.

11. Landay AL, Jessop C, Lennette ET, et al. Chronic fatigue syndrome: clinical condition associated with immune activation. Lancet 1991; 338:707–12.

12. Buchwald D, Cheney P, Peterson, et al. A chronic illness characterized by fatigue, neurologic and immunologic disorders, and active human herpesvirus type 6 infection. Ann Intern Med 1992; 116:103–13.

13. Gow J, Simpson K, Rethwilm A, et al. Search for retrovirus in the chronic fatigue syndrome. J Clin Pathol 1992; 45:1058–61.

14. Flugel RM, Mahnke C, Geiger A, et al. Absence of antibody to human spuma-retrovirus in patients with chronic fatigue syndrome [letter]. Clin Infect Dis 1992; 14:623–4.

15. Heneine W, Woods TC, Saswati DS, et al. Absence of evidence for infection with known human and animal retroviruses in patients with chronic fatigue syndrome. Clin Infect Dis (in press).

16. Palca J. On the track of an elusive disease. Science 1991; 254:1726–8.

17. Centers for Disease Control and Prevention. Inability of retroviral tests to identify persons with chronic fatigue syndrome, 1992. MMWR 1993; 42:183.

18. DeFreitas E, Hilliard B, Cheney PR, et al. Retroviral sequences related to human T-lymphotropic virus type II in patients with chronic fatigue immune dysfunction syndrome. Proc Natl Acad Sci USA 1991; 88:2922–6.

19. Levine PH, Jacobson S, Pocinki AG, et al. Clinical, epidemiologic, and virologic studies in four clusters of the chronic fatigue syndrome. Arch Intern Med 1992; 152:1611–6.

20. Khan AS, Heneine WM, Chapman LE, et al. Assessment of a retrovirus sequence and other possible risk factors for the chronic fatigue syndrome in adults. Ann Intern Med 1993; 118:241–5.

21. Folks TM, Heneine W, Khan AS, et al. Investigation of retroviral involvement in chronic fatigue syndrome. In: Whelan J, ed. Chronic fatigue syndrome. CBA Found Symp 1993; 173:160–75.

22. Bohannon RC, Donehower LA, Ford RJ. Isolation of a type D retrovirus from B-cell lymphomas of a patient with AIDS. J Virol 1991; 65:5663–72.

23. Khabbaz RF, Heneine W, George JR, et al. First isolation of a simian immunodeficiency virus from a human. Fourth International Conference on AIDS, Berlin, June 7–11, 1993.

24. Fuqua SA, Naso RB. A comparison of the intracellular precursor polyproteins of simian sarcoma-associated virus [SiSV(SiAV)] and three human virus isolates: HL23V, HEL12V and A1476V. J Gen Virol 1982; 62:49–63.

25. Jarrett O, Laird HM, Hay D. Determinants of the host range of feline leukaemia viruses. J Gen Virol 1973; 20:169–75

8

Immunological Function in Chronic Fatigue Syndrome

Warren Strober
National Institute of Allergy and Infectious Diseases, National Institutes of Health, Bethesda, Maryland

INTRODUCTION

Immunological function in chronic fatigue syndrome (CFS) has been the focus of intense study by numerous investigators (1–5). One aim of such study has been to define a primary immunological abnormality that is responsible for what is widely assumed to be the cause of the manifestations of the syndrome, infection due to one or another organism. Another aim is to discover and characterize secondary immune abnormalities that are in reality responses to an underlying infection and that cause the manifestations of the syndrome as an unintended side effect. Regardless of which of these aims more accurately captures the order of pathophysiological events in CFS, studies that identify specific immunological abnormalities in the syndrome have become increasingly important to its definition. This, because in the absence of a single causative infectious agent, the CFS-associated immunological abnormalities have become the common denominator that allows one to think of CFS as a consistent disease entity. In addition, any infection that is present in CFS is likely to be due to an intracellular organism that could be present in a latent or an active state; thus, it is only the presence of associated immunological findings that allows one to postulate that the latter, not the former, is present. These reasons for the centrality of immunological study of CFS can also be stated more provocatively by saying that in the absence of a specific infection as a cause of CFS, the presence of immunological abnormalities in the syndrome has become a major way of establishing a physical basis for the disorder and, thus, differentiating CFS from purely psychiatric/psychological syndromes. This has value to many CFS patients and their physicians because it moves the understanding of the syndrome beyond mere speculation and interpretation and opens the door to new and novel forms of therapy.

In the following review of the immunological findings in CFS, we will try to separate fact from fancy in this area and thus attempt to identify the abnormalities that can now be considered reasonably established. Our approach will be to consider what is known of the phenotype and/or function of each of the various types of cells in the lymphoid system, from the point of view of both in vitro and in vivo cell function. The latter, of course, relates to the circulating levels of immune cell products such as immunoglobulins and cytokines. In the context of describing each abnormality, we will discuss its possible relation to persistent infection in CFS as well as its possible relation to symptom formation. Later, in a summary section, we will explain how various abnormalities described earlier may relate to one another and thus form a framework for the view that CFS is, at least in part, an immunological disorder.

Before we begin our discussion, it is well to mention certain problems with assessing immunological function in CFS that confront anyone who attempts to analyze the now rather extensive studies in this area. First, the abnormalities identified generally consist of relatively subtle shifts in populations of immunological values, so that differences between CFS patients and normal controls are only established by application of stringent statistical tests. In this situation, the differences—although significant—are of uncertain physiological importance. In addition, the differences do not allow one to clearly identify whether CFS patient populations are made up of several subgroups, only one (or some) of which is truly abnormal, or whether they comprise a homogeneous group that differs from normal individuals by a small degree. These possibilities could, in theory, be distinguished by examination of the distribution of immunological values; however, in practice, this is difficult because of the large populations required. Second, in comparing results obtained by different investigators, the results are frequently inconsistent. This could arise from a variety of factors such as different criteria of case definition, different types of control patients or values, and different methods of performing tests. This inconsistency means that only those findings found by a variety of investigators under a variety of conditions can be said to be definite features of CFS; other findings are, at best, suggestive clues to the immunological status of CFS patients that require additional verification. Third and finally, the CFS patient group may itself be a dynamic and changing body of individuals whose disease manifestations are subject to change with respect to time. Overall, then, the study and analysis of immunological dysfunction in CFS is a somewhat perilous task and one that should be approached with a good deal of skepticism.

LYMPHOCYTE MASS IN CFS

To place our subsequent discussion of lymphoid cell phenotype and function in CFS into an appropriate context, it is useful to first consider the size of the lymphoid cell population in patients, as revealed by lymphocyte counts in the peripheral blood. As reported by Buchwald and Komaroff (1), such counts (as well as those of total leukocytes) disclose that a sizable proportion of the CFS patient population (20–30%) manifest abnormal lymphocyte counts, usually lymphocytosis. These figures, however, probably overstate lymphocyte count abnormalities in CFS, since the data extant provides little indication that abnormalities in individual patients are severe or persistent. In addition, the data are derived from studies of relatively small groups of patients that are unlikely to be representative of the CFS patient population as a whole. Indeed, in several studies of large patient groups in which this was done, mean lymphocyte counts did not differ from those of control individuals and patients with frankly abnormal values were rare (4–7). On this basis, it seems reasonable to speculate that those relatively few CFS patients in whom lymphocyte count abnormalities do occur are part of the small subgroup of patients with more tangible evidence of subacute infection. In addition, one can say that since mean lymphocyte counts in CFS are normal, abnormalities of lymphocyte subset levels expressed as percentage values (such as those discussed later on) can be generally considered an accurate mirror of lymphocyte subset absolute values.

Another finding in CFS relevant to the issue of lymphocyte mass is the rather frequent occurrence of lymphadenopathy in patients with the syndrome. However, although this abnormality is reported in some 30–50% of patients, the extent of the lymph node enlargement is rarely if ever consistent with a gross increase in lymphoid mass. In addition, it is not clear that the lymphadenopathy is more than a rather transient phenomenon that is not present throughout the much longer period during which the patient experiences fatigue.

T-CELL FUNCTION IN CFS

We will start our analysis of immunological function in CFS with a discussion of T cells, subdividing the latter into studies of T-cell phenotype and studies of T-cell function. This will, quite naturally, encompass a discussion of cytokine/lymphokine abnormalities in CFS since for the most part the latter are produced by T cells. For convenience, however, cytokines produced by macrophages—and perhaps other cells—will also be discussed in this section.

T-Cell Phenotype in CFS

The advent of monoclonal antibodies that define subsets of circulating lymphocytes has led to the identification of lymphocyte subset abnormalities associated with particular immunological diseases. A number of studies of this type have been conducted in CFS and have disclosed that this syndrome is, in fact, associated with phenotypic abnormalities of one sort or another.

The most fundamental of the T-cell phenotype studies in CFS, or indeed in other diseases of immunological interest, are those that focus on CD4/CD8 enumeration (1–14). Unfortunately, the data relating to CFS in this area are anything but straightforward, undoubtedly owing to some of the difficulties mentioned earlier regarding immunological studies of CFS generally. Thus, while total T-cell percentages in patients, as defined by quantitation of peripheral T cells bearing a pan T-cell marker such as CD3, is almost always normal in CFS (4–6,11),* there have been reports of normal, high, and low CD4 or CD8 T-cell levels (percentages) in patient groups with the syndrome. In one recent study (involving some 259 patients) of CD4 and CD8 T-cell levels in CFS, Buchwald et al. found that CD4 levels (percentages) are high and CD8 levels are low in the patient population, so that the patients as a group manifested an increased CD4/CD8 ratio (~3.2 in patients vs. 2.3 in controls); however, examination of these data shows that the control group was poorly defined and the patient group was quite heterogeneous; futhermore, it is not clear that the patient values were obtained under the same conditions as the control values. Unfortunately, other studies of CD4 and CD8 T cells in CFS, although conducted under somewhat more careful conditions, do not lead to a clearer picture of patient CD4/CD8 T-cell status. Thus, in studies conducted by Kibler et al. (11 patients) (9), Subira et al. (20 patients) (8), Chao et al. (10 patients) (10), Gupta and Vayuvegula (20 patients) (4), Landay et al. (147 patients) (11), and Tirelli et al. (40 patients) (6), normal CD4 and CD8 T-cell levels and normal CD4/CD8 ratios were observed; in contrast, in the studies conducted by Klimas et al. (30 patients) (3) and Ho Yen et al. (50 patients) (12), normal CD4 T-cell levels were accompanied by raised CD8 T-cell levels, although both Behan et al. (40 patients) (2) and Straus et al. (18 patients) (5) found reduced CD4 T-cell levels and slightly but nonsignificantly increased CD8 T-cell levels. Finally, Gold et al. (26 patients) (13) found high CD4 T-cell levels associated with normal CD8 T-cell levels and Lloyd et al. (20 patients) (14) found reductions in both CD4 and CD8 T-cell levels.

In assessing the significance of these mixed CD4/CD8 T-cell results, it is fair to say that the most striking finding is the *absence* of a striking finding, particularly the absence of a clearly raised CD8 T-cell level. To understand why this is so, one must first realize that CD8 T cells, by virtue of their capacity to recognize "endogenous" antigens in the context of MHC class I antigens, are the main lymphoid effector cells that react with and eliminate (lyse) host cells

---

*One curious exception to this rule was the finding of Subira et al. (8), who reported that CFS patient T cells contained a decreased percentage of CD3 T cells, but a normal percentage of CD2 or CD5 T cells. Thus it appeared that one pan T-cell marker was decreased (CD3) but others (CD2 and CD5) were normal. This finding, however, was not corroborated by Straus et al. (5) or by numerous other investigators.

infected with intracellular pathogens. It is not surprising then that in diseases characterized by intracellular infection, especially of a chronic variety (such as HIV infection or other viral infections), one invariably sees persistent elevations of CD8 T-cell levels and reversed CD4/CD8 ratios (15,16); in effect, in these diseases qualitative and quantitative changes in CD8 T cells are "footprints" of the chronic infection. On this basis, if one argues that infection is ongoing in CFS in spite of an essentially normal CD4/CD8 T-cell status, one must presume that the infection is so mild that it does not arouse a major host defense mechanism designed specifically to counter such infection. In addition, one takes on the obligation to demonstrate the presence of a more subtle abnormality of immunological function that mirrors the subtle nature of the infection.

A subtle abnormality of this sort may have indeed been found in the study of T-cell subsets defined by the CD45RA and CD45RO cell surface markers. Such an abnormality was first observed in a study by Klimas et al. (3), and then reported on independently and more definitively by Straus et al. (5). The latter authors determined the CD45RA/RO phenotype in 18 patients with CFS meeting the Centers for Disease Control and Prevention (CDC) case definition criteria and in 10 clinically similar, fatigued patients not fully meeting the CDC criteria who were, nevertheless, similar to the CDC-defined group. The control group consisted of a group of individuals carefully matched for age, sex, and other criteria; in addition, neither patients nor controls were on medication during the study. The data were as follows: (1) the percentage of T cells bearing both the CD4 and CD45RA markers (CD4/CD45RA T cells) was significantly reduced in CFS (16.7% vs. 28.0%, $p = 0.005$); (2) while the number of T cells bearing both CD4 and CD45RO (CD4)/CD45RO T cells), the reciprocal T-cell population since CD4 T cells bear either CD45RA or CD45RO, was not increased, the CD4/CD45RO T cells were qualitatively abnormal in that T cells bearing CD45RO had a significantly increased expression of three cell surface adhesion markers [CD29, CD54 (ICAM-1), and CD58 (LFA-3) as well as a nonsignificant increase in a fourth adhesion marker [CD11 (LFA-1)]. That the CD45RO T cells expressing increased amounts of adhesion markers were CD4 T cells (and not other kinds of cells) was shown in three-color FACS analysis in which it was found, for example, that 25.3% ± 2.4% of patients' CD4 T cells bore both CD45RO and CD29, whereas only 14.4% ± 1.1% of control CD4 T cells bore these markers. Finally, increased numbers of cells bearing adhesion markers were not found on CD4 T cells as a whole, nor on CD45RA-bearing T cells. Largely similar findings were obtained in the second group of patients not meeting the CDC criteria for CFS.

The data relating to reduced CD4/CD45RA T cells are shown in Fig. 1. It is apparent that the patient group and the control group show considerable overlap, which can be due to either small changes that are not discernible in small patient groups owing to "experimental noise" or to the fact that the patients consist of several subgroups, only one of which has the CD4/CD45RA phenotypic abnormality; these subgroups could consist of different forms of CFS or patients with the same form of CFS at different stages of disease. Despite the statistical nature of the findings, several factors suggest that differences between patients and controls are real. First, the findings are self-consistent in that there was a significant inverse correlation between the percentage of CD4/CD45RA T cells and the percentage of T cells bearing both CD45RO and adhesion markers, suggesting that the two abnormalities are reciprocally interrelated. In addition, despite the qualitative change in CD4/CD45RO T cells, the number of CD4/CD45RO T cells was not increased and the total number of CD4 T cells was decreased; these data fit nicely with the fact that CD4/CD45RO T cells bearing adhesion markers are likely to become tissue-bound cells that leave the circulation once formed. Finally, while the number of CD8 T cells bearing CD45RA was not decreased, the number of CD8/CD45RO T cells was increased, indicating that a related abnormality of CD8 cells exists in CFS.

Second, the data of Straus et al. (5) have been corroborated by other investigators. Thus, both in the aforementioned study by Klimas et al. and in a subsequent study by Tirelli et al., involving some 40 patients and matched controls, a decreased number of CD45RA T cells was also found. In the latter study, as in the study of Straus et al., decreased numbers of CD4/CD45RA T cells were not accompanied by increased numbers of CD4/CD45RO T cells. In addition, in this study, increased levels of CD4 T cells bearing the adhesion

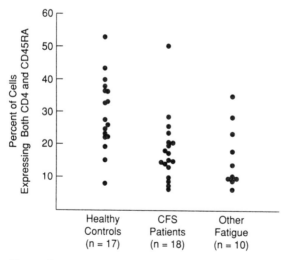

Figure 1   Cells expressing both CD4 and CD45RA in CFS and other patients with fatigue. Differences significant at the $p < 0.005$ level.

marker CD54 (ICAM-1) were found, although it was not determined whether the latter was present on CD45RA or CD45RO T cells. Third and finally, in an as-yet-incomplete follow-up study of T-cell phenotype in CFS conducted by Fritz, Strober, and Straus (unpublished), the same kind of phenotypic findings are again being found; that is, the CFS patient group tends to have an altered ratio of CD45RA to CD45RO T cells.

What is the possible cause of the decreased number of CD4/CD45RA T cells in CFS? To begin to answer this question, one must first discuss what is known of the function of these cells or the cells that bear these surface markers. CD45RA is a member of a family of proteins encoded by tandem genes on chromosome 1 that undergo alternative RNA splicing to produce RNAs responsible for the various family members (17,18). Each isoform comprises a unique extracellular domain coupled with a common intracellular domain, with the latter influencing T-cell signaling via its phosphatase activity and, hence, its ability to influence the phosphorylation of the tyrosine kinase, *lck* (19,20). The CD45RA (high molecular weight) and the CD45RO (low molecular weight) isoforms of CD45 define virtually nonoverlapping populations of T cells that differ in a number of important ways (21,22). First, the RA$^+$ T-cell population manifests a greater proliferative response to mitogens than the RO$^+$ population, whereas the reverse is true with respect to recall antigens. In addition, newborn T cells are composed mainly of RA$^+$ T cells, but with age, the number of RO$^+$ T cells increases as a fraction of the total T-cell population, first rapidly and then more gradually. These facts have led to the concept that the CD45RA$^+$ T cells are mainly "naive" T cells whereas the CD45RO$^+$ T cells are mainly "memory" T cells, or at least contain the memory T-cell subpopulation. Second, when T cells are activated, they rapidly gain RO expression and gradually lose RA expression. Moreover, unstimulated RO$^+$ T cell populations contain cells that express activation markers whereas RA$^+$ T cells do not, and RO$^+$ T cells are larger than RA$^+$ T cells and appear to contain subpopulations of rapidly dividing, more short-lived cells. These facts have given rise to the view that RO$^+$ T cells are, in reality, a type of activated T cell (albeit not necessarily a dividing T cell) that arises from RA$^+$ T cells as a result of exposure to antigens; this fits well with the view that although RO$^+$ T cells appear to be a stable, differentiated T-cell form, they are, in fact, capable of reverting back to CD45RA T cells. In the latter sense, CD45RA T cells may contain a small but definite subpopulation of memory cells. Third, CD45RA and CD45RO T cells differ in their capacity to produce cytokines: although both cell types produce IL-2, only CD45RO T cells produce large amounts of other cytokines such as IFN-γ, IL-4, and GM-CFS. This fact helps to explain why CD4/CD45RO T cells are the classic helper T cells that support B-cell differentiation and immunoglobulin production; however, it does not explain why CD4/CD45RA T cells act as suppressor/inducer T cells or direct suppressor cells. In the latter regard, it may be that RA$^+$ cells produce a range of cytokines whose net effect is inhibition of B-cell responses, but this remains to be proven. Fourth and finally, CD45RA T cells express far fewer adhesion markers on their surface than CD45RO T cells. This has the important consequence that RO$^+$ cells have a greater capacity to interact with vascular epithelium in both normal and inflamed tissue sites. Recently, it has been shown that the capacity to do so may be dependent on arrays of adhesion markers that are tissue-specific (23).

On the basis of these background facts, one compelling explanation of the reduced CD4/CD45RA T cells in CFS is that patients are being exposed on a chronic (ongoing) basis to an antigen stimulus inducing conversion of CD45RA to CD45RO T cells and/or maintaining CD45RO T cells in the RO$^+$ state. The fact that CD45RO T cells were not increased, as one might expect if this population arose from CD45RA T cells, is not against this hypothesis since it is possible that CD45RO T cells, once formed, leave the circulation and enter tissues, as mentioned previously. It should be noted, however, that the CD45RO T cells in CFS contained a larger subset of cells bearing adhesion markers than "ordinary" CD45RO T cells. Thus, the case can be made that there are two manifestations of increased antigen exposure in CFS, one the increased conversion of CD45RA into CD45RO T cells, and the second the increased induction of adhesion markers on CD45RO T cells.

Additional support for the view that reduced CD45RA T-cell levels in CFS are due to chronic antigenic stimulation comes from the fact that in several autoimmune states such as multiple sclerosis, systemic lupus erythematosus, and rheumatoid arthritis, one also sees reductions in CD45RA T cells, particularly during periods of disease exacerbation (22). Furthermore, diminished numbers of CD45RA T cells are observed in an immunodeficiency state such as common variable immunodeficiency, a disease in which one assumes that chronic infection with a variety of organisms may be present (24). Finally, decreased numbers of CD45RA T cells are seen in patients following bone marrow transplantation, where the allogeneic environment of the host provides a chronic antigenic stimulus to the immune system (25).

A decreased number of CD45RA T cells and an altered population of CD45RO T cells in CFS should also be manifest in the ability of CFS T cells to proliferate to various stimuli and to produce cytokines. We shall, therefore, return to a discussion of the functional consequences of a shift in the ratio of CD45RA/CD45RO T cells, when we discuss other immunological abnormalities present in CFS.

T-Cell Activation in CFS

In view of the finding that T-cell populations in CFS show evidence of having undergone antigen exposure and differentiation into a more mature (memory)

T-cell phenotype, it is of some interest to know if T cells in CFS patients express activation antigens as more immediate markers of antigenic exposure. The data on this question are equivocal. Tirelli et al. reported that CD3 T cell of CFS patients contained a significantly increased subset of cells expressing HLA-DR (MHC class II) antigens (6), while Klimas et al. (3) and Landy et al. (11) reported increased percentages of CD8 T cells (but not of CD4 T cells) bearing HLA-DR antigens. In the Landay study, the increased HLA-DR expression on CD8 T cells was accompanied by increased expression of CD38 (another surface antigen occuring on cells after cell activation), but not by increased expression of CD25, the IL-2 receptor. This constellation of markers suggests that the CD8 T cells are in a chronically rather than an acutely activated state. Another finding in this study was that the CD8 T cell manifested reduced co-expression of CD11b, at least in those patients with severe disease; this suggested that the CD8 T cells belonged to a subset of cytolytic rather than suppressor T cells. However, this does not fit with the fact that in this study and other studies (5), the CD8 T cells in the mononuclear cell population as a whole did not manifest increased expression of CD57, the latter molecule being one that also appears on suppressor CD8 T cells (26). Thus, the data is unclear with relation to whether CD8 T cells in CFS show evidence of abnormal differentiation into active cytolytic cells.

Overall, the evidence presented by Landy suggesting increased CD8 T-cell activation in CFS does correlate with the findings discussed earlier relating to the decreased CD45RA T cells and increased CD45RO T cells displaying adhesion markers in CFS; however, in the major study in which the CD45RA/RO abnormality was observed, the study of Straus et al. (5), no increase in HLA-DR, CD25, or CD38 expression was noted. Thus, additional study will be necessary to clarify the phenotype of CD8 T cells in CFS.

T-Cell Function in CFS

T-cell function in CFS has been evaluated using a variety of in vivo and in vitro assays. Turning first to in vivo assays, both Murdoch (27) and Lloyd et al. (14) reported that patients with CFS manifest cutaneous anergy. Thus, in the study of Lloyd et al., involving some 20 patients as well as equal numbers of normal controls and patients with depression, 10 of the 20 patients had "abnormal" delayed hypersensitivity skin tests, as evaluated with seven commercially available skin test antigens (14). More particularly, 6/20 were "hypoergic", i.e., had reduced responses, and 4/20 had full-blown cutaneous anergy; in comparison, only 2/20 normal controls and 2/20 depressed patients were hypoergic and none were anergic. These differences were statistically significant and suggest that patients with CFS manifest deficient in vivo T-cell function. Very similar findings were obtained in an earlier study by Murdoch, involving 33 patients (27). However, DuBois et al. (28) in a study of 6 patients and the study of Straus et al., involving 20 patients (5), found essentially no cutaneous anergy, albeit under less stringent conditions than that of Murdoch (27) and Lloyd et al. (14).

The preceding somewhat equivocal evidence that CFS patients manifest in vivo abnormalities of T-cell function finds corroboration in several studies of the capacity of patients' cells to undergo proliferation upon stimulation with mitogens in vitro. In these studies, CFS lymphocytes have usually (but not always) been shown to manifest reduced proliferation compared to normals using a spectrum of mitogens including PHA, Con A, and pokeweed mitogen (2,3,5,10,13). In addition, in one study the proliferative response to *Staphylococcus* enterotoxin B (SEB), a so-called superantigen that interacts with T cells via nonpolymorphic determinants present on the variable region of the β chain of one of the T-cell receptor families, was also reduced (5). The response to SEB is of considerable interest because it shows that T-cell signaling via the T-cell receptor, rather than the variety of receptors potentially acted upon by mitogens, may be abnormal in CFS patients. In confirmation of this conclusion, it has also been shown that patient responses to anti-CD3 antibodies capable of reacting directly with a component of the T-cell receptor are also reduced (29).

As in other areas of the immunological study of CFS, the data on T-cell proliferation are not entirely consistent. Thus, in studies by Jones et al. (30), Milton et al. (31), and Borysiewicz et al. (34), normal proliferative responses to mitogens were observed. This could conceivably be explained by the relatively small size of the patient groups in these studies, coupled with the fact that in the positive studies cited earlier, the difference between the patient group and the control group was small, albeit significant. More difficult to explain are the results of Gupta and Vayuvegula, who reported on proliferative responses to mitogens in a group of some 20 patients and matched controls (4). In this case, however, the investigators found that stimulation of patient cells with a variety of soluble antigens (*Candida albicans*, mumps, tetanus toxoid, and *Escherichia coli* antigens) was mildly to moderately reduced. This may indicate that in this patient group, the lymphocyte proliferation defect was more subtle and thus only discernible with a lesser (antigenic) stimulus.

A second and more functionally relevant assay of T-cell function is the measurement of the capacity of stimulated T cells to secrete cytokines. Using this test, CFS patient groups have again shown abnormalities, usually decreased lymphokine production. Specifically, in a series of studies, it was found that patient cells (peripheral blood lymphocytes) produce less IL-2 and IFN-γ when stimulated by lectin mitogens (PHA, Con A, and pokeweed mitogen) or with the "biochemical mitogen," PMA (2,3,5,9,10,13,31). In one of these studies, that conducted by Kibler et al. (9), there was a good correlation between the IFN-γ and IL-2 abnormality in individual patients in linear regression analysis; this indicates that the lymphokine production defect, when present, tends to affect several lymphokines at once, rather than one or another lymphokine randomly.

These findings are counterbalanced by those of Morte et al. (32), who found normal interferon production, and Altmann et al. (33), who found increased interferon production in CFS. However, these latter studies were performed with relatively small groups of patients and with generally less specific assay techniques, so they must necessarily carry less weight than the other studies of IFN-γ production cited.

As for cellular production of other cytokines, Chao et al. showed that mononuclear cells of CFS patients stimulated with LPS or PHA produced increased amounts of IL-6, and cells stimulated with LPS also produced increased amounts of TNF-α and IL-1β (10). In addition, while patients had elevated TGF-β levels in their serum (see below), LPS-stimulated mononuclear cells of CFS patients produced less TGF-β than controls, and PHA-stimulated cells produced normal amounts of TGF-β.

A final assay of in vitro T-cell function in CFS involves the evaluation of T-cell cytolytic and suppressor function, generally but not exclusively the function of activated CD8 T cells. In a study of T-cell cytolytic function, Borysiewicz et al. (34) found that in four CFS patients, the ability of cytolytic T cells to retard/prevent the outgrowth of Epstein-Barr virus-transformed B cells was markedly diminished in the so-called Epstein-Barr virus regression assay devised by Rickinson et al. (35). Of interest, such specific cytolytic T-cell dysfunction was not associated with general cytolytic T-cell dysfunction, inasmuch as patient cells could be induced to lyse HLA-mismatched target cells following stimulation by the latter in a mixed lymphocyte reaction. This interesting finding has not been followed up in a large group of CFS patients, and it remains unclear if it is found in patients generally, or only in a subgroup who have had a prior and/or recent Epstein-Barr virus infection.

In a corresponding study of suppressor T-cell function in CFS, Tosato et al. showed that T cells of CFS patients have a normal capacity to "help" autologous B cells to differentiate into immunoglobulin-producing plasma cells in a pokeweed mitogen-induced culture system; nevertheless, when CFS T cells (particularly those obtained from patients with high Epstein-Barr virus antibody titers) were admixed with normal (allogeneic) B cells, they suppressed the latter's ability to differentiate (36). To put these findings into perspective, Tosato et al. showed that while patients with acute infectious mononucleosis had T cells that exert excessive suppression of autologous B cells, those recently recovered from acute infectious mononucleosis have T cells that exert excessive suppression on allogeneic B cells, but not autologous B cells. Thus, CFS patients appear to be "frozen" in a functional state normally occurring during recovery from acute Epstein-Barr virus infection.

Several possible explanations can be put forward to explain the T-cell function and lymphokine production abnormalities noted above. The simplest of these is that CFS patients have a mild, but definite immunodeficiency state characterized by a reduced T-cell capacity to become activated by various stimuli. The mechanism underlying such hypothetical immunodeficiency is quite unclear, but it can be said that reduced IL-2 production is not its cause, since IL-2 production in CFS is quite adequate to support normal T-cell proliferation. Another possible explanation of the T-cell dysfunction is that the T cells present in peripheral blood in CFS are enriched for a cellular subset that manifests reduced responses to mitogens. This explanation, at first glance, would fit with the fact that CD45RA T cells are known to respond to mitogens more vigorously than CD45RO T cells and, as we have seen, the former are reduced in CFS (22). However, T cells in CFS patients also respond less well to anti-CD3 antibodies (i.e., antibodies capable of crosslinking an integral component of the T-cell receptor) and also less well to superantigen (SEB) or recall antigens, which preferentially activate CD45RO T cells, a cell type not reduced in CFS. Furthermore, CD45RA T cells are poor producers of IFN-γ, yet this is one of the lymphokines whose production is deficient in CFS. An alternative, and perhaps more viable, explanation of the T-cell dysfunction based on the presence of an altered T-cell subset involves the fact that the CD45RO T cell subset in CFS is abnormal in the sense that it contains an increased number of cells bearing adhesion markers. Thus, while "normal" CD45RO T cells may indeed manifest increased responses to various stimuli (in comparison with CD45RA T cells), the CD45RO T cells in CFS may actually be hyporesponsive to these stimuli, because they are in a hyper-differentiated state. This concept is of particular interest because it leaves open the possibility that while CFS T cells are deficient in their capacity to produce certain lymphokines (IL-2 and IFN-γ), they may have an increased capacity to secrete as yet unidentified lymphokines that play a role in disease patho-genesis.

A final possible explanation for the decreased proliferative and lymphokine responses in CFS is that the T cells are under the influence of suppressor T cells that squelch responses. Some evidence for this possibility is inherent in a study by Tosato et al., who, as mentioned previously, found that at least certain patients with CFS have increased suppressor T-cell activity (36). However, in the Tosato studies suppression was seen when the T cells were stimulated by pokeweed mitogen-activated allogeneic cells and not seen in an autologous cell culture system in which they were stimulated by pokeweed mitogen-activated autologous cells. Thus, if suppression is indeed occuring in cultures where proliferation is being measured in response to mitogens, one would have to postulate that in the latter situation a strong T-cell stimulus (PHA or Con A) is inducing one T-cell population (? a $CD8^+$ T-cell population) to suppress another autologous T-cell population (? a $CD4^+$ T-cell population). One way to test this possibility is to perform cell-mixing studies with CFS T cells and normal T cells to determine if the former reduce the responses of the latter.

Circulating Cytokines in CFS

The studies of lymphokine/cytokine production by CFS T cells stimulated in culture, as discussed before, have been complemented by studies of circulating serum or plasma cytokine levels in CFS patients. Considering circulating IL-2 and IFN-γ levels first (the lymphokines produced in decreased amounts by lymphocytes stimulated in vitro), Straus et al. found that IL-2 levels in 25 patients were measurable and normal, while Chao et al. found that levels in 10 patients and 10 controls were undetectable (10,37). In addition, Linde et al. found measurable and normal levels of IFN-γ in 35 patients, while Lloyd et al. found undetectable IFN-γ levels in both serum and cerebrospinal fluid in 25 patients and 28 controls (38,39). Of interest, in the latter study low but detectable levels of IFN-γ were found in patients with CNS infection. These studies showing no difference between patients and controls are in contrast with a single study of some 104 patients conducted by Cheney et al., who found very high circulating IL-2 levels in CFS patients compared with controls (40); however, these data can be safely discounted in view of the Straus and Chao studies. Turning next to circulating IFN-α levels, Straus et al., in the study cited before, as well as in an earlier study, found undetectable levels in both patients and controls using two types of assay procedures (37,41). On the other hand, Ho-Yen et al. found an increase in the mean level of IFN-α in 15 patients (0.76 ± 1.08 IU/ml in CFS patients vs. 0.20 ± 0.21 IU/ml in controls), whereas Lloyd et al. found no difference in serum IFN-α levels between patients and controls and a nonsignificant increase in patient cerebrospinal fluid IFN-α levels; as in the case of IFN-γ, cerebrospinal fluid levels of IFN-α in CFS patients were lower than those in patients with CNS infection (39,42).

Taken together, the above data relating to IFN levels in CFS (both IFN-γ and IFN-α) suggest that these levels are essentially normal. However, one piece of information discordant with this conclusion should be mentioned: circulating levels of an enzyme activated by exposure of cells to interferons, $2',5'$-oligoadenylate synthetase, has been shown to be increased in two separate (but small) groups of CFS patients (43,44). Thus, normal IFN levels in CFS are paradoxically associated with a possible cellular footprint of increased IFN secretion. How this finding relates to decreased mitogen-induced IFN-γ secretion in vitro is unknown.

A variety of studies have focused on the level of inflammatory cytokines in CFS, including IL-1α, IL-1β, IL-6, TNF-α, IL-10, and TGF-β. One provocative observation made in this area is that of Linde et al., who showed that IL-1α levels were increased about twofold in 35 CFS patients, as compared with levels in 18 healthy controls (38). Of interest, an equal increase in IL-1α levels was seen in patients with primary Epstein-Barr virus infection, but not in patients who were 6 months postinfection; thus, CFS patients differed from those recovering from Epstein-Barr virus infection, in contradistinction to those patients studied by Tosato et al. (36) with respect to suppressor cells. Unfortunately, the finding of Linde et al. regarding a raised IL-1α level in CFS has not yet been corroborated and, in fact, in unpublished studies by Fritz et al. (29), IL-α levels were undetectable in the plasma of 20 CFS patients.

As for levels of other inflammatory cytokines, Chao et al. and Fritz et al. found that TNF-α and IL-10 levels in both CFS patients and controls were usually undetectable, whereas Lloyd found that TNF-α levels in CFS patients and controls were measurable and equivalent in both serum and cerebrospinal fluid (10,29). In addition, circulating IL-β levels were found to be mostly undetectable in both CFS patients and controls (10,29,38), while circulating IL-6 levels, although found to be increased in a distinct subset of CFS patients by Chao et al. in an initial study, were found to be normal in a follow-up study (10,45); other data on serum IL-6 levels were in agreement with the second study; i.e., levels were undetectable in both CFS patients and controls (29).

An interesting exception to the preceding generally negative data on circulating cytokine levels in CFS is the finding of Chao et al. of distinctly raised circulating TGF-β levels (290 ± 46 pg/ml in CFS patients vs. 104 ± 18 pg/ml in controls) (10). In follow-up studies, these investigators have also shown that following mild exercise, CFS patients manifested even higher TGF-β levels (>400 pg/ml) (46). These data are somewhat suspect, however, since they were not normally distributed. In addition, the data were obtained with the use of a bioassay whose specificity was not completely validated, despite the fact that addition of anti-TGF-β to the assay abolished positive results. In addition, Fritz et al., using a specific ELISA assay, found no evidence of raised TGF-β levels in CFS patients (29).

Finally, it is important to mention that serum levels of various immunological products associated with the presence of activated lymphoid cells on macrophages have been determined, including sIL2-R (29,38,40), CD8 antigens (38), IL-2 receptor antagonist (29), and neopterin (38,39,45). The levels of all of these have been normal with the exception of neopterin, which was increased in one of the three studies (45).

Overall, the preceding studies on circulating levels of various lymphokines and cytokines in CFS have not yielded evidence of a clear-cut and reproducible abnormality of lymphokine/cytokine secretion in CFS. Taken at face value, this is an important negative finding since, if one assumes that an abnormality of immune function is the basis of the manifestations of CFS, one would also assume that lymphokine/cytokine effects on various organs, particularly the central nervous system, is the main mechanism involved. The data on lymphokine/cytokine secretion in CSF, however, cannot be taken at face value. The fact is that in many cases, circulating levels were below the level of detectability with the methods available, and it is thus possible that with more sensitive methods, abnormalities will be found. In addition, the serum may be a poor place to look for lymphokine/cytokine abnormalities, because of the rapid clearance of such substances from the circulation; one may have to look in tissue fluids to find abnormalities. Rapid clearance may also explain the fact that although subtle abnormalities of IL-2 and IFN-γ secretion can be detected in vitro, they cannot be detected in vivo. Finally, it is fair to point out that the set of cytokines so far identified is incomplete; thus it remains possible that an as yet unrecognized lymphocyte/monocyte product may yet be identified as a cause of symptoms in CFS.

B-CELL PHENOTYPE AND FUNCTION IN CFS

B cells, no less than T cells, have been subjected to considerable scrutiny in CFS, from both a phenotypic and functional perspective. B-cell numbers, as quantitated by a variety of B-cell-specific monoclonal antibodies, have generally been normal in CFS (4,5,9) or, at most, mildly increased (3) or decreased (47), the latter in patients with recent-onset disease. In addition, in two studies the fraction of B cells expressing CD5, an antigen associated with B cells capable of producing polyspecific antibodies (autoantibodies), was increased (3,6), but this was not found in a third study by Straus et al. (5). Finally, there has been no phenotypic evidence of B-cell activation in CFS, inasmuch as B cells in patients with the disease do not express CD23, a B-cell activation marker (5).

B-cell function in CFS, as disclosed by in vitro responses of patients' mononuclear cells to pokeweed mitogen, has usually, but not always, been normal. Thus, both Tosato et al., in a study discussed previously (36), and Chao et al. (10) have shown that peripheral cells from CFS patients produce normal amounts of Ig when stimulated with pokeweed mitogen in the presence of autologous or allogeneic T cells, whereas Borysiewicz et al. (34) and Hamblin et al. (48) found reduced Ig production by pokeweed mitogen-stimulated B cells. The finding that CFS B cells perform normally in vitro finds corroboration in numerous studies of spontaneous antibody responses in vivo. In this regard, patients' responses to various naturally occurring viral pathogens, such as Coxsackie virus and Epstein-Barr virus, are, if anything, quite robust; it was these responses that first drew attention to the possibility of chronic infection as a cause of CFS.

Unfortunately, this evidence of normal B-cell function, both in vitro and in vivo, does not rule out the possibility that CFS patients have a qualitative B-cell function defect involving the ability to produce one or another Ig class or subclass. Evidence that such a defect does in fact exist in CFS comes mainly from Lloyd and his colleagues, who have reported extensively on Ig class and subclass levels in patients with CFS (49). In an initial study (involving some 69 patients), these investigators reported that a substantial fraction of CFS patients (23%) had decreased IgM levels, a small fraction (4%) had decreased IgA levels, and a surprisingly high fraction (56%) had IgG subclass deficiencies, especially IgG3 subclass (44%) and IgG1 subclass deficiencies (17%). The IgG3 and IgG1 deficiencies were statistically significant in comparison to a simultaneously studied control group. In a later study conducted by the same investigators, this time comprising 78 patients and 71 controls (probably encompassing the original patient group), total IgG levels were found to be decreased (11.3 ± 3.2 g/L in CFS patients vs. 13.2 ± 3.1 g/L in controls; $p < 0.05$) as were IgG1, IgG2, and IgG3 subclass levels (IgG4 levels were normal) (49). The most severe of the subclass abnormalities was the IgG3 deficiency (0.49 ± 0.27 g/L in CFS patients vs. 0.63 ± 3.1 g/L in controls; $p < 0.01$). Of interest, these Ig subclass abnormalities did not correlate with age, sex, or disease duration.

The findings of Lloyd et al. are partially supported by studies of other large groups of CFS patients in which abnormalities of Ig levels involving one or another Ig class has been found in some individuals (28,43,50–53). In addition, there are sporadic reports of cases of CFS with IgG1, IgG3, and IgG4 deficiency, alone or in combination (1,53,54). It is not clear, however, that such abnormalities represent anything more than normal variation in Ig level since, in contrast to the data of Lloyd et al., the data were not clearly related to normal control values. Then, too, the findings of Lloyd et al. can be questioned as to physiological meaning, since the magnitude of the deficiencies found was not impressive and the data required large numbers of patients to reach statistical significance. In addition, it is not clear that the abnormalities identified by Lloyd et al. are reproducible over time, a critical question in view of the many vagaries of measuring IgG subclass levels. Finally, abnormalities of Ig levels in CFS have not been verified with studies of the capacity of patients to respond to de novo antigen challenge with the production of class- and subclass-specific antibodies to the challenge antigens.

Assuming, for the moment, that the class and subclass deficiencies are real, one can reasonably inquire as to their provenance. One possibility is based on the now considerable evidence that Ig class and subclass synthesis depends on lymphokine/cytokine levels, which control Ig production at the level of either isotype switch differentiation or terminal differentiation. Thus, the abnormalities could reflect the more fundamental lymphokine/cytokine defect. However, the fact that the patients as a group manifest a number of different Ig abnormalities would force one to postulate that CFS is associated with a number of different cytokine abnormalities, which vary from patient to patient. In addition, one would expect that if indeed a cytokine deficiency underlies the Ig abnormality, the deficiency would be quite apparent given the levels of cytokine known to be necessary to affect Ig expression in vitro. Overall, therefore, it is difficult to ascribe the Ig abnormalities to an underlying cytokine abnormality, and one must, at the moment, admit that the cause of this abnormality, if it exists in CFS, is unknown.

Despite the uncertain significance of Ig-level abnormalities in CFS, two double-blind, placebo-controlled trials, testing the effect of treating CFS patients with intravenous gammaglobulin, have been conducted, one with a group of 49 patients (study 1) and a second with a group of 49 patients (study 2) (55,56). In both studies a substantial number of patients had Ig deficiency, but in study 1 the type of deficiency was variable as to class and subclass, and in study 2 the type of deficiency was unstated. One difference in the studies was the IVIG dose; in study 1, 1 g/kg was administered (once per month for 6 months) and in study 2, 2 g/kg was given (once per month for 3 months). A second difference was treatment assessment; in study 1, a self-assessment examination was used exclusively, whereas in study 2, both blind-physician assessment and self-assessment were used.

The results of the two studies led to opposite conclusions (55,56). In study 1 (the lower-dose study), no significant improvement in symptoms was seen, whereas in study 2 (the high-dose study), a significant improvement was seen: 43% of patients on IVIG improved vs. 11% on placebo. This improvement correlated with simultaneous improvement in CD4 T-cell levels, PHA responses, and delayed hypersensitivity (skin test) responses. In fact, patients with these cell-mediated defects (and with Ig abnormalities) at the start of the study, were said to be more likely to respond to IVIG than those without abnormalities. This suggested that an immune defect does underlie many cases of CFS and that the immune defect is reversed by IVIG therapy. However, it is difficult to understand how the correction of a manifestation of a B-cell defect (Ig level) could actually improve T-cell function, and it seems likely that additional confirmatory data will be necessary to really substantiate the role of IVIG therapy in CFS.

Autoantibodies in CFS

A final abnormality to consider under the heading of altered B-cell function is the occurrence of autoantibodies in CFS, although such antibodies might also owe their origin to T-cell abnormalities.

As already mentioned, the presence of increased numbers of CD5 B cells in CFS, i.e., B cells associated with autoimmunity, is claimed by some, but not all, investigators to be elevated in CFS. Somewhat more convincing evidence of autoimmune abnormalities has been the rather frequent finding of antinuclear antibodies and rheumatoid factor in CFS patients, although these are present in low concentration and then only in a small subset of patients (1). In addition, other antibodies such as antithyroid antibody, antismooth muscle antibody and antigastric parietal cell antibody, anti-insulin and -insulin receptor antibody have been reported by several investigators in a variable proportion of patients (1). Finally, findings not infrequently associated with the presence of autoantibodies, cryoglobulins, cold agglutinins, and immune complexes have been found in patients by various investigators (2,43,47). It is difficult to assess the significance of these findings because they have generally been obtained in the absence of evaluation of control groups, are present only in a minority of patients, and have occurred in the absence of frank autoimmune disease. Thus, it seems most likely that these findings are best explained as secondary manifestations of an underlying immunological disturbance, perhaps due to the increased T-cell maturation and/or activation, as discussed before, which leads to stimulation of B-cell subsets capable of producing autoantibodies.

NATURAL KILLER CELLS IN CFS

Another cell type extensively studied in CFS is the natural killer (NK) cell, a non-MHC-restricted cytolytic cell thought to be important in immune surveillance against tumor cells or virally infected cells (57). Generally speaking, NK cells are large cells containing granules and bear on their surface both the CD16 (Leu-11) and CD56 (NKH-1) antigens. These markers, plus the absence of the CD3 marker, differentiate these cells from T cells. NK cells mediate cytotoxicity by at least two mechanisms. First, they bind to and lyse antibody-coated target cells via interaction of their Fc receptor (the CD16 molecule) with the Fc portion of the coating antibody. This interaction is known as antibody-dependent cellular cytotoxicity (ADCC). Second, they bind directly to and lyse certain target cells, even in the absence of antibody, via as yet poorly characterized receptor molecules.

NK Cell Phenotype in CFS

The impetus to study NK cells in CFS has come from the presumed association of the syndrome with Epstein-Barr virus infection or other viral infections. In the most extensive study of NK cells in CFS, that conducted by Caliguri et al. and initially involving 12 patients and six matched controls, NK cells (identified by the simultaneous presence of CD56 and CD16 and the absence of CD3) were reduced in patients (4.9% ± 3.1% in patients vs. 10.4% ± 5.2% in controls) (58). Similar results were obtained by the same investigators in a second, independent study of 29 patients and 17 controls. In both studies, the percentages of CD56$^+$ cells also bearing CD3$^+$ cells in patients were normal. These findings were subsequently corroborated by those of Gupta and Vayuvegula, who, in a study of 20 patients and matched controls, also noted an approximately 50% decrease in the number of CD16 and CD56 cells (4). However, Kibler et al. found normal numbers of NK cells in a study of 13 patients, when such cells were identified by morphological characteristics (9).

A somewhat different abnormality of NK cell phenotype was found by Morrison et al. (59). In the study conducted by these investigators (involving 23 patients), the percentage of mononuclear cells bearing CD56 was increased (26.5% in CFS patients vs. 18.1% in controls); in addition, the cells expressing CD56 at a high density (CD56^{bright}) were particularly increased (7.6% in CFS patients vs. 0.4 in controls), suggesting that the increase in the CD56^{+} population as a whole was actually due to an increase in the CD56^{bright} subpopulation. The CD56^{bright} cell population appeared to be activated cells, since most coexpressed CD71 (the transferrin receptor) and CD25 (the α chain of the IL-2 receptor). Whether or not these cells are conventional NK cells is unclear since coexpression of CD16 on these cells was not directly measured. However, the percentage of total CD56^{+} cells coexpressing CD3, a T-cell marker, was increased (42.2% in CFS patients vs. 21.8% in controls) and the percentage of CD56^{+} cells bearing CD16 (a marker found exclusively on NK cells) was decreased (54.1% in CFS patients vs. 86.5% in controls). If one assumes that these changes are due to the presence of CD56^{bright} cells, then the latter would appear to be a T-cell subset that also bears a marker (CD56) more usually found on NK cells. Indeed, it is known that CD56 is normally expressed on a small subpopulation of T cells, which may, in fact, have NK-like function under some circumstances. Increased numbers of CD56 cells in CFS were also found in patients studies by Klimas et al., Tirelli et al., and Chao et al. (3,6,10). The data obtained by Tirelli et al., in concert with the previously described data of Morrison, showed that the percentage of CD16^{+}/CD3– cells was decreased and the percentage of CD56^{+}/CD16^{-} cells was increased, as were CD56^{+}/CD8^{+} cells in CFS.

Finally, Ho-Yen et al. determined the number of CD56^{+} cells in patients with "postviral" fatigue syndrome, a variant of CFS in which symptoms can be clearly related to an initiating viral illness (12). These authors found that CD56^{+} cells were substantially increased in 20/50 patients, decreased in 8/50 patients, normal in 17/50 patients and low initially and then normal in 5/50 patients. In addition, CD8^{+} T cells were elevated in the patients with either high or low CD56^{+} cells. These data suggest first that CD56^{+} cell levels may vary during the course of disease and second that CFS is a heterogeneous patient group with respect to CD56^{+} cells, even within a single study group. One possible cause of this heterogeneity is that CD56^{+} cells, as implied earlier, may be increased in some patients because of a T-cell defect and decreased in others because of an NK-cell defect.

Functional Studies of NK Activity in CFS

Studies of the functional activity of NK cells in CFS complement the above-described phenotype studies. The most complete of such studies was that of Caliguri et al., who showed that whether NK activity is measured using a conventional target cell (the erythroleukemic cell K-562) or with an EBV-transformed B-cell target (LAZ 388), NK-induced lysis mediated by CFS patient cells is only about one-third that of control cells (58) (see Fig. 2). NK cells from many patients did, however, respond to IL-2 with increased NK activity (as do NK cells from normal individuals), and the fraction of patients with abnormal values fell after IL-2 preincubation. Since such preincubation blocks that portion of NK activity mediated by CD56$^+$ T cells, i.e., the cells mentioned previously that may be increased in CFS patients, this form of nonspecific cytolytic activity may be normal, or even increased, in CFS.

Decreased NK activity has also been observed by Klimas et al. (3) and Kibler et al. (9), but not by Gold et al. (13), in each case using K-562 target cells. In the Klimas study (30 patients and 73 controls), cytolytic activity was 9% in CFS patients versus 25% in controls, and patients displayed a decrease in maximal killing velocity (cells killed in 4 hr). In this study, decreased NK functional activity was associated with increased levels of CD56 cells. This paradox is resolved if it is assumed, as implied above, that the CD56 cells do not in fact represent NK cells. In the Kibler study, NK activity of unfractionated cells was clearly decreased in CFS patients compared to controls, whereas isolated large granular lymphocytes were only marginally decreased. This too can be explained

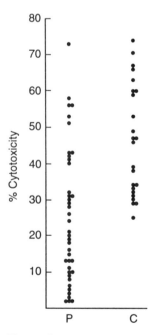

Figure 2 NK activity of CFS patients and controls. P, patients; C, controls. K-562 target cells used.

on the assumption that the large granular lymphocyte population contained large numbers of $CD56^+$ noncytolytic cells.

Also relevant to NK function in CFS is a report by Aoki et al., who reported on 23 patients with "low natural killer syndrome" (LNKS), who clinically resembled those CFS patients in that they manifested prolonged fatigue and low-grade fever (60). While T-cell phenotyping (CD4/CD8 ratios) and T-cell proliferative function in these patients was normal, as were cells bearing the CD16 (NK cell) marker, the patients had reduced NK cytolytic function in assays based on the lysis of K-562 target cells. These patients thus differed from those of Caliguri, who had reduced numbers of $CD16^+$ cells. In the absence of an obvious infectious or neoplastic cause of this abnormality, the authors felt justified in postulating the existence of a new syndrome. However, closer examination of the data discloses that many patients with the same symptoms did not have low NK cytolytic capacity and that the patients studied seem similar, if not identical, to CFS patients. If this is the case, however, it is not clear why these patients have normal $CD16^+$ cell levels, whereas CFS patients have low $CD16^+$ cell levels.

In summary of the data relating to NK cells in CFS, it now seems fairly well established that the number of NK cells defined by CD16 is reduced, whereas the number of NK cells defined by CD56 is reduced, normal, or even increased. This discrepancy can be resolved by assuming that the $CD56^+$ cells are, in many cases, $CD8^+$ T cells (with or without NK cytolytic activity) rather than conventional NK cells. In future studies it will be of interest to focus on the $CD56^+$ cell population to verify that they are in fact T cells and to determine their cytolytic capacity. Finally, it also seems well established that NK cytolytic function is decreased in patients with CFS, but the relation of this abnormality to other immunological aberrancies in CFS is unknown.

MONOCYTE PHENOTYPE AND FUNCTION IN CFS

Monocytes and macrophages have rarely been studied in CFS despite the fact that these cells can also reflect the presence of covert primary or secondary immune abnormalities. Evidence of monocyte abnormalities is inherent in the claim by Buchwald and Komaroff that monocytosis occurs in their cohort of CFS patients (1); however, this is not the case in several studies in which monocytes were quantitated by staining with monocyte-specific antibodies (10,11,61). More solid evidence of a monocyte abnormality comes from a study conducted by Gupta and Vayuvegula (involving 20 patients and matched controls), in which the proportion of monocytes expressing adhesion markers (LFA-1 and ICAM-1) was found to be normal, but the density of these markers on positive cells was significantly increased (4). In addition, while IFN-γ augmented the density of these markers in both CFS patients and controls, the increase was less in the patients, suggesting that monocytes were already at a maximal or near-maximal level of expression of these markers.

This evidence of macrophage activation was also seen in another study of macrophage function in CFS, conducted by Prieto et al (61). In this study (involving 35 "consecutive" patients and 25 healthy controls), the number of monocytes in peripheral blood (as detected with the Leu-M3 antibody) was normal; however, patients could be segregated into two groups with respect to macrophage phenotype and function. One group, comprising 85% of the patients (30 of 35), had markedly reduced numbers of cells displaying the DR antigen (MHC class II), the CR-1 and FcR receptors, and cytoskeletal vimentin filaments (the latter detected with antivimentin antibody); in addition, macrophage-mediated phagocytosis of *Candida albicans* and latex particles was markedly reduced. A second group, containing 15% of patients (five of 35), had normal parameters. These defects were not found in patients with acute infection or with various autoimmune diseases.

Curiously, this monocyte/macrophage abnormality was partially reversed when cells were exposed to the opioid antagonist naloxone, suggesting that the effect was due to the action of opioids on monocytes; however, serum β-endorphin levels were normal and serum enkephalins were not measured. The authors speculated that chronic viral infection, or simply stress, leads to increased opioid production and the observed changes in macrophage function. If this is so, one should see similar macrophage abnormalities in other states characterized by these putative factors, and this has yet to be reported. Finally, whatever its cause, the effect of the observed macrophage abnormality may be responsible for certain aspects of T-cell dysfunction. For instance, the proliferative and lymphokine production defects discussed earlier could, in reality, be secondary to reduced macrophage function. At the moment, however, this seems unlikely since relatively few macrophages and monocytes are necessary to support normal lymphocyte responses to mitogens and antigens.

ALLERGY IN CFS

Allergies are a common complaint in CFS and are said to occur more frequently in the syndrome than in control individuals. It is yet to be established, however, that this symptom complex is due to an abnormality of IgE-mediated immune function. Evidence in favor of the latter is the observation that CFS patients manifest increased rates of cutaneous reactivity to allergens and increased levels of circulating IgE (62,63); in addition, patients with allergies have lymphocytes that undergo proliferative responses upon exposure to allergens (62). Finally, in one study, stimulation of CFS patient cells with an antigen or with allergens caused a significant increase in the numbers of B cells bearing Epstein-Barr virus-associated antigens (EBNA) (64). During the era when Epstein-Barr virus infection was considered to play a major role in CFS, this interesting finding suggested that allergic reactivity might in fact account for the syndrome. Later, however, when this concept was no longer tenable (41), this finding became more difficult to explain. One possibility is that B cells in CFS undergo a type of activation upon stimulation in vitro that is better able to support reactivation of latent Epstein-Barr virus; thus the finding is an indication of altered potential of CFS B cells to react generally, not just with respect to Epstein-Barr virus. In any case, the above findings fall short of proving that IgE-mediated allergy is truly increased in CFS. This conclusion arises from the fact that an undefined hypersensitivity is not infrequently seen in patients with somatic disorders. That this may be the case in CFS is suggested by the findings of a recent study in which CFS patients with and without food intolerance were compared and found to be similar with respect to various psychological factors, except for the fact that patients with food intolerance had a far greater frequency of functional somatic symptoms (65).

CONCLUSION

Immunological findings in CFS, as we have seen, involve virtually every aspect of lymphoid cell function. Yet in most cases, these findings are less than definitive because they are generally not found in all patients and all studies, or because they do not represent sharp departures from normality. On the contrary, much of the data is characterized by small, albeit statistically significant, shifts in cell population values. It remains to be established that these shifts are etiologically important as either primary or secondary factors in disease pathogenesis.

One important abnormality that has been seen by several investigators is a relatively subtle change in circulating CD4 T-cell subpopulations characterized by a reduced subpopulation of CD45RA T cells. This change is strongly reminiscent of clinical and experimental situations in which T cells are subjected to antigenic stimulation and thus induced to undergo transformation from "naïve" CD45RA to "memory" CD45RO T cells. By its very nature, the CD45RA "defect" in CFS is likely to be a secondary abnormality that has arisen from chronic infection rather than being a primary cause of the latter. Nevertheless, one cannot conclude that this abnormality is necessarily the immediate cause of symptomatology in CFS. Thus, one may argue that the presence of an expanded population of mature CD45RO T cells that bear adhesion markers (and therefore have the capability of entering tissues and releasing cytokines at tissue sites) provides at least circumstantial evidence that immunologically mediated processes are responsible for the clinical picture of CFS. Thus far, however, the best available data is that CFS T cells manifest reduced proliferation and lymphokine production (IL-2 and IFN-γ) upon stimulation in vitro. Moreover, there is no convincing evidence that such cells are producing disease-causing cytokines in vivo, inasmuch as the evidence for the presence of abnormal levels of circulating cytokines is generally negative. In the latter regard, reports of increased serum TGF-β levels in CFS have not been confirmed and, in any case, these are found in only a subset of patients. In addition, the major source of TGF-β is not the T cell, but rather the macrophages and other accessory cells. The only other positive data relative to abnormal circulating cytokine levels is the finding of elevated 2'-5'-oligo-adenylate synthetase, a marker of cell stimulation by interferon; however, direct measurement of interferon levels in CFS have yielded normal levels. Overall, these considerations indicate that much remains to be done to complete the circle of proof necessary to establish a link between the T-cell abnormality and production of symptoms in CFS. At the moment, we have only the fact that an abnormality may exist, not that the abnormality is more than an epiphenomenon having little to do with disease pathogenesis.

An immunological abnormality that is of a piece with the T-cell phenotype abnormality in CFS is the finding of Tosato et al. that T cells of CFS patients have an abnormal propensity, when appropriately stimulated, to suppress B-cell synthesis. The nature of the T cell mediating such suppression or, indeed, the mechanism of the suppression itself has not yet been defined. Nevertheless, it is not too much of a stretch to postulate that such suppression is a direct result of the presence in the circulation of memory cells that either induce suppressor cells or mediate suppressor function themselves. One possibility that needs to be explored in this context is that suppression is due to CD8$^+$ T cells bearing CD45RO and adhesion markers.

The findings of Tosato et al. are also important because they establish a relationship between an immune abnormality (immune suppression) and virus antibody titer. This relationship suggests, in turn, that many, or most, of the immune abnormalities in CFS patients are limited to those patients with CFS whose disease began with a more or less clear-cut infectious episode (a mononucleosis-like illness) and who thus may have ongoing disease because of difficulties with clearing the infection. This view is also favored by several reports of individuals who, after an acute infectious illness, develop chronic fatigue syndrome accompanied by a rather obvious immune abnormality, such as lymphocytosis, activated B cells, or lymphadenopathy. Such cases may be a "forme fruste" of CFS that are an extreme example of a large, if not all-encompassing, CFS group (66,67). As a corollary to this, one must also consider the possibility that certain other subgroups of patients with CFS do not fall into this category and thus presumably have chronic fatigue not due to, or associated with, immunological abnormalities. This, of course, would explain why patients differ in their immunological profile, and why averaged immunological values in the group as a whole are generally not particularly impressive. A final point to be made here is that the type of postinfectious immune abnormality found in CFS may well occur in many individuals without symptoms of CFS. Such a group, for instance, could be found among those with high viral antibody titers found in large surveys of "normal" individuals. Thus, the possibility emerges that factors other than immunological abnormalities may be necessary for the development of CFS. We shall return to this possibility later.

One finding in CFS that is contrary to the notion that chronic infection is the cause of the immunological abnormality is the absence of a clear-cut elevation in CD8 T cells and/or the presence of CD8 T cells bearing markers indicative of cell activation, such as CD57. Such cells are commonly found in the presence of chronic viral infection, such as chronic infection with cytomegalovirus, or the human immunodeficiency virus, HIV-1 (26). While elevated numbers of CD8 T cells or CD8 T cells with a clearly altered phenotype were not found, CFS patients do manifest, at least in some studies, elevated numbers of CD56$^+$ cells. Such cells may well be a new, hitherto incompletely appreciated form of activated or differentiated CD8 T cell, which are sentinels of the peculiar, chronic infection characteristic of CFS. This being the case, it would be worthwhile to further define the function and specificity of such CD56$^+$ cells.

A second type of immunological finding in CFS, and one that is considerably different from those involving some aspect of T-cell phenotype or function, is the abnormality of NK cells. On the one hand, it is possible that this abnormality, like the T-cell abnormality, is secondary to an underlying chronic infection. One mechanism that could account for this is a direct cytotoxic effect of the infecting organism on NK cells. A theoretical basis for this possibility is the recent observation that human herpes virus 6 (HHV-6) has been shown to be able to infect and lyse an NK cell line in vitro (68). When it was reported that these CFS patients were infected with HHV-6, this possibility seemed to move from the theoretical to the actual; however, follow-up studies failed to confirm the presence of HHV-6 infection in CFS, and HHV-6 killing of NK cells returned to the status of disease model.

The possibility that the abnormality of NK function is a secondary abnormality relates to the T-cell defects discussed previously. In this regard, NK cell function is augmented by IFN-γ and IL-2, and thus the reduced production of these lymphokines by CFS T cells could be a cause of decreased NK-cell differentiation. This seems unlikely, however, since the IL-2/IFN-γ secretion defect observed in CFS does not seem severe enough to cause the NK disfunction.

It is also possible that the NK abnormality in CFS is a de novo abnormality that is primary to chronic infection, rather than secondary. However, reduced NK activity is actually an unusual finding in clinical immunology, and when it is seen in the context of infection, the latter is usually severe and obvious (60). It is true that in HIV infection one sees reduced NK function; however, in this case NK cells are not reduced as in CFS, and the problem appears to be a qualitative rather than a quantitative NK-cell defect (69). It is of some interest that in one report, treatment of CFS with an immunomodulator (a polysaccharide known as lantinan), which results in considerably increased NK function, has been found to be an effective form of treatment for a small group of patients with CFS (60). This finding would also support a primary role for NK function in CFS were it not for the fact that, in addition, lantinan could and does affect other immune functions, not just NK function. However, the effects of lantinan on the CFS have never been verified.

Whatever the origin or defect in NK function in CFS, this defect remains the most documented and reproducible immunological disorder in the syndrome. As such, it deserves additional and more sophisticated study with the view of gaining a better definition of the precise NK-cell type that is abnormal in CFS, as well as a more complete understanding of the kind of NK-cell target that fails to be lysed in the disease.

Finally, any consideration of whether the various immunological abnormalities in CFS are primary or secondary must ultimately confront the question of whether these abnormalities are an outgrowth of psychological abnormalities that are associated with the disorder. To state this issue more directly: are the immunological findings a result of a chronic stress syndrome, or are they the cause of such a syndrome? The best way to answer this question, short of defining the precise links between immunological abnormalities on the one hand and chronic fatigue and associated symptoms on the other, is to determine whether immunological abnormalities of the types found in CFS are also found in other more classic forms of psychological disease. If, in fact, immunological findings of the type found in CFS are not found in these other disorders, then it may be possible to conclude that the immunological findings in CFS are not simply the result of psychological stress.

Unfortunately, the data available to address this question are equivocal at best (70,73). Thus, in a large study of patients with classical depression, no clear-cut differences between patients and controls could be found with respect to T-cell proliferation or limited studies of T-cell phenotype and NK function (66). However, the patients did manifest a decline in T-cell function with increasing age, whereas controls, if anything, experienced an increase in such function. In another study of a very small number of patients with various forms of depression, findings not unlike those in CFS were found, including phenotypic findings indicative of altered CD4/CD8 ratios, T-cell activation, and T-cell maturation (increased CD45RA⁻ cells) (67). Clearly, these data relating, or not relating, to clear-cut psychological disease and immunological abnormalities are simply not strong enough to prove the hypothesis that the immunological findings in CFS are unique to CFS, and thus that they are not secondary to psychological stress. On the contrary, the possibility that the immunological findings in CFS are also found in more classic psychological diseases remains very much alive. In this context, it is possible that these immunological abnormalities in CFS are secondary to subtle endocrine changes, characteristic of certain abnormal psychological states that transcend the arbitrary diagnostic categories that have been conceived for various psychological diseases.

To conclude, we have discussed at length the immunological data in CFS, and whether the immunological abnormalities found are a primary or secondary manifestation of chronic infection with one or more unknown organisms. In addition, we have discussed the possibility that these abnormalities are primary or secondary to a chronic stress syndrome and possible endocrine changes that occur as a result of the latter. Overall, while one can point to real evidence that immunological abnormalities exist in CFS, one is hard put to relate such abnormalities to genesis of the disease syndrome. If we assume (without a surfeit evidence) that the immunological findings in CFS (and possibly other psychological diseases) are in some way responsible for the symptom complex, what theoretical construct of disease pathogenesis can be imagined? To this observer, the best possibility is that chronic infection of a rather borderline or subclinical nature occurs in individuals with CFS, as well as in individuals without disease, which results in relatively minor abnormalities in the immune system and ultimately the secretion of potentially harmful cytokines. In many, or indeed most, individuals with such infection, these immunological abnormalities do not result in symptoms; however, in patients who eventually develop CFS, the same abnormalities are sensed differently and symptoms do develop. In a variation on this theme, a subtle abnormality of the immune system is preexistent to, and necessary for, the onset and continuance of chronic infection; the infection then introduces new immunological abnormalities and the same pathway of disease pathogenesis indicated above ensues. An important, indeed a key, feature of this hypothesis of CFS is that immunological abnormalities in the syndrome may be necessary for its occurrence, but they are never sufficient: one must have other abnormalities before the immunological deflections of chronic fatigue syndrome will cause disease.

REFERENCES

1. Buchwald D, Komaroff AL. Review of laboratory findings for patients with chronic fatigue syndrome. Rev Infect Dis 1991; 13(Suppl 1):S12–18.
2. Behan PO, Behan WMH, Bell J. The postviral fatigue syndrome—an analysis of the findings in 50 cases. J Infect 1985; 10:211–222.
3. Klimas N, Salvato F, Morgan R, Fletcher MA. Immunologic abnormalities in chronic fatigue syndrome. J Clin Microbiol 1990; 28(6):1403–1410.
4. Gupta S, Vayuvegula B. A comprehensive immunological analysis in chronic fatigue syndrome. Scand J Immunol 1991; 33:319–327.

5. Straus SE, Fritz S, Dale JK, Gould B, Strober W. Lymphocyte phenotype and function in the chronic fatigue syndrome. J Clin Immunol 1993; 13(1):30–40.

6. Tirelli V, Pinto A, Marotta G, Crovato M, Quaia M, De Paoli P, Galligioni E, Santini G. Clinical and immunological study of patients with chronic fatigue syndrome: a case study from Italy. Arch Intern Med 1993; 153:116–117.

7. Buchwald D, Cheney PR, Peterson DL, Henry B, Wormsley SB, Geiger A, Ablashi DV, Salahuddin SZ, Saxinger C, Biddle R, Kikinis R, Jolesz FA, Folks T, Balachandran N, Peter JB, Gallo RC, Komaroff AL. A chronic illness characterized by fatigue, neurologic and immunologic disorders, and active human herpesvirus type 6 infection. Ann Intern Med 1992; 116:103–113.

8. Subira ML, Castilla A, Maria-Pilar C, Prieto J. Deficient display of CD3 on lymphocytes of patients with chronic fatigue syndrome. J Infect Dis 1989; 160:165–166.

9. Kibler R, Lucas D, Hicks MJ, Poulos BT, Jones JF. Immune function in chronic active Epstein-Barr virus infection. J Clin Invest 1985; 5:46–54.

10. Chao CC, Janoff EN, Hu Shuxian, Thomas K, Gallagher M, Tsang M, Peterson PK. Altered cytokine release in peripheral blood mononuclear cell cultures from patients with the chronic fatigue syndrome. Cytokine 1991; 3:292–298.

11. Landay AL, Jessop C, Lennette ET, Levy JA. Chronic fatigue syndrome: clinical condition associated with immune activation. Lancet 1991; 338:707–712.

12. Ho-Yen DO, Billington RW, Urquhart J. Natural killer cells and the postviral fatigue syndrome. Scand J Infect Dis 1991; 23:711–716.

13. Gold D, Bowden R, Sixbey J, Riggs R, Katon WJ, Ashley R, Obrigervitch R, Corey L. Chronic fatigue: a prospective clinical and virologic study. JAMA 1990; 264:48–53.

14. Lloyd A, Hickie I, Hickie C, Dwyer J, Wakefield D. Cell-mediated immunity in patients with chronic fatigue syndrome, healthy control subjects and patients with major depression. Clin Exp Immunol 1992; 87:76–79.

15. Edelman AS, Zolla-Pazner S. AIDS: a syndrome of immune dysregulation, dysfunction, and deficiency. FASEB J 1989; 3:22–30.

16. Reinherz EL, O'Brian C, Rosenthal P, Schlossman SF. The cellular basis of viral-induced immunodeficiency: analysis by monoclonal antibodies. J Immunol 1980; 125:1269–1275.

17. Streuli M, Hall LR, Saga Y, Schlossman SF, Saito H. Differential usage of three exons generates at least five different mRNAs encoding human leukocyte common antigens. J Exp Med 1987; 166:1548–1566.

18. Seldin MF, Morse HC, LeBoeuf RC, Steinberg AD. Establishment of a molecular genetic map of distal mouse chromosome 1: further definition of a conserved linkage group syntenic with human chromosome 1 q. Genomics 1988; 2:41–56.

19. Tonks NK, Charbonneau H, Diltz CD, Fischer EH, Walsh KA. Demonstration that the leukocyte common antigen CD45 is a protein tyrosine phosphatase. Biochemistry 1988; 27:8698–8701.

20. Mustelin T, Coggeshall KM, Altman A. Rapid activation of the T cell tyrosine protein kinase $pp56^{lck}$ by the CD45 phosphotyrosine phosphatase. Proc Natl Acad Sci USA 1989; 86:6302–6308.

21. Beverley PCL. Functional analysis of human T cell subsets defined by CD45 isoform expression. Semin Immunol 1992; 4:35–41.
22. Clement LT. Isoforms of the CD45 common leukocyte antigen family: markers for human T cell differentiation. J Clin Immunol 1992; 12:1–10.
23. Mackay CR. Migration pathways and immunologic memory among T lymphocytes. Semin Immunol 1992; 4:51–58.
24. LeBranchu Y, Thibault G, Degenne C, Bardos P. Deficiency of CD4$^+$CD45R$^+$ T lymphocytes in common variable immunodeficiency. N Engl J Med 1990; 323:276–277.
25. Clement LT, Isacescu I, Champlin R, Giorgi JV, Bradley G. Differentiation of CD4$^+$ T cell subpopulations after allogeneic bone marrow transplantation. Clin Res 1990; 38:432A.
26. Wang ECY, Taylor-Wiedeman J, Perera P, Fisher J, Borysiewicz LK. Subsets of CD8$^+$, CD57$^+$ cells in normal, healthy individuals: correlations with human cytomegalovirus (HCMV) carrier status, phenotypic and functional analysis. Clin Exp Immunol 1993; 94(2):297–305.
27. Murdoch JC. Cell-mediated immunity in patients with myalgic encephalomyelitis syndrome. NZ Med J 1988; 101:511–512.
28. DuBois RE, Seeley JK, Brus I, Sakamoto K, Ballow M, Harada S, Bechtold TA, Pearson G, Purtillo DT. Chronic mononucleosis syndrome. South Med J 1984; 77:1376–1382.
29. Fritz D, Strober W, Dale JK, Straus SE. Unpublished observations.
30. Jones JF, Ray G, Minnich LL, Hicks MJ, Kibler R, Lucas DO. Evidence for active Epstein-Barr virus infection in patients with persistent, unexplained illnesses: elevated anti-early antigen antibodies. Ann Intern Med 1985; 102:1–7.
31. Milton JD, Clements GB, Edwards RH. Immune responsiveness in chronic fatigue syndrome. Postgrad Med J 1991; 67:532–537.
32. Morte S, Castilla A, Civeira M-P, Serrano M, Prieto J. Gamma-interferon and chronic fatigue syndrome [letter]. Lancet 1988; 2:623–624.
33. Altmann C, Larratt K, Golubjatnikov R, Kirmani N, Rytel M. Immunologic markers in the chronic fatigue syndrome. Clin Res 1988; 36:845A.
34. Borysiewicz LK, Haworth SJ, Cohen J, Mundin J, Rickinson A, Sissons JGP. Epstein-Barr virus-specific immune defects in patients with persistent symptoms following infectious mononucleosis. Q J Med 1986; 58:111–121.
35. Rickinson AB, Moss DJ, Pope JH. Long-term T cell mediated immunity to Epstein-Barr virus in man. I. Complete regression of virus-induced transformation in cultures of seropositive donor leukocytes. Int J Cancer 1978; 22:662–668.
36. Tosato G, Straus SE, Henle W, Pike SE, Blease RM. Characteristic T cell dysfunction in patients with chronic active Epstein-Barr virus infection (chronic infectious mononucleosis). J Immunol 1985; 134:3082–3088.
37. Straus SE, Dale JK, Peter JB and Dinarello CA. Circulating lymphokine levels in the chronic fatigue syndrome. J Infect Dis 1989; 160:1085.
38. Linde A, Andersson B, Svensen SB, Ahrne H, Carlsson M, Forsberg P, Hugo H, Kerstorp A, Lenkei R, Lindwall A, Loftenius A, Salb C, Andersson J. Serum levels of lymphokine and soluble cellular receptors in primary Epstein-Barr virus infection and in patients with chronic fatigue syndrome. J Infect Dis 1992; 165:994–1000.

39. Lloyd A, Hickie I, Brockman A, Dwyer J, Wakefield D. Cytokine levels in serum and cerebrospinal fluid in patients with chronic fatigue syndrome and control subjects. J Infect Dis 1991; 164:1023–1024.

40. Cheney PR, Dorman SE, Bell DS. Il-2 and the chronic fatigue syndrome. Ann Intern Med 1989; 110:321.

41. Straus SE, Dale JK, Tobi M, Lawley T, Preble O, Blease RM, Hallahan C, Henle W. Acyclovir treatment of the chronic fatigue syndrome: lack of efficacy in a placebo-controlled trial. N Engl J Med 1988; 319:1692–1698.

42. Ho-Yen DO, Carrington D, Armstrong AA. Myalgic encephalomyelitis and alpha-interferon. Lancet 1988; 1:125.

43. Straus SE, Tosato G, Armstrong G, Lawley T, Preble OT, Henle W, Davey R, Pearson G, Epstein J, Brus I, Blease RM. Persisting illness and fatigue in adults with evidence of Epstein-Barr virus infection. Ann Intern Med 1985; 102:7–16.

44. Morag A, Tobi M, Ravid Z, Revel M, Shattner A. Increased (2'-5')-oligo-adenylate synthetase activity in patients with prolonged illness associated with serological evidence of persistent Epstein-Barr virus infection [letter]. Lancet 1982; 1:744.

45. Chao CC, Gallagher M, Phair J, Peterson PK. Serum neopterin and interleukin 6 levels in chronic fatigue syndrome. J Infect Dis 1990; 162:1412–1413.

46. Peterson PK, Sivi SA, Grammith FC, Schenck CH, Pheley AM, Hu S, Chao CC. Effects of mild exercise on cytokines and cerebral blood flow in chronic fatigue syndrome patients. Clin Diagn Lab Immunol 1994; 1:222–226.

47. Miller NA, Carmichael HA, Calder BD, Behan PO, Bell EJ, McCartney RA, Hall FC. Antibody to coxsackie B virus in diagnosing postviral fatigue syndrome. Br Med J 1991; 302:140–143.

48. Hamblin TJ, Hussain J, Akbar AN, Tang YC, Smith JL, Jones DB. Immunological reason for chronic ill health after infectious mononeucleosis. Br Med J 1983; 287:85–88.

49. Lloyd AR, Wakefield D, Boughton CR, Dwyer JM. Immunological abnormalities in the chronic fatigue syndrome. Med J Aust 1989; 151:122–124.

50. Wakefield D, Lloyd A, Brockman A. Immunoglobulin subclass abnormalities in patients with chronic fatigue syndrome. Pediatr Infect Dis J 1990; 8(Suppl):S50–53.

51. Salit IE. Sporadic postinfectious neuromyasthenia. Can Med Assoc J 1985; 133:659–663.

52. Roubalova K, Roubal J, Skopovy P, Fucikova T, Domorazkova E, Vonka V. Antibody response to Epstein-Barr virus antigens in patients with chronic viral infection. J Med Virol 1988; 25:115–122.

53. Read R, Spickett G, Harvey J, Edwards AJ, Larson HE. IgG1 subclass deficiency in patients with chronic fatigue syndrome [letter]. Lancet 1988; 1:241–242.

54. Linde A, Hammerstrom L, Smith CIE. IgG subclass deficiency and chronic fatigue syndrome [letter]. Lancet 1988; 1:885–886.

55. Peterson PK, Shepard J, Macres M, Schenck C, Crosson J, Rechtman D, Lurie N. A controlled trial of intravenous immunoglobulin G in chronic fatigue syndrome. Am J Med 1990; 5:554–560.

56. Lloyd AR, Hickie I, Brockman A, Hickie C, Wilson A, Dwyer J, Wakefield D. Immunologic and psychologic therapy for patients with chronic fatigue syndrome: a double blind, placebo-controlled trial. Am J Med 1993; 2:197–203.

57. Trinchieri G, Perussia B. Human natural killer cells: biologic and pathologic aspects. Lab Invest 1984; 50:489–494.

58. Caliguri M, Murray C, Buchwald D, Levine H, Cheney P, Peterson D, Komaroff AL, Ritz J. Phenotypic and functional deficiency of natural killer cells in patients with chronic fatigue syndrome. J Immunol 1987; 139:3303–3313.

59. Morrison LJ, Behan WH, Behan PO. Changes in natural killer cell phenotype in patients with post-viral fatigue syndrome. Clin Exp Immunol 1991; 83:441–446.

60. Aoki T, Usuda Y, Miyakoshi H, Tamura K, Herberman RB. Low natural killer syndrome: clinical and immunologic features. Nat Immun Cell Growth Regul 1987; 6:116–128.

61. Prieto J, Subira ML, Castilla A, Serrano M. Naloxone—reversible monocyte dysfunction in patients with chronic fatigue syndrome. Scand J Immunol 1989; 30:13–20.

62. Olson GB, Kanaan MN, Geoffrey MG, Kelley LM, Jones JF. Correlation between allergy and persistent Epstein-Barr virus infections in chronic-active Epstein-Barr virus-infected patients. J Allergy Clin Immunol 1986; 78:308–320.

63. Straus SE, Dale JK, Wright R, Metcalfe DD. Allergy and the chronic fatigue syndrome. J Allergy Clin Immunol 1988; 81:791–795.

64. Olson GB, Kanaan MN, Kelley LM, Jones JF. Specific allergen-induced Epstein-Barr nuclear antigen-positive B cells from patients with chronic-active Epstein-Barr virus infection. J Allergy Clin Immunol 1986; 78:315–320.

65. Manu P, Matthews DA, Lane TJ. Food intolerance in patients with chronic fatigue. Int J Eat Disord 1993; 13:203–209.

66. Ablashi DV, Sullivan JL, Caliguri M, Weinberg DS, Hall CG, Ashley RL, Saxinger C, Balachandran, et al. A chronic "postinfectious" fatigue syndrome associated with benign lymphoproliferation, B-cell proliferation, and active replication of human herpesvirus 6. J Clin Invest 1990; 10:335–344.

67. Marshall GS, Starr SE, Witzleben CL, Gonczol E, Plotkin SA. Protracted mononucleosis-like illness associated with acquired cytomegalovirus infection in a previously healthy child: transient cellular immune defects and chronic hepatopathy. Pediatrics 1991; 87(4)556–562.

68. Lusso P, Malnati MS, Garzino-Demo A, Crowley RW, Long EO, Gallo RC. Infection of natural killer cells by human herpesvirus 6. Nature 1993; 362:458–462.

69. Sirianni MC, Soddus S, Malorni W, Arancia G, Aiuti F. Mechanism of defective natural killer cell activity in patients with AIDS associated with defective distribution of tubulin. J Immunol 1988; 140:2565–2568.

70. Schiefer SJ, Keller SE, Bond RN, Cohen J, Stein M. Major depressive disorder and immunity. Arch Gen Psych 1989; 46:81–87.

71. Maes M, Lambrechts J, Bosmans E, Jacobs J, Suy E, Vandervorst C, DeJonckheere C, Minner B, Raus J. Evidence for a systemic immune activation during depression: results of leukocyte enumeration by flow cytometry in conjunction with monoclonal antibody staining. Psych Med 1992; 22:45–53.

72. Hickie I, Silove D, Hickie C, Wakefield D, Lloyd A. Is there immune dysfunction in depressive disorders? Psych Med 1990; 20:755–761.

73. Ur E, White PD, Grossman A. Hypothesis: cytokines may be activated to cause depressive illness and chronic fatigue syndrome. Eur Arch Psych Clin Neurosci 1992; 241:317–322.

III

NEUROLOGICAL, PSYCHOLOGICAL, AND PSYCHIATRIC ISSUES

9

Muscle Metabolism, Histopathology, and Physiology in Chronic Fatigue Syndrome

Richard H. T. Edwards, John E. Clague, Henry Gibson, and Timothy R. Helliwell
University of Liverpool, Liverpool, England

Chronic fatigue syndrome (CFS) consists of a constellation of symptoms with physical and mental fatigue as major features [1,2]. Patients frequently complain of fatigue and myalgia at rest, which are exacerbated by exercise and also complain of the inability to reach their previous exercise performance. Similar symptom constellations have been described over the years under various names including irritable heart [3], neurocirculatory asthenia [4], effort syndrome [5,6], and autonomic imbalance [7].

The prominence of muscle symptoms in CFS has led understandably to the assessment of muscle function and structure in this condition. In physiological terms, *fatigue* can be defined as the failure to sustain force or power output [8]. Fatigue can be classified according to its site of origin as either central or peripheral, and objective electrophysiological assessment can further identify high- and low-frequency fatigue (Table 1). If fatigue in CFS is peripheral in origin, then it should be possible to demonstrate an abnormality by these well-established methods. However, patients with CFS may be using the term "fatigue" in a different, more subjective, sense of tiredness or weariness.

In this chapter we review previous histopathological and physiological investigations in CFS. Some studies have been poorly documented, or have failed to distinguish abnormalities that might be explained by disuse, that occur in normal subjects, or that reflect a primary myopathic cause of CFS. We also summarize the histopathological and electrophysiological changes seen in patients

Table 1 Neurophysiological Classification of Skeletal Muscle Fatigue

Type of fatigue	Possible mechanism
Central (failure of neural drive)	Failure to sustain maximal recruitment of motor units or firing frequency
Peripheral (failure of force generation in whole muscle)	
High-frequency fatigue	Impaired neuromuscular transmission or conduction of action potential
Low-frequency fatigue	Impaired excitation–contraction coupling

Source: After Ref. 1.

who present with CFS in our clinic. Our findings support the view that the symptom of fatigue in CFS results from abnormal central drive, rather than a peripheral defect in muscle function, and are consistent with a role for psychological factors in this condition.

MUSCLE METABOLIC STUDIES

Examination of patients with CFS invariably reveals normal muscle bulk, and measurements of muscle enzymes in blood, as markers of muscle damage, are usually normal [9] or mildly elevated [10]. Interest was aroused in defects in muscle metabolism as a cause of CFS by the report of Arnold et al [11], who described abnormal nuclear magnetic resonance (NMR) spectroscopy findings in a single patient with myalgic encephalomyelitis (ME) 4 years after varicella–zoster infection. Early severe intracellular acidosis was described, pH in the forearm muscles falling to 6.3 after 5 min of mild exercise (normal pH > 6.8). Although recovery after exercise was normal, suggesting that aerobic lactate metabolism or elimination was normal, the recovery time course of phosphocreatine recovery was slow. In addition, low postexercise ADP was observed, and it has been suggested that these changes might occur with defective muscle adenylate and creatine kinase activity, although no additional information was provided [12]. Subsequent communication with the authors suggested that these findings were not a consistent feature in other suspected ME patients [12]. Yonge reported details of six patients with postviral syndrome whose NMR spectroscopy findings were more variable, showing abnormalities similar to the initial case report in only two patients [13]. No details of patient activity levels were included, but the patient described by Arnold et al. [11] had been less active for 4 years and physical deconditioning, resulting in reduced mitochondrial enzyme activity, may account for the NMR spectroscopy findings.

MUSCLE MITOCHONDRIAL FUNCTION

In 1985, Byrne et al. reported abnormal mitochondrial respiration rates in two patients with relapsing myalgia [14], and ultrastructural studies of muscle have reported abnormal mitochondria [14–17] in patients with postviral (chronic) fatigue syndrome (PVFS). In animal models, persistent viral infections are described that lead to cell dysfunction (e.g., mice infected with lymphocytic choriomeningitis virus develop pituitary dysfunction [17]). Behan has suggested that persistent virus in mitochondria might interfere with the specialized "luxury" functions of muscle, without leading to cell death [18]. However, in muscle, functional measurements (i.e., force generation) are normal, and a further report found no abnormalities in glycolytic or mitochondrial function in a larger series of CFS patients [19]. Moreover, the significance of mitochondrial abnormalities has been revealed in the work of Wagenmakers et al. [20,21]. This group has reported mitochondrial enzyme activities in patients with muscle disease, including metabolic myopathy and also patients with "effort syndrome," which is believed to be very similar physiologically and psychiatrically to CFS [22,23]. Mitochondrial function was related to activity level, as well-trained normal controls and active patients with muscle disease had higher enzyme activity than more sedentary subjects. It was suggested that the findings in the effort syndrome patients reflected disuse and lack of exercise, as exercise training increases or inactivity decreases mitochondrial enzyme activity in muscle [24]. Therefore, it appears that the abnormalities of mitochondria and of mitochondrial function described in CFS are not causal, but more likely, represent a consequence of the inactivity produced by this condition. The abnormalities seen using magnetic resonance spectroscopy [11,13] can be explained by reduced mitochondrial activity through physical inactivity.

MUSCLE HISTOPATHOLOGY
A Review of Previous Reports

Histological examinations have revealed a variety of apparent abnormalities in CFS. However, many studies were not controlled, and patient details were poorly documented, including their activity level and disease duration. Consequently, it is difficult to decide whether the abnormalities described reflect a primary process, or arose as a consequence of behavioral change, since immobility can rapidly lead to changes in skeletal muscle [25–27]. It is also important when determining changes in muscle to define the criteria used to quantify changes. Many reports are descriptive and difficult to standardize.

In 1985, Behan et al. described abnormal muscle biopsies from unspecified sites in 20 subjects with PVFS [15]. Fifteen of the biopsies contained scattered necrotic fibers and "moderately increased size, and number" of type II fibers were observed, without reference to quantitative measurement. Increased numbers of mitochondria and occasional tubular inclusions were reported from electron microscopy studies. In the two cases reported by Byrne et al. [14], initial biopsies were normal, but those taken after 3 and 5 years, respectively showed type II fiber atrophy. Teahon et al. reported normal histological findings in 18 patients seen at a primary referral center [28]. The numbers were later expanded to 30 patients, and reported by Peters and Preedy, and again no consistent histological abnormalities were seen [9]. Detailed histomorphometric examination revealed no evidence of type I fiber atrophy, four subjects showed type II fiber atrophy, which was marked in only one subject. Five cases revealed type II fiber hypertrophy. Histochemical staining was normal.

More recently Behan et al. reported the results of biopsy in 50 patients with postviral fatigue following a viral illness that was unspecified in 70% of patients [16]. In these patients, type II fiber atrophy was described in 78% of patients, ranging from mild and focal (6 patients), to moderate and diffuse in 33 patients, again no quantification was provided, and these findings are in contrast to their earlier report [15]. Four patients, had mild type I atrophy. Prominent mitochondria were revealed by Gomori staining in 25 cases and, in 80% of cases, mitochondrial abnormalities were seen with electron microscopy, including branching and fusion of cristae and "compartmentalization." No similar abnormalities were seen in control subjects. The authors suggest that persistent viral infection may produce changes in mitochondria in PVFS that then lead to cell dysfunction similar to that seen in mitochondrial myopathies. This work has been criticized in that the changes could reflect the consequence of type II fiber atrophy, which was not present in the control subjects and may be a consequence of inactivity. Moreover, mitochondrial function studies were not performed to see if these morphological changes were of functional significance. A report from the same unit by Doyle did not support these suggestions either [29]. He reported the results of 100 biopsies in patients with myalgic encephalomyelitis (ME) and, although the study was not quantitative, type II fiber atrophy was reported in only one biopsy, electron microscopy was reported as normal in 70% of biopsies, and no evidence of "mitochondrial hyperactivity" was noted. In the remaining 30% of biopsies, diverse abnormalities affecting small numbers of biopsies were described, including cytoplasmic inclusions (six cases), central cores (four cases), and mitochondrial crystalline inclusions (one case).

We have examined the muscle histologically, including histochemical staining, morphometry and electron microscopy of biopsies from patients presenting to our clinic. We examined biopsies from 74 patients who fulfilled the United Kingdom diagnostic criteria for CFS [2], 34 patients who presented with muscle pain or myalgia, but with no fatigue symptoms, and 22 normal volunteers [30]. Our CFS patient group consisted of patients who had been symptomatic for up to 17 years. Biopsies were obtained using the conchotome method [31] from the tibialis anterior muscle and sometimes from the quadriceps or from the medial head of gastrocnemius (Table 2). Twenty nine (39%) of the CFS patients gave a history of preceding viral illness. At the time of biopsy, each subject's daily physical activity level was graded into three categories: normal daily physical activity, reduced daily activity, and severely reduced physical activity.

Morphological Abnormalities Evaluated

The morphological changes we examined were grouped into changes in fiber type prevalence and fiber size, degenerative and regenerative changes, changes in the lipid and glycogen contents of fibers, mitochondrial abnormalities, and enzyme deficiencies (Table 3). Most of the morphological changes affected less than 1% of fibers in a biopsy. The normal prevalence of type 1 fibers is between 67 and 85% in tibialis anterior and between 35 and 55% in calf and quadriceps [32–34]. The areas of 100 type 1 and type 2 fibers were measured on sections stained for myosin ATPase at pH 9.4 [34], and atrophy and hypertrophy factors were calculated from the smaller fiber diameters [33].

Mitochondrial hyperplasia was defined as the presence of ragged-red fibers or prominent subsarcolemmal aggregates in most fibers but did not include cases with small, subsarcolemmal mitochondrial aggregates in a few fibers.

No cases of deficiency of myophosphorylase or phosphofructokinase were identified.

Table 2 Patients and Muscles Studied

	Normal	CFS	Myalgia
Patients studied			
Male	11	34	17
Female	11	40	17
Total	22	74	34
Mean age	31.2	40.1	40.3
Median age	32	42	40
Range	26–60	16–64	20–64
Muscles biopsied			
Tibialis anterior	22	69	28
Quadriceps		4	3
Calf		1	2
Tibialis anterior and quadriceps			1

Source: After Ref. 20.

Table 3 Morphological Features Evaluated, the Possible Significance of Abnormalities Identified, and Their Prevalence in Normal Biopsies

Feature	Significance	No. of abnormal control biopsies
Fiber type prevalence	Individual variation, altered neural input	2
Fiber size	Atrophy and hypertrophy reflect demand on fibers	0
Degenerative changes (necrosis, granular degeneration rimmed vacuoles, cytoplasmic bodies, nemaline rods, targeted fibers, lymphocytic infiltration	Active muscle damage	1
Regenerative changes		
Basophilic, type 2C fibers >5% fibers with internal nuclei	Recovery from recent damages; later or incomplete regeneration; incomplete or abnormal regeneration	2
Split and ringed fibers		
Lipid and glycogen content		
Increased lipid or glycogen	Nonspecific substrate storage owing to inactivity; metabolic defect	
Single-fiber glycogen depletion	Increased single fiber activity	1
Mitochondrial hyperplasia	Increased demand on normal fibers; mitochondrial enzyme defect	1
Enzyme defects		
Partial cytochrome c oxidase	Mitochondrial myopathy; normal muscle with increasing age	1
Myoadenylate deaminase	Significance uncertain	0

Source: After Ref. 20.

Morphological Findings

Abnormalities were present in 32% of control biopsies. Two biopsies had fiber type prevalences outside the normal range, one with a high and one with a low type 1 fiber prevalence. Two biopsies showed occasional, scattered atrophic fibers. One biopsy showed focal necrosis, regeneration, and lymphocytic infiltration, with mitochondrial hyperplasia and partial cytochrome *c* oxidase deficiency. Other changes seen in single biopsies only are shown in Table 3.

Abnormalities were present in 81% of biopsies in patients with CFS and a wide range of changes were encountered (see Table 4).

Changes in Fiber Type Prevalence and Grouping. Only one biopsy showed fiber type grouping, and all other biopsies showed a normal dispersed pattern of fiber type. For tibialis anterior biopsies, there was no significant difference between the mean type 1 fiber prevalence in control and in CFS patients. However, 20 (27%) biopsies did show a low type 1 fiber prevalence, and 9 (12%) a high type 1 fiber prevalence. The difference between the control and CFS groups was not statistically significant.

Although a low type 1 fiber prevalence in CFS has been observed by others [15], its significance is uncertain, and any possibility of changes in fiber type prevalence must be viewed with caution owing to the small size of a biopsy sample in relation to the size of the whole muscle, to the variations seen between sites within a muscle in normal individuals, and to variation between individuals [35].

Abnormalities of Fiber Size. All the CFS patients had mean fiber areas within the normal ranges, which are broad owing to individual variation in fiber size [32,34]. Occasional, scattered atrophic fibers were seen in 12 biopsies, but only 5 biopsies had abnormal atrophy or hypertrophy factors (see Table 4). No overall tendency toward fiber atrophy, which might be expected because of the reduced physical activity, was found in our patients. Two patients showed type 2 fiber atrophy, one showed type 2 fiber hypertrophy, and two showed hypertrophy of both type 1 and 2 fibers. All these features have been reported previously: scattered atrophic fibers [10], type 2 fiber atrophy [9,14,36], and type 1 or 2 fiber hypertrophy [9,10,14,15]. Our data support the view that there are no consistent changes in fiber size.

Degeneration and Regeneration. Degenerative or regenerative features were seen in 32 (43%) CFS patients (see Table 4). There was no correlation with a history of viral infection. Necrosis was an uncommon finding, and other abnormalities occurred only in a few biopsies. Scattered necrotic fibers have been described in 75% of CFS biopsies [15] and in occasional fibers by others [10]. Since necrosis was uncommon and can be seen in asymptomatic individuals, it is unlikely to be a significant abnormality in CFS.

Basophilic regenerating fibers were rarely encountered, but ringed fibers,

Table 4 Prevalence of Various Abnormalities in Normal Volunteers, CFS Patients with or Without Myalgia, and Myalgia Patients

No. of patients	Normal 22	CFS – myalgia 18	CFS + myalgia 56	Myalgia 34
Fiber type prevalence				
Mean % type 1 (SEM)	74.3(6)	72.5(10)	72.5(14)	75.1(10)
Low % type 1	1	6	14	6
High % type 1	1	2	7	3
Fiber size				
Scattered atrophy	2	2	10	4
Type 1 atrophy				1
Type 2 atrophy		1	1	2
Type 2 hypertrophy			1	3
Type 1 + 2 hypertrophy			2	2
Degenerative features (total)	1	2	10	3
Necrosis	1		2	
Degeneration			4	1
Cytoplasmic bodies			4	2
Rimmed vacuoles				1
Nemaline rods			1	
Targetoid fibers		1		
Lymphocytes	1	1		
Regenerative features (total)	2	7	18	7
Basophilic fibers	2			
Ring fibers	1	6	18	7
Fiber splitting		1	1	1
>5% internal nuclei	1		2	3
Miscellaneous features				
Increased glycogen		2		
Decreased glycogen	1	6	10	7
Increased lipid			1	
Increased mitochondria	1	2	3	3
MAD deficiency			3	3
Fibrosis		1	2	

Source: After Ref. 20.

usually one or two per section, were seen in 32% of patients. In one patient a cluster of several small ringed fibers was observed. Ringed fibers are frequently observed, along with other myopathic features, in myotonic and limb-girdle dystrophies, after experimental tenotomy, occasionally in neuropathic disorders, and in normal autopsy material [37]. Ringed fibers may form when contact between the origin and insertion of a muscle is interrupted [37] and may reflect regeneration under tangential stress [38].

Miscellaneous Histological Changes.   Increased lipid was seen in the fibers of only one biopsy, and two biopsies showed focally increased glycogen, but no biochemical abnormalities were detected in these patients. Decreased glycogen was present in occasional fibers in 22% of patients and may reflect differences in the functional activity of a few fibers, with increased activity possibly leading to anaerobic metabolism and the local production of pain-inducing metabolites (see Table 4).

Myoadenylate deaminase deficiency was found in three CFS patients who complained of myalgia.

Five biopsies had increased numbers of mitochondria, accompanied by partial cytochrome *c* oxidase deficiency in two patients. The increased mitochondrial number was confirmed on electron microscopy, but no structural abnormalities of mitochondria were identified.

Partial deficiency of cytochrome *c* oxidase is a feature of chronic progressive external ophthalmoplegia with proximal myopathy [39] and has been identified in other neuromuscular disorders, including dystrophies and neuropathies [40]. The prevalence of enzyme-negative fibers has been found to increase with age in a necropsy study [41]. The low frequency of mitochondrial abnormalities in our patients and their occurrence in normal individuals suggests that mitochondrial abnormalities are not a consistent feature of CFS, as suggested by others [16,18].

Electron Microscopy.   Twenty biopsies were processed for electron microscopy. The observations supported the light microscopic findings in the few cases with increased mitochondrial number or increased glycogen or lipid levels on light microscopy. Most biopsies included occassional fibers with minor sarcomeric changes such as Z-band streaming and A-band disorganization. One biopsy included a fiber with a filamentous aggregate beneath the sarcolemma. None of these abnormalities could be considered diagnostic of any specific muscle disease, and most are occasionally found in normal individuals.

Morphological Abnormalities in Relation to Symptoms.   We have compared the incidence of morphological abnormalities in four groups of biopsies. Those from the 22 asymptomatic controls, from 18 CFS patients without myalgia, from 56 CFS patients with myalgia, and from 34 patients with myalgia alone and no fatigue (see Table 4). Abnormalities were seen in 82% of myalgia patients, a very similar incidence to that in CFS patients, and again a wide range of changes occurred.

For male and female patients, mean fiber sizes were larger for both type 1 and type 2 fibers in the myalgia group than in the normal or CFS groups (Fig. 1), but these differences were not significant except for type 2 fibers in female patients ($p = 0.03$). Type 1 fibers were larger in CFS patients with myalgia than in those without myalgia ($p = 0.05$). The absence of a significant trend in male

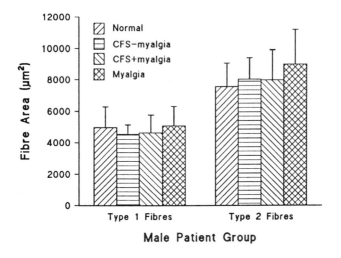

Male Patient Group

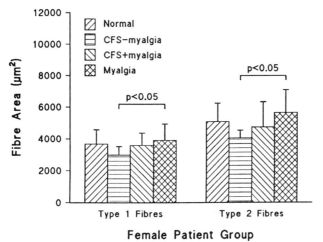

Female Patient Group

Figure 1   Mean (SEM) fiber areas in controls and CFS patients with or without myalgia and those patients with myalgia alone. (After Ref. 20.)

CFS patients suggests this is unlikely to be of pathogenetic significance. Biopsies from eight myalgia patients had abnormal atrophy or hypertrophy factors: the fiber types affected were similar to those of CFS patients.

Degenerative or regenerative features were seen in eight myalgia patients. There is no correlation between the prevalence of these changes and symptoms. Two myalgia patients had clusters of several small ringed fibers, as were seen in one CFS patient. A decreased glycogen concentration was present in occasional fibers in 21% of myalgia patients, and 9% showed mitochondrial hyperplasia, similar prevalences to CFS patients.

Myoadenylate deaminase (MAD) deficiency was found in 5.5% of the biopsies, three CFS patients with myalgia and three other myalgia patients. This is greater than the prevalence of 2–3% in other series [42]. MAD deficiency was originally described in association with exercise-related muscle cramps and myalgia [43], but later work has revealed MAD deficiency in a range of neuromuscular diseases (including neuropathies, dystrophies, and polymyositis), as well as those with myalgia or cramps [42]. Kelemen et al. considered that MAD deficiency was eight times more frequent in patients with exertional myalgia (3 of 36 patients) than in patients with associated diseases [44], yet none of 35 patients with exertional myalgia in the series of Mercelis et al. [42] had MAD deficiency. In our experience of 920 biopsies over a 6-year period, we have seen 11 cases, 6 with myalgia and 1 each accompanying Becker's dystrophy, facioscapulohumeral dystrophy, hypothyroidism, hyperthyroidism, polymyositis, and viral myositis. MAD deficiency, therefore, seems to occur more frequently in patients with myalgia, with or without fatigue, but it can occur in other muscle diseases when myalgia is not a prominent symptom. Therefore, MAD deficiency, by itself, is not the cause of myalgia in CFS.

No relation was observed between duration of symptoms and morphological abnormality. Similarly no relation was observed between physical activity category at the time of biopsy and histopathological abnormalities.

PHYSIOLOGICAL FUNCTION OF SKELETAL MUSCLE
Physiology of Muscle

The initiation of a contraction relies on the successful integration of a chain of functions originating in the brain and ending with the interaction of the contractile proteins within muscle to generate force (see Table 1). Any failure of this command chain will ultimately result in loss of force-generating capacity of the muscle. Most commonly loss of force generation producing weakness is seen when there is loss of muscle bulk, such as the dystrophies or polymyositis. Muscle bulk is usually normal in CFS in the early stages, although prolonged immobilization or a significant reduction in activity may produce profound effects on muscle (25–27).

Reduced motor drive (central fatigue mechanisms) may similarly have profound effects on strength. Consequently, subjective or clinical assessments of strength are unreliable, as they are unable to distinguish reduced central drive from failure of peripheral mechanisms. An objective approach to the testing of muscle function is thus essential if the site of weakness or fatigue is to be determined, and whether factors that are *central* (within the central nervous system) or *peripheral* (within the muscle) are influencing muscle performance.

Most patients examined who had effort syndrome [45], postviral fatigue [46,47], and chronic fatigue syndrome have been able to generate normal force using several muscle groups, with or without verbal encouragement (Fig. 2). In

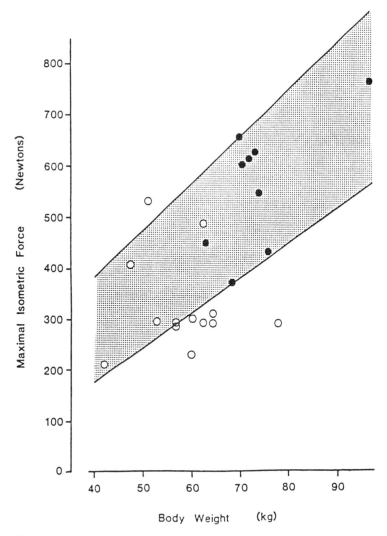

Figure 2 Strength of quadriceps in relation to body weight in patients with effort syndrome. Open circles females, closed circles males; shaded area represents normal range from Edwards et al. [43]. (After Ref. 35.)

those subjects unable to generate normal force, the technique of twitch interpolation, has permitted the central component of force generation to be objectively assessed [47–49]. This technique involves electrical stimulation of muscle through its motor nerve or motor end points using percutaneous stimulation during isometric voluntary activity. An increase in force production on stimulation with single impulses during a maximal voluntary contraction indicates incomplete central drive activation (i.e., not all motor units are recruited). In CFS patients, this technique has shown that the ability to generate force is normal. In patients with proved viral infection [47], this technique has also shown no abnormality in the muscle's ability to generate force. Failure of force generation owing to central factors may occur because of motivational factors, failure to understand the maneuvers, apprehension, fear of pain, or reflex inhibition of motor units because of pain. [50].

Electrophysiological Assessment of Muscle

Jamal et al. have reported abnormal jitter using single-fiber electromyography (EMG) in patients with postviral fatigue [51,52]. No evidence of impulse blocking (i.e., effective failure of a neuromuscular junction) was found, and the authors suggested that this represents possible abnormalities in muscle membrane. The physiological significance of EMG jitter is whether a reduction in force occurs, as is seen in patients with myasthenia gravis, caused by impulse blocking, in whom jitter is prominent, but this is not seen in patients with CFS and this finding is of doubtful significance and cannot explain the fatigue experienced by patients.

Electrical stimulation of muscle permits additional analysis of function, independent of volition. The methods used are well documented [53,54]. A computer-controlled delivery of a train of impulses is used over a range of 1–100 Hz to document frequency/force characteristics that permit the assessment of types of fatigue (see Table 1). This stimulation train of frequencies is known as a *programmed stimulation myogram* (PSM). One possible explanation of the prolonged symptoms of excessive fatigue in CFS is the persistence of "low-frequency fatigue" [55], which is thought to arise from a failure in excitation–contraction coupling and is associated with the need for greater central drive to overcome the likely reduction in force per impulse [56]. Moreover, the resulting mismatch of afferent–efferent activity may explain the further increase in sensation of effort [47]. However, Stokes et al. found no difference in the frequency/force curve or the rate at which force declined during repetitive stimulation of the adductor pollicis when compared with controls (Fig. 3). The persistence of low-frequency fatigue [55], as reflected by a lower 20:50 Hz tetanic force ratio, therefore, cannot be offered as a possible explanation of the symptom of prolonged fatigue, nor can failure of neuromuscular transmission or failure of

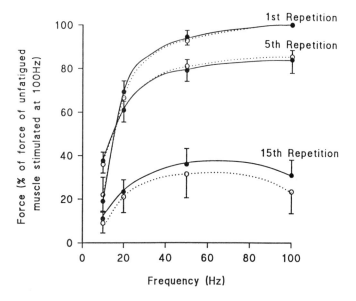

Figure 3 Frequency/force curves for adductor pollicis during fatiguing contractions (repeated PSMs) with circulatory occlusion in patients with effort syndrome (closed circles) and controls (open circles). (After Ref. 35.)

sarcolemmal excitation, providing further evidence that EMG abnormalities cannot adequately explain the symptom of excessive fatigue.

Exercise Testing

Exercise testing is used both diagnostically and as a functional assessment in patients with muscle disease. Some metabolic muscle diseases are characterized by exertional myalgia, for example, McArdle's disease, and exercise testing is used in the investigation of this condition. Riley et al. observed reduced aerobic work capacity during treadmill exercise in CFS patients with higher heart rates and higher blood lactate concentrations at peak exercise, similar to the pattern seen in deconditioned normal subjects [58]. Montague et al. found reduced peak heart rates and exercise capacity in CFS patients [59]. They suggested that there might be a defect in the cardiac pacemaker function. However, their study did not account for symptoms limiting exercise that might explain why only more fit subjects with lower heart rates continued at higher levels of exercise and, therefore, produced the disparity in peak heart rates compared with controls. In a study of 12 CFS patients fulfilling the UK criteria for the diagnosis of CFS [2] and 12 age- and sex-matched controls, we found no differences in exercise capacity. Only three of our CFS patients and none of the control subjects were taking regular exercise at the time of the study, and there were wide differences in exercise capacity in both our CFS patients and the control group [49]. Unlike Riley et al. [48] we observed lower peak heart rates and levels of blood lactates in CFS patients, which suggest that patients were not exercising to their physiological capacity (Table 5). The heart rate/work rate response during exercise was identical in our patients and controls, suggest a similar degree of fitness in both groups. We believe that the differences observed between our study and that of Riley et al. [58] are explained by the different degrees of fitness within the general population and varying periods of inactivity in the patient groups (i.e., their patients were more deconditioned than those we studied). Our results suggest that physical deconditioning is not the sole cause of exercise limitation in CFS patients.

Endurance studies that have examined fatigability with repetitive muscle exercise until exhaustion have been unable to find differences in force generation in CFS patients [46–48]. Lloyd et al. even reexamined their patients after a 3-hr rest interval to see if failure of force generation occurred when patients complained of symptoms after exercise, again no differences were found [46].

Exercise testing, in addition to being an important assessment, can be therapeutic, in that it can be the first convincing demonstration to the patients

Table 5 Resting, Peak Exercise, and Recovery Physiological Characteristics of Muscle Function Data for CFS Patients and Controls

	Patients mean (95% Cl) 6 m, 6 f	Controls mean (95% Cl) 6 m, 6 f	p
Resting heart rate (b min^{-1})	81.5 (72–92)	76.8 (66–84)	NS
Peak heart rate (b min^{-1})	162.7 (144–178)	190 (180–198)	0.0
Resting PE	7.1 (5.9–8.3)	6.2 (5.9–6.4)	NS
Peak PE	19.2 (18.4–20.0)	19.1 (18.5–19.7)	NS
Peak work rate (watts)	155.0 (120–210)	175.0 (150–210)	NS
Exercise duration (min)	11.7 (8–16.5)	13.5 (10.8–16.5)	NS
Resting lactate (mmol/L)	1.93 (1.13–2.42)	1.82 (0.93–3.01)	NS
5-min postexercise lactate (mmol/L)	8.01 (6.2–10.1)	10.43 (9.0–12.9)	NS

Source: After Ref. 39.

that their capabilities are indeed greater than they believe from their tiredness at rest or on minimal exertion.

Muscle Physiology Following Exercise

Of several studies, only Lloyd et al. [46] have noted a delay in recovery of force in the male patients studied over a 4-hr recovery period following repetitive submaximal activity; however, twitch interpolation was not used in the recovery period, so effort at this time may have been submaximal. Stokes et al. found no difference in the immediate rates of recovery of stimulated force after stimulated activity followed for 15 min, [45], nor did Gibson et al., who followed recovery for up to 48 hr in 12 patients after exhaustive incremental cycle ergometry [49]. The evidence points to no alteration in physiological recovery of muscle function, suggesting that the delayed sensation of fatigue experienced in CFS cannot be due to a delay in physiological recovery.

Patients frequently experience postexercise pain. As already demonstrated, it is unrelated to physiological fatigue processes, and it is possible that the discomfort may arise from the well-documented postexercise pain following unaccustomed exercise or eccentric contractions, during which the muscle lengthens while contracting. Pain usually peaks at about 48 hr [56], but the discomfort may be prolonged in some patients in view of their reduced exercise level before commencing the exercise procedure.

Perception of Effort

In view of the findings of normal muscle function at rest and no demonstrable abnormalities during the recovery period following exercise, an alternative explanation for the symptoms of excessive fatigue experienced in CFS must be offered. Lloyd et al. first suggested that the fatigue of postinfectious fatigue syndrome is associated with an abnormality of perception of muscle force and effort [46]. Several studies have since documented effort perception using the well-established technique of scoring effort perception with a Borg scale [60]. Effort sensation has been assessed during various forms of activity, including isometric contractions [47], treadmill exercise [58], and cycle ergometry [49]. Gibson et al. [49] and Riley et al. [58] both showed a disproportionate increase in perception for the level of exercise. In addition, Gibson et al. demonstrated that, unlike control subjects, who show a threshold in effort perception at about 20–30% of maximum capacity and then a linear increase with increasing exercise [61], the effort perception of CFS patients increased linearly immediately from the onset of exercise (Fig. 4). These findings suggest either that CFS patients have a lower threshold for sensation during exercise, or that CFS patients have an additional perception of fatigue at rest over and above that experienced from exercise. In contrast with these findings, Lloyd et al. were unable to demonstrate any differences in effort perception between controls and CFS patients using repetitive submaximal exercise of the elbow flexors to more closely mimic routine daily activity [47]. This finding may reflect the differences in experimental design in which one muscle is active compared with the integration of "whole-body" activity during cycle ergometry or treadmill exercise. However, the authors suggest that the normal effort perception in CFS patients, which reflects the central "motor command," provides further suppport for disturbances in higher brain function above executive pathways for movement.

CONCLUSIONS

This review of the histopathological changes in muscle, muscle metabolism, and muscle physiology in CFS patients supports the view that the symptoms of CFS are not explicable by changes in muscle structure or function.

The wide range of histopathological abnormalities of muscle seen in CFS are not consistent, and they may occur in normal subjects, or may reflect secondary changes owing to reduced activity. None of the histopathological changes found in CFS are consistently related to the symptom of myalgia. Although mitochondrial abnormalities have been described, mitochondrial function tests have been normal or reflected the level of physical activity in patients.

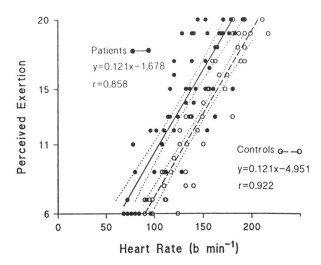

Figure 4 Relation between perceived exertion measured using a Borg scale and heart rate during incremental exercise. A parallel shift in slope to the left is seen for the CFS patient group (closed circles) demonstrating a change in threshold for greater perception of effort compared with the control subjects (open circles). Data pooled, regression lines and 95% confidence intervals shown for $n = 12$ in each group. (After Ref. 39.)

Physiological investigations consistently reveal normal muscle function in CFS, and exercise performance is normal, or compatible with physical deconditioning. Differences in individual studies reflect the variability in physical fitness in the general population. The fatigue experienced by patients with CFS is centrally mediated and is not due to peripheral failure of force generation. These findings support the view that CFS is not a myopathy, and current findings support the importance of perceptual and possibly other psychological factors in this condition [62].

REFERENCES

1. Holmes GP, Kaplan JE, Gantz NM, Komaroff AL. Chronic fatigue syndrome: a working case definition. Ann Intern Med 1988; 108:387–9.
2. Sharpe MC. A report—chronic fatigue syndrome: guidelines for research. J R Soc Med 1991; 84:118–21.
3. Da Costa JKM. On irritable heart: a clinical study of a form of functional cardiac disorder and its consequences. Am J Med Sci 1871; 61:17–52.
4. Oppenheimer B, Levine SA, Moneson RA, Rothechild MA, St Lawrence W, Wilson FN. Appendix of illustrative cases of neurocirculatory asthenia. Milit Surg 1918; 42:409.
5. Lewis T. Soldier's heart and effort syndrome. London: Shaw & Sons, 1918.
6. Wood P. Da Costa's syndrome or (effort syndrome). Br Med J 1941; 1:767.
7. Kessel L, Hyman HT. The clinical manifestations of disturbances of the involuntary nervous system (autonomic imbalance). Am J Med Sci 1923; 165:513.
8. Edwards RHT. Human muscle function and fatigue. In: Porter R, Whelan J, eds. Human muscle fatigue: physiological mechanisms. Ciba Found Symp. London: Pitman Medical, 1981:1–18.
9. Peters TJ, Preedy VR. Pathological changes in skeletal muscle in ME: implications for management. In: Jenkens R, Mowbray J, eds. Postviral fatigue syndrome. London: John Wiley & Sons, 1991:137–46.
10. Archard LC, Bowles NE, Behan PO, Bell EJ, Doyle D. Postviral fatigue syndrome: persistence of enterovirus RNA in muscle and elevated creatine kinase. J R Soc Med 1988; 81:326–9.
11. Arnold DL, Radda GK, Bore PJ, Styles P, Taylor DJ. Excessive intracellular acidosis of skeletal muscle on exercise in a patient with post-viral exhaustion/fatigue syndrome. Lancet 1984; i:1367–9.
12. Edwards RHT, Newham DJ, and Peters TJ. Muscle biochemistry and pathophysiology in postviral fatigue syndrome. Br Med Bull 1991; 47:826–37.
13. Yonge RP. Magnetic resonance studies: implications for psychiatry. J R Soc Med 1988; 81:322–5.
14. Byrne E, Trounce I, Dennett X. Chronic relapsing myalgia (? post viral): clinical, histological and biochemical studies. Aust NZ J Med 1985; 15:305–8.
15. Behan PO, Behan WMH, Bell EJ. The postviral fatigue syndrome—an analysis of the findings in 50 cases. J Infect 1985; 10:211–22.

16. Behan WMH, More IAR, Behan PO. Mitochondrial abnormalities in the postviral fatigue syndrome. Acta Neuropathol 1991; 83:61–5.
17. de la Torre JC, Borrow P, Oldstone MBA. Viral persistence and disease: cytopathology in the absence of cytolysis. Br Med Bull 1991; 47:838–51.
18. Behan WMH. Editorial: muscles, mitochondria and myalgia. J Pathol 1992; 166:213–4.
19. Byrne E, Trounce I. Chronic fatigue and myalgia syndrome: mitochondrial and glycolytic studies in skeletal muscle. J Neurol Neurosurg Psychiatry 1987; 50:743–6.
20. Wagenmakers AJM, Kaur N, Coakley JH, Griffiths RD, Edwards RHT. Mitochondrial metabolism in myopathy and myalgia. Adv Myochem 1987; 1:219–30.
21. Wagenmakers AJM, Coakley JH, Edwards RHT. The metabolic consequences of reduced habitual activities in patients with muscle pain and disease. Ergonomics 1988; 31:1519–27.
22. Wessely S, Powell R. Fatigue syndromes: a comparison of chronic "post-viral" fatigue with neuromuscular and affective disorders. J Neurol Neurosurg Psychiatry 1989; 52:940–8.
23. Rosen SD, King JC, Wilkinson JB, Nixon PGF. Is chronic fatigue syndrome synonymous with effort syndrome? J R Soc Med 1990; 83:761–4.
24. Henrikson J, Reitman JS. Time course of changes in human skeletal muscle succinate dehydrogenase and cytochrome oxidase activities and maximal oxygen uptake with physical activity and inactivity. Acta Physiol Scand 1977; 99:91–7.
25. Jaffe DM, Terry RD, Spiro AJ. Disuse atrophy of skeletal muscle. J Neurol Sci 1978; 35:189–200.
26. Sargeant AJ, Davies CTM, Edwards RHT, Maunder C, Young A. Functional and structural changes after disuse in humans. Clin Sci 1977; 52:337–42.
27. Gibson JNA, Halliday D, Morrison WL, Stoward PJ, Hornsby GA, Watt RW, Murdoch G, Rennie MJ. Decrease in human quadriceps muscle protein turnover consequent upon leg immobilization. Clin Sci 1987; 72:503–9.
28. Teahon K, Preedy RV, Smith DG, Peters TJ. Clinical studies of the post-viral fatigue syndrome (PVFS) with special reference to skeletal muscle function. Clin Sci 1988; 75:45P.
29. Doyle D. An account of 100 muscle biopsies in epidemic myalgic encephalomyelitis (EME). In: Hyde BM, Goldstein J, Levine P, eds. The clinical and scientific basis of myalgic encephalomyelitis/chronic fatigue syndrome. Ottawa: Nightingale Research Foundation, 1991:352–6.
30. Edwards RHT, Gibson H, Clague JE, Helliwell TR. Muscle histopathology and physiology in the chronic fatigue syndrome. In: Edwards RHT, ed. London: Ciba Foundation, 1993; 173:102–131.
31. Dietrichson P, Coakley J, Smith PEM, Griffiths RD, Helliwell TR, Edwards RHT. Conchotome and needle percutaneous biopsy of skeletal muscle. J Neurol Neurosurg Psychiatry 1987; 50:1461–7.
32. Sandstedt P, Nordell L-E, Henriksson K. Quantitative analysis of muscle biopsies from volunteers and patients with neuromuscular disorders. Acta Neurol Scand 1982; 66:130–44
33. Dubowitz V. Muscle biopsy: a practical approach. 2nd ed. Eastbourne: Bailliere-Tindall, 1985.

34. Helliwell TR, Coakley J, Smith PEM, Edwards RHT. The morphology and morphometry of the normal human tibialis anterior muscle. Neuropathol Appl Neurobiol 1987; 13:297–307.
35. Sandstedt PER. Representativeness of a muscle biopsy specimen for the whole muscle. Acta Neurol Scand 1981; 64:427–37.
36. Gow JW, Behan WMN, Clements GB, Woodall C, Riding M, Behan PO. Enteroviral RNA sequences detected by polymerase change chain reaction in muscle of patients with postviral fatigue syndrome. Br Med J 1991; 302:692–6.
37. Bethlem J, van Wijngaarden GK. The incidence of ringed fibres and sarcoplasmic masses in normal and diseased muscle. J Neurol Neurosurg Psychiatry 1963; 26:326–32.
38. Mastaglia FL, Walton J. Skeletal muscle pathology. Edinburgh: Churchill Livingstone, 1982:245.
39. Johnson MA, Turnbull DM, Dick DJ, Sherratt HSA. A partial deficiency of cytochrome c oxidase in chronic progressive ophthalmoplegia. J Neurol Sci 1983; 60:31–53.
40. Yamamoto M, Koga Y, Ohtaki E, Nonaka I. Focal cytochrome c oxidase deficiency in various neuromuscular diseases. J Neurol Sci 1989; 91:207–13.
41. Müller-Höcker J. Cytochrome c oxidase deficient fibres in the limb muscle and diaphragm of man without muscular disease: an age-related phenomenon. J Neurol Sci 1990; 100:14–21.
42. Mercelis R, Martin J-J, de Barsy T, Van den Berghe G. Myoadenylate deaminase deficiency: absence of correlation with exercise intolerance in 452 muscle biopsies. J Neurol 1987; 234:385–9.
43. Fishbein WN, Armbrustmacher VW, Griffin JL. Myoadenylate deaminase deficiency: a new disease of muscle. Science 1978; 200:545–8.
44. Kelemen J, Rice DR, Bradley WG, Munsat TL, DiMauro S, Hogan EL. Familial adenylate deaminase deficiency and exertional myalgia. Neurology 1982; 32:857–63.
45. Stokes MJ, Cooper RG, Edwards RHT. Normal muscle strength and fatigability in patients with effort syndromes. Br Med J 1988; 297:1014–17.
46. Lloyd A, Hales J, Gandevia S. Muscle strength, endurance and recovery in the post infectious fatigue syndrome. J Neurol Neurosurg Psychiatry 1988; 51:1316–22.
47. Rutherford O, White PD. Human quadriceps strength and fatigability in patients with postviral fatigue. J Neurol Neurosurg Psychiatry 1991; 54:961–4.
48. Lloyd AR, Gandevia SC, Hales JP. Muscle performance, voluntary activation, twitch properties and perceived effort in normal subjects and patients with the chronic fatigue syndrome. Brain 1991; 114:85–8.
49. Gibson H, Carroll N, Clague JE, Edwards RHT. Exercise performance and fatigability in patients with chronic fatigue syndrome. J Neurol Neurosurg Psychiatry 1993; 56:993–8.
50. Stokes MJ, Young A. The contribution of reflex inhibition to arthrogenous muscle weakness. Clin Sci 1984; 67:7–14.
51. Jamal GA, Hansen S. Electrophysiological studies in the post-viral syndrome. J Neurol Neurosurg Psychiatry 1985; 48:691–4.

52. Jamal GA, Hansen S. Post-viral fatigue syndrome: evidence for underlying organic disturbance in the muscle fibre. Eur Neurol 1989; 29:273–6.
53. Edwards RHT, Young A, Hosking GP, Jones DA. Human skeletal muscle function: description of tests and normal values. Clin Sci Mol Med 1977; 52:283–90.
54. Cooper RG, Edwards RHT, Gibson H, Stokes MJ. Human muscle fatigue: frequency dependence of excitation and force generation. J Physiol 1988; 397:585–99.
55. Edwards RHT, Hill DK, Jones DA, Merton PA. Fatigue of long duration in human skeletal muscle after exercise. J Physiol 1977; 272:769–8.
56. Newham DJ, Mills KR, Quigley BM, Edwards RHT. Pain and fatigue after concentric and eccentric muscle contractions. Clin Sci 1983; 64:55–62.
57. Gandevia SC, McClosky DI. Changes in motor commands, as shown by changes in perceived heaviness, during partial curarization and peripheral anaesthesia in man. J Physiol 1977; 283:673–99.
58. Riley MS, O'Brien CJ, McCluskey DR, Bell NP, Nicholls DP. Aerobic work capacity in patients with chronic fatigue syndrome. Br Med J 1990; 301:953–6.
59. Montague TR, Marrie TJ, Klassen GA, Bewick DK, Horacek BM. Cardiac function at rest and with exercise in the chronic fatigue syndrome. Chest 1989; 95:779–84.
60. Borg GAV. Perceived exertion as an indicator of somatic stress. Scand J Rehabil Med 1970; 2:92–8.
61. Jones NL. Clinical exercise testing. 3rd ed. Philadelphia: WB Saunders, 1988:75–109.
62. Wood GC, Bentall RP, Gopfert M, Edwards RHT. A comparative psychiatric assessment of patients with chronic fatigue syndrome and muscle disease. Psychol Med 1991; 21:619–28.

10

Neuropsychological Features of Chronic Fatigue Syndrome

Jordan Grafman
National Institute of Neurological Disorders and Stroke,
National Institutes of Health, Bethesda, Maryland

Neuropsychological complaints are among the defining features of chronic fatigue syndrome (CFS). For example, Komaroff estimates that 50–85% of patients with CFS in published studies report impaired cognitive functioning [1]. Despite their frequent complaints of cognitive impairment, very few peer-reviewed neuropsychological studies of CFS patients have yet appeared in print. Those that have, vary in their assessment techniques, subject selection methods, and conclusions. The remaining neuropsychological reports in the literature are anecdotal or worse, clearly belie the a priori biases of their source.

In this chapter I briefly review those aspects of CFS that could conceivably lead to neuropsychological deficits. More detailed coverage of this topic can be found elsewhere [2]. Next, I describe the neuropsychological profile of CFS patients, based on the extant literature. This is followed by suggestions for a neuropsychological assessment targeted to the CFS patient. The chapter concludes with some comments about the value of neuropsychological assessment in CFS.

THE NEUROLOGICAL EXAMINATION

The neurological examination of CFS patients is typically completely normal, although patients commonly report problems with strength, sleep, balance, cognition, and mood. There have been relatively few reports giving precise information on neurological findings in CFS [2]. Chronic fatigue syndrome rarely presents with objective changes in muscle functions [see Chapter 9] or with hard neurological symptoms or signs [3]. Between 10 and 20% of CFS patients have an abnormal Romberg test and 15–25% of CFS patients demonstrate an impaired tandem gait [1].

Magnetic resonance imaging (MRI) studies of CFS patients are occasionally positive, yet controversy persists. For example, one recent study indicated that 70% of the CFS patients associated with an outbreak of the disorder in Lake Tahoe, Nevada, had punctate bright signals on their MRIs [4]. Such MRI abnormalities appear to resemble the hyperintensities reported in leukoariosis. On the other hand, in the National Institutes of Health (NIH) CFS patient population, bright signals were uncommon in patients' MRIs [Straus SE, personal communication].

Few metabolic-imaging studies have been attempted with CFS patients. Several recent studies using single-photon emission computed tomography (SPECT) found abnormalities in the basal ganglia in these patients [5].

The presence of neurological findings in some CFS patients and controversial imaging studies reporting subcortical lesions or dysfunction require the neuropsychologist to be especially cautious in interpreting the results of neuropsychological testing in CFS patients. Nevertheless, the observation that many patients with CFS tend to improve over time, in conjunction with the lack of evidence of any significant progressive neurological deterioration, argues against portraying CFS as a neurodegenerative disorder.

THE NEUROPSYCHOLOGICAL EVALUATION

Neuropsychological evaluations are an integral part of the clinical neuroscience workup of patients with suspected central nervous system (CNS) disease and, thus, can play an important role in the assessment of patients considered to have CFS. Neuropsychological evaluations provide the referral source with critical information about the patients' cognitive processes and mood state. The broad-based neuropsychological evaluation typically examines motor coordination and strength, simple sensory functions, general intellectual functioning, information-processing speed, attention, language, perception, reasoning and problem-solving, memory, mood state, and personality. The neuropsychological evaluation may be conducted by a trained technician, student-in-training, or a psychologist. Clinical neuropsychologists interpreting the test results should, at a minimum, have received specialized training as a postdoctoral fellow in clinical neuropsychology. Certification is available for clinical neuropsychologists from the American Board of Professional Psychology.

The neurospsychological evaluation of patients with CFS can aid in interpreting the effects of pharmacological intervention, estimating the progression of symptoms or rate of patient recovery, and in the experimental evaluation of specific cognitive processes in selected single-cases or subgroups of CFS patients [2,6,7]. It is particularly important when a diagnosis is one of exclusion, as it is with CFS, to establish a neuropsychological baseline by which subsequent clinical changes could be judged.

A SUMMARY OF THE NEUROPSYCHOLOGICAL FINDINGS

Self-Report

Patients with CFS routinely complain of problems in concentration and memory. Up to 85% of patients complain of impaired cognition. Until recently, these problems had been unsystematically recorded. A similar situation existed some 40 years ago for the syndrome known then as chronic brucellosis, in which nonspecific symptoms of nervousness and difficulty in concentrating were frequently reported to clinicians. An objective study of these patients by Imboden and his colleagues found no evidence of cognitive deficits [8].

A recent study by Grafman et al. [9] investigated patient self-report of cognitive status by mailing out surveys to a sample of CFS patients being followed at the National Institutes of Health (Table 1 gives a description of the survey scales). About two-thirds of the sample returned the forms (Table 2 describes the responders). There was no relation between selected laboratory findings and self-report (Table 3 outlines a description of the laboratory findings). A large

Table 1 Self-Rating Scales Used in a Survey of NIH Patients with CFS

Scales	Description of scale
Beck Depression Inventory	Measures number of depressive symptoms
Neuropsychology Self-Rating Scale	
Memory scale	Memory complaints
Knowledge scale	Remote memory complaints
Language scale	Problems in understanding or expressing language
Spatial scale	Route-finding and spatial location problems
Perception scale	Difficulty in recognizing people or objects
Praxis scale	Difficulty in simple and complex motor control
Emotional scale	Disturbances in mood regulation
Memory Self-Rating Scale	
Verbal scale	Verbal learning and memory complaints
Nonverbal scale	Nonverbal learning and memory complaints
Temporal scale	Problems in remembering order and recency

Table 2 Characteristics of CFS Patients in the NIH
Study: Historical and Demographic Features in 54
Responding Study Patients

Patient characteristics	
Age (yr)	38.8 (9.3)
Disease duration (yr)	9.1 (6.4)
Females/males	36/18
Pattern of illness onset	
Infectious mononucleosis	25%
Mononucleosislike illness	23%
Acute febrile illness	34%
Insidious onset	18%

proportion of CFS patients complained about verbal memory and mood state
changes, whereas problems in perceptual, linguistic, spatial, and nonverbal
memory functions were rarely endorsed (Fig. 1).

The memory complaints of CFS patients were occasionally so severe that they
were comparable with those reported by patients with definitely diagnosed central
nervous system disorders and amnesia. Although indicating that their memory
and mood state impairment was very bothersome, the respondents reported that
during the worst state of their illness, their memory and mood state problems
were even more severe. With a Beck Depression Inventory Total Score of 15 as
a clinical cut-off for depression, more than 50% of the sample were currently
depressed, whereas up to 90% of the sample recall having been depressed during

Table 3 Selected Laboratory Findings in CFS Patients
Participating in an NIH Survey

Selective laboratory findings that were correlated with cognitive and mood scales	Subjects with finding (%)
Immunoglobulin deficiency	
IgG	5
IgA	2
IgM	1
White blood cell count ($<3500/\mu^3$)	2
Sedimentation rate (>20 mm/h)	2
Heterophile antibodies (Monospot test)	6
EBV Serology	
IgG Anti-VCA ($\geq 1:40$)	93
IgA Anti-VCA ($\geq 1:10$)	25
EA-R ($\geq 1:10$)	74
EB nuclear antigen ($\geq 1:2$)	93

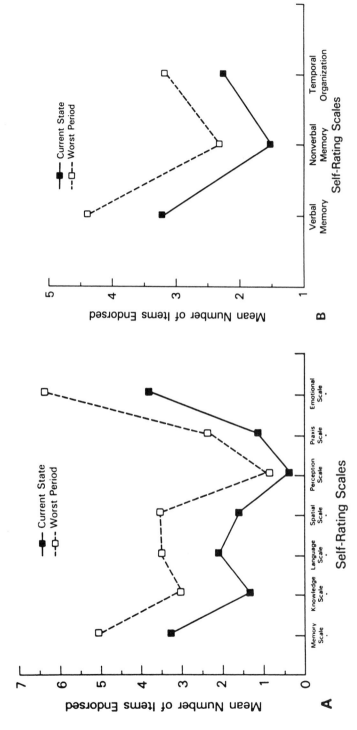

Figure 1 Survey results from the NIH CFS patients study. (A) CFS neuropsychology self-rating inventory: asterisks under the scale name indicate a significant difference between the current and worst-period ratings. (B) CFS memory self-rating scale: there were no significant differences noted on these scales between the current and worst-period reports. Note the relatively greater number of verbal memory complaints.

the worst period of their illness (Fig. 2). In general, women had more complaints than men. Importantly, there was a strong correlation between the degree of depression and severity of these memory complaints (Table 4).

ISSUES RELATING TO THE NEUROPSYCHOLOGICAL EVALUATION

The issue of concurrent affective disease has emerged as a polarizing and confounding issue in studies of neuropsychological function in CFS. Most published studies have shown a higher proportion of mood state changes and psychiatric diagnoses in CFS than in the population at large [10]. In the context of the neuropsychological evaluation, it is important to take this observation into consideration. It is known, for example, that depression may affect cognitive

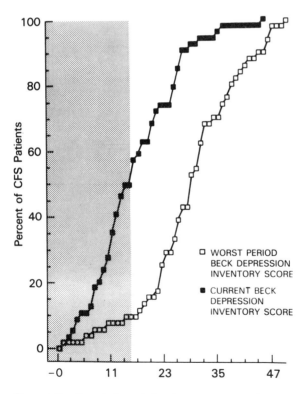

Figure 2 Cumulative relative frequency count of survey-respondent Beck Depression Inventory scores. The shaded area indicate scores that fall within the normal range.

processes, such as divergent thinking, which is required on those neuro-psychological tests that demand more effort (e.g., certain free-recall tasks) [11]. Thus, the cognitive deficits reported or found in CFS could be secondary to a primary psychiatric disorder [12,13]. Critics of this interpretation point to a lack of diagnosable affective disorder in a large enough minority of CFS patients to argue against it playing an etiological role [1]. They prefer to consider an alternative possibility that the mood state changes arise from the social and physical limitations imposed on these patients by their illness. Yet a third possibility is that both depression and cognitive deficits cooccur and are the result of single or multiple central nervous system lesions or dysfunctions [2].

Some patients initially considered to have CFS may, in fact, be misdiagnosed and have another disorder that affects the central nervous system, such as multiple sclerosis or a definable acute viral infection [14–17]. There is evidence that colds and influenza, for example, may acutely and selectively affect cognitive performance [2]. What distinguishes CFS patients from patients with these other illnesses is the chronicity of their neuropsychological complaints in conjunction with negative neurological and physical findings.

Neuropsychological Studies

Few neuropsychological studies of CFS patients have been published in peer-reviewed scientific journals. The reader should be aware that a much larger number of reports have appeared in support-group newsletters, at professional and CFS advocacy group meetings, or have been conveyed by personal correspondence. It is probable that at least some of these reports will eventually reach the scientific literature. However, until such time as they do, the reader should be very cautious in the interpretation of these non–peer-reviewed reports, since their methodology may be poor, subject selection biased, and interpretation of the results questionable, no matter the direction of the results. This often happens in the first generation of investigations into a newly established disorder. Eventually, the wheat is separated from the chaff and a balanced picture of the disorder emerges.

The first published neuropsychological study of CFS was from the Toronto group. Altay et al. studied 21 subjects (who met CFS criteria) with what was termed postinfectious neuromyasthenia [18]. Seventeen of the 21 subjects were women. The average age of the subjects was 36 years old, and they had a mean education level of slightly over 16 years (college graduates). They were administered the following tests: Trail Making Test A and B (which measures attention and the ability to shift concepts); Digit Symbol Subtest of the Wechsler Adult Intelligence Scale–Revised [WAIS-R (measures speed of information processing and short-term memory)]; Similarities Subtest from the WAIS-R (measures verbal reasoning and concept formation); and the Shipley Institute of Living Scale (measures vocabulary knowledge and abstract reasoning). The

Table 4 Interscale Correlations in the NIH CFS Patient Survey

	Spearman rank order correlations										
	Beck Depression Inventory (A)	Beck Depression Inventory (B)	Emotional scale (A)	Emotional scale (B)	Memory scale (A)	Memory scale (B)	Verbal memory (A)	Verbal memory (B)	Non-verbal memory (A)	Non-verbal memory (B)	Temporal organization (A)
Beck Depression Inventory (B)	0.5638 (54) 0.0001										
Neuropsychology Self-Rating Inventory											
Emotional scale (A)	0.7613 (54) 0.0000	0.4435 (51) 0.0017									
Emotional scale (B)	0.3259 (54) 0.0212	0.6379 (51) 0.0000	0.4367 (54) 0.0020								
Memory scale (A)	0.5792 (54) 0.0000	0.4753 (51) 0.0008	0.4867 (54) 0.0004	0.3604 (52) 0.0108							
Memory scale (B)	0.5347 (54) 0.0002	0.5546 (51) 0.0001	0.4971 (54) 0.0004	0.4903 (52) 0.0005	0.7600 (54) 0.0001						

Memory Self-Rating Scale

	Memory Self-Rating Scale	Verbal memory (A)	Verbal memory (B)	Nonverbal memory (A)	Nonverbal memory (B)	Temporal organization (A)
Verbal memory (A)	-0.5726 (54) 0.0000					
Verbal memory (B)	-0.5498 (54) 0.0001	-0.4748 (51) 0.0008				
Nonverbal memory (A)	-0.5832 (54) 0.0000	-0.6224 (51) 0.0000	-0.5897 (54) 0.0000			
Nonverbal memory (B)	-0.4344 (54) 0.0024	-0.4506 (51) 0.0014	-0.5841 (54) 0.0000	-0.4421 (52) 0.0018		
Temporal organization (A)	-0.5220 (54) 0.0001	-0.5524 (51) 0.0001	-0.5885 (54) 0.0000	-0.6653 (52) 0.0000	-0.8108 (54) 0.0000	
Temporal organization (B)	-0.5960 (54) 0.0000	-0.5107 (51) 0.0003	-0.5071 (54) 0.0000	-0.3039 (52) 0.0317	-0.6569 (54) 0.0000	-0.6313 (52) 0.0000

results were compared with the most recently revised normative data available on each test, matched for age. The results demonstrated that the CFS subjects performed at or above the age-matched normative sample, despite that 20 of the 21 subjects in this study felt that they performed quite poorly and nowhere near their premorbid standard.

In contrast, Riccio et al. found some significant abnormalities in memory in a sample of CFS patients they studied [19]. Nine patients (median age 30; four women) who fulfilled the operational criteria for a diagnosis of myalgic encephalomyelitis (ME) were compared with a matched control group on a set of neuropsychological and psychiatric tests. All the patients reported problems in concentrating before the testing. Subjects were assessed with (1) The National Adult Reading Test; (2) WAIS-R; (3) Wechsler Memory Scale (WMS), which measures various aspects of verbal and nonverbal memory; (4) Sentence Verification Test (measures speeded semantic processing); (5) Letter and Category Verbal Fluency Tests (requires subjects to generate as many words as they can within 1 min that begin with a specific letter or belong to a specific semantic category, such as animals); (6) Grooved Pegboard Test, which evaluates fine motor coordination; (7) Wisconsin Card Sorting Test (WCST), which measures concept formation and shifting; (8) Trailmaking Test A and B; (9) Present State Examination (PSE), which is a standardized psychiatric interview; (10) Hospital Anxiety and Depression Questionnaire; (11) State–Trait Anxiety Scale; (12) Profile of Mood States; (13) Illness Behavior Questionnaire; and (14) Eysenck Personality Questionnaire.

The ME patients had a significantly lower score on the WMS subtest that measures story memory and a modest decline in paired-associate learning compared with the matched control group. No other significant differences emerged from the neuropsychological comparisons. No substantial differences between groups were found on the psychiatric interview or objective personality inventories.

Smith examined self-report of cognitive deficits in a set of 232 ME patients [20–22]. He found that ME patients reported a higher level of cognitive complaints than controls, but that their complaints largely reflected their higher levels of psychopathology, as estimated by objective inventories.

Smith then went on to study differing subsets of these patients on a variety of performance measures. He found that ME patients were substantially slower than controls on a simple response time task (409 > 253 ms, respectively), as well as on a five-choice serial response time task. The ME patients were also shown a spatial pattern that is known to induce visual discomfort and illusions. The ME patients were more likely than controls to report visual illusions and feel dizzy after observing the pattern. In a task that required subjects to visually search for a target among distractors, ME patients were slower and less accurate than controls. On the Stroop Color–Word Test (which requires selective attention and inhibition of competing information), ME patients performed more slowly and were more prone to distraction from competing stimuli than controls. In a story memory task, ME patients were poorer than controls in recalling both gist and detailed information.

Smith also administered other memory tasks. He found no difference between ME patients and controls on a digit span test. The ME patients demonstrated a problem in learning words from a list on the early trials, but by the later trials, overall recall was similar to controls. On a word recognition test, ME patients developed a yes strategy in saying whether words were seen before or not—thus, they had a large number of hits and a very large number of false-alarms. So large, in fact, that Smith compared their performance with patients with Korsakoff syndrome, who have a rather profound amnesia. On a sentence verification task (requiring semantic-processing speed), ME patients completed fewer items than controls. The ME patients also produced fewer words on a verbal fluency test. Importantly, the number of subjects completing each task varied, and no significance levels were reported. The pattern of deficits held whether patients were viewed as mildly or severely affected.

Krupp et al. found that neuropsychological differences between CFS patients ($N = 45$) and controls disappeared when self-report of depression was adjusted for [23]. DeLuca et al. studied 12 CFS patients on the Paced Auditory Serial Addition Test (PASAT), which measures information-processing speed and parallel-processing of information [24]. The CFS patients were significantly worse than controls on this task, but performed similarly to MS patients. The CFS patients' Beck Depression Inventory Scores were not correlated with their performance on the PASAT.

The studies reviewed so far provide a mixed picture of the cognitive status of CFS patients. Some studies found normal to near-normal cognitive status in CFS patients or could account for the mild neuropsychological deficits on the basis of severity of depression. One of the studies found mainly memory deficits. One study with British ME patients identified delays in information-processing speed and response times in addition to memory deficits. Did these disparate results arise because the subject samples were not comparable among studies? All the samples seemed to involve relatively young, mostly female, and well-educated subjects who had met either the CFS or ME criteria that describe rather similar, but not necessarily identical, cohorts. The term ME emphasizes the neurological features of the syndrome and, in doing so, may have biased the selection of individuals with a predisposition for more significant neurological deficits. In light of the mixed results just reviewed, the studies we have conducted at the NIH may shed some light on the fundamental cognitive problems experienced by CFS patients.

The National Institutes of Health Studies

When self-reporting, CFS patients preponderantly complain about problems in concentration, memory, and mood [2,22,25]. If their concentration were impaired, it might be expected that designing a study that would require CFS subjects to keep their attention focused for several hours would exacerbate their concentration problems. Our first study was designed to examine this simple hypothesis. We adapted a paradigm that requires sustained attention [26]. In this task, subjects are asked to look at a computer monitor and determine when a target letter appears among a set of distractor letters. The target and distractors either remain similar over trials, or they can change, and the distractors can be targets from previous trials or totally new items. This task requires both controlled processing (when the target and distractor relations shift) or relatively automatic processing (when the target and distractor relations remain the same). We required subjects to press a key as quickly as possible when they saw a target (targets were not present on all trials). In addition, we recorded the patients event-related brain-evoked potentials (ERP) during their performance. The event-related brain potential is a sensitive measure of "central-processing time" and is independent of response execution. It allows a subtle evaluation of the integrity of brain mechanisms involved in the perception of, and reasoning about, stimuli. Both the latency and amplitude of the various event-related brain potentials can be measured and, when altered, have different implications for brain functions.

Besides the main attention task just described, we also administered a standard visual "odd-ball" task in which the subject has to respond with a key press when a target stimulus appeared. The target stimuli could appear with different probabilities—the one most often used is the 20% probability, which led investigators to describe this task as the oddball. We administered this task briefly before and after the main attention task. The whole testing session took approximately 4 hr. We were particularly interested in seeing whether we could observe objective changes in test performance, reaction times (rt), or ERPs, over the 4-hr period of testing.

The results were rather surprising. There were no overall between-group differences in performance accuracy nor ERP latency or amplitude on any of the tasks. Performance and ERP similarities were maintained across the 4-hr session. Interestingly, despite normal performance accuracy and ERPs, the CFS patients response times were significantly slower than controls in both tasks. These response time differences were not exacerbated across the 4-hr session. Furthermore, patients complained both during the session (despite normal accuracy and central-processing times) and the following day about how tired the testing made them.

These results suggest that CFS patients can adequately and selectively attend to information over a long period, even when that information is presented rapidly and requires sustained focused attention. We also can report that the brain mechanisms required for this attentiveness appear to be normally operating (but see Prasher et al. for a contrary finding [27]). We did not measure motor preparation with the ERP and, therefore, we have no clear explanation for the delayed response times we observed, nor for the severity of the patients' complaints (in light of their adequate performance accuracy).

Given their other major complaints about memory and problem-solving, we next attempted to evaluate the memory and reasoning capacity of CFS patients [9]. We studied 20 CFS patients and 17 normal volunteers. Although we focused on memory measures, tests of planning, response time, and intellectual capacity were also included. Two "tower" planning tasks were selected because they represented different difficulty levels in planning. Thus, this battery not only measured those domains of cognition noted by CFS patients to be taxing, but included measures known to be sensitive to "subcortical dementia," such as time perception, response speed, and planning. The following battery of tests and scales were administered over a total of 8 hr on 2 consecutive days of study. A more detailed descripton of these tests (and all others mentioned in this chapter), except where noted, is available in Lezak [28].

All patients and controls demonstrated excellent effort and motivation during the evaluation. All of the patients remarked that the examination was tiring for them. Some patients complained of debilitating fatigue only on the day following the completion of the evaluation.

General Intellectual Performance

1. Wechsler Adult Intelligence Scale–Revised: This is a standard intelligence test composed of 11 subtests assessing verbal and nonverbal abilities.

Timing and Reaction Time Tasks

1. Simple reaction time: Subjects were instructed to press the space bar on a computer keyboard as quickly as possible every time a stimulus appeared on a computer monitor.
2. Serial reaction time test: Stimuli would appear at one of four positions, one at a time, and subjects were to press the key that was underneath the position where the stimulus would appear as quickly as possible. There were seven blocks of 100 trials each. The first two blocks were composed of random presentations, the next four blocks were composed of ten repetitions of a fixed sequence of ten stimuli, and the last block was another random presentation. Familiarity with the task itself should be reflected by a slight decrease in rt across the first two blocks. The further expected *decline* in rt across blocks 3 through 6 indicates the procedural learning of the repeated sequence. The expected *increase* in rt on block

7 (composed of random trials) *compared* with block 6 (the last repeated trial block) is an indication of visuomotor procedural learning (the difference score that we use subtracts the rt of block 7 from block 6).

3. Time wall: This task measures elapsed time perception based on encoding the speed of a visual stimulus that falls behind an opaque mask.

4. Time clock: This task requires the subject to make 60 taps at 1-sec intervals each.

Problem-Solving and Planning

1. Tower of London: Subjects were shown a collection of three colored disks placed upon a set of different-sized pegs in a certain pattern, defined as the *initial state*. They were then shown a card indicating the *final state* that the disks should be in. Subjects were then told to move the disks one at a time until they reached the final state. Only one disk could be moved at a time, there was a limit on how many disks could be placed on the pegs, and there was a time limit of 2 min by the end of which a move had to be made.

2. Tower of Hanoi: This is a more demanding task than the Tower of London, but measures similar planning and procedural knowledge skills. Subjects were shown the graphic image of a collection of five disks placed upon a set of pegs on a computer screen. From this initial state, subjects were asked to use the numerical keys on the keyboard to shift disks to different pegs to reach a final state. Subjects had to solve the problem within 2 mins. The number correct out of nine problems was recorded. Each problem had a different initial state, but a constant final state.

3. Twenty questions: Subjects had to identify the correct object from a set of 24 objects by asking questions. Two problems (each with a specific target object) are given with the type of question (e.g., deductive) asked by the subject and whether the subject identified the object or not recorded by the test examiner. This test measured reasoning ability the question development (e.g., divergent vs convergent).

Memory

1. Wechsler Memory Scale–Revised: This is a standardized test that includes several subtests that measure short-term memory, verbal and nonverbal learning and immediate and delayed recall, mental control, and attention.

2. Experimental Paired-Associate Test: Subjects were asked to remember several types of paired items (either word–word, word–picture, picture–word, or picture–picture pairs). Subjects were next given a visual cued-recall test using the first item in each pair, followed by a verbal free-recall test and an incidental learning task that required subjects to indicate whether each item was presented originally as a picture or a word.

3. Hasher Frequency Monitoring Task: Subjects were read a set of words that they were told to remember. Some of the words were repeated up to seven times. Following the presentation of this list, subjects were asked to recall as many of the items as they could from the original list. Then, subjects were read all the items from the original list and some items that were never presented before and asked to estimate how many times they had heard these words.
4. Story memory: Subjects were read two stories and asked to recall as much information as they could about each story following its presentation. The number of story idea units recalled were recorded.
5. Word fluency: Subjects were asked to generate words for 90 sec that belonged to various categories (e.g., animals, countries, things you can buy in supermarkets) or began with a specific letter (e.g. F,A,S).

Mood State and Physical Condition
1. Beck Depression Inventory: This scale was completed by the subject who indicated the number and severity of symptoms associated with depression that they were currently experiencing. A score of 15 or higher is suggestive of at least mild depression.
2. Somatization scale: This questionnaire is completed by the subject who indicates whether he or she is currently experiencing unusual symptoms that are typically associated with somatization.
3. Neurobehavioral rating scale: This scale is completed by the test *examiner* and indicates the severity of behavioral symptoms (e.g., depressed affect) observed by the examiner during the test examination.
4. Fatigue scale: Subjects rated their fatigue on an unpublished analog scale, developed by the Centers for Disease Control, reflecting the degree of fatigue they were experiencing on the day of testing, the month before the testing, and the month before their illness.

These scales and questionnaires were used for screening purposes only. A psychiatric diagnosis requires a formal psychiatric interview, which was not completed on any of the patients or controls in conjunction with this specific evaluation.

There were no significant between-group differences in performance on tests of intelligence, response time, planning, time perception, or problem-solving, with two exceptions. The CFS patients demonstrated greater variability than the controls in the timing of their tapping on the Time Clock task [$F (1,33) = 4.62, p < 0.03$], although the overall mean tapping times of the CFS patients and controls were similar. The CFS patients solved *more* problems than did the controls on the Tower of London task [$F (1,33) = 4.04, p < 0.05$]. On the other hand, CFS patients tended to make more errors in correctly solving the Tower of London problems [F (1,30) = 7.38, $p < 0.01$]. The essentially normal performance of CFS patients on these measures was in accord with expectations, given that their cognitive complaints primarily revolved around memory functions.

Several different components of memory functioning were evaluated. There were no between-group differences on the digit span task, indicating that short-term memory span was intact in the CFS group. There were also no between-group differences in retrieval of category exemplars suggesting that at least some aspects of semantic memory search and retrieval were intact. The CFS patients also demonstrated normal reaction times and visuomotor procedural learning on the Serial Reaction Time Task.

Despite normal functioning on these memory measures, CFS patients had a significantly lower score than controls on the General Memory Index of the Wechsler Memory Scale [F (1,34) = 5.05, p < 0.03], suggesting that some aspects of their current memory functioning were impaired. Specific subtest raw score comparisons revealed that the CFS patients were impaired only on the immediate [F (1,34) = 5.94, $p < 0.02$] and delayed [F (1,34) = 5.15, $p <$ 0.02] visual reproduction subtests that require the subject to reproduce complex geometric designs. Other subtests requiring attention and orientation, immediate and delayed verbal cued and free-recall, and nonverbal recognition memory were all performed within normal limits. On two measures of free- and incidental-recall (from the Experimental Paired-Associates and Hasher Frequency tasks), CFS patient recall and judgment were similar to those of the controls. On the first of two experimental stories, the CFS patients recalled as many story idea units as did the controls. However, following the second story, patients recalled significantly fewer idea units than did controls [F (1,33) = 15.26, $p < 0.0004$]. Furthermore, on the Experimental Paired-Associates Test (see Fig. 1), CFS patients recalled fewer words in the cued-retrieval condition than did controls [F (1,35) = 4.81, $p < 0.03$].

Thus, CFS patients appeared to have generally normal memory functioning, yet paradoxically, they demonstrated specific difficulties in recalling information under conditions of greater semantic structure and context (e.g., cued, as opposed to free-recall, and recall of story propositions, as opposed to isolated words) and in reproducing geometric designs. This is the opposite of the common finding in which normal subjects *and* patients with various types of central nervous system impairments are generally helped by increasing stimulus structure (as seen in story memory or cued-recall tasks). Correlational analysis was not particularly helpful in identifying associations between other variables (e.g., age, education, degree of fatigue, mood state), and these unusual memory deficits in the CFS patients, although verbal IQ was significantly correlated with the number of propositions retrieved on story two ($r = 0.46$), suggesting that the general verbal skills of these patients were partially responsible for their poorer performance.

In this particular study, there were no significant differences in the number of depressive symptoms reported by the CFS patients and controls on the Beck Depression Inventory. Scores from an examiner-rating scale showed that about a quarter of the CFS patients we tested demonstrated mild to moderately impaired attention and memory in their interactions with the examiner. As expected, CFS patients reported being significantly more fatigued on the day of testing than controls [F (1,30) = 46.37, $p < 0.0001$], and their fatigue on the testing day was compatible with their general level of fatigue throughout the illness. However, there were no differences between the level of pre-illness fatigue in the CFS patients and the current level of fatigue in the controls. Furthermore, there was no relation between any of these fatigue measures and cognitive performance in the CFS group.

Our neuropsychological evaluation demonstrated that CFS patients have mild selective deficits in memory-processing arising against a background of relatively normal cognitive functioning. Curiously, they had greater problems recalling material when the material or retrieval measure was the most structured. There was no relation between performance on these specific memory measures and mood state, fatigue level, age, or education, although verbal intelligence was correlated with story memory performance.

Summary of Neuropsychological Studies

In reviewing the few neuropsychological studies published in peer-reviewed journals, a few general observations can be made. Most CFS patients have *complaints* of cognitive deficits, particularly in the domains of attention and concentration, memory, and problem-solving. Most patients will also have *complaints* of emotional distress. In some studies, the severity of the cognitive and mood-state complaints tend to be correlated. Objective neuropsychological testing does not substantiate the range and severity of the cognitive complaints of CFS patients. However, some areas of cognitive deficit emerge, with memory and concentration problems most frequently identified. The severity of the objectively recorded cognitive deficits range from mild to severe, although most cases fall into the mild range. There is some evidence that CFS patients have more difficulty remembering well-structured, as opposed to loosely structured, information—a somewhat unusual finding. Furthermore, on most tests of sustained attention, CFS patient performance remains accurate over time, shows normal brain processing, and no change in response times (which although slowed, were stable over 4 hr time).

THE DILEMMA FOR THE NEUROPSYCHOLOGIST

What should determine whether or not a CFS patient is to be neuropsychologically evaluated? It is always possible that another neurological disorder may be masquerading as CFS—for example, multiple sclerosis. Furthermore, the complaints of CFS patients must be addressed. Therefore, a standard neuropsychological screening evaluation should include tasks that focus on attentional processes, response times, memory, and problem-solving. Some attempt to estimate premorbid cognitive abilities would be useful. Some personality scales measuring anxiety, depression, somatization, and level of fatigue and its effect on interpersonal functioning should also be included. A scale that measures the cognitive complaints of CFS patients should be used in conjunction with their objective test performance. Table 5 can serve as a guide for domains and types of tests useful in the examination of CFS patients. When possible, a formal psychiatric diagnostic interview should be conducted with each patient. Since the patient may have cycles of fatigue, testing should be scheduled to optimize test performance [29].

Given the disparity between the severity of cognitive complaints and objective test performance reported so far in the CFS literature, neuropsychologists must

Table 5 The Domains of Cognitive Functioning to Be Evaluated in CFS

Intelligence
     Measure of global intellectual ability
Reasoning and problem solving
     Measure of concept formation
     Measure of planning
     Measure of analogic reasoning
     Measure of feeling of knowing
Attention
     Measure of sustained attention
     Measure of selective attention
     Measure of divided attention
Memory
     Measure of short-term memory span
     Measure of learning
     Measures of recall and recognition
     Measure of implicit/automatic memory
Response time
     Measures of motor speed and coordination
     Measures of simple and choice response times
Mood state and personality
     Measure of fatigue
     Measure of somatization
     Measure of personality traits
     Measures of depression and anxiety
     Measure of self-report of cognitive status
     Psychiatric interview

refrain from the kind of skepticism that would blind them to interesting patterns of deficits and strengths in CFS patients. For the time being, given their complaints, all CFS patients should be carefully examined for neuropsychological deficits.

There are several possible explanations for impaired cognitive performance in CFS patients. For example, CFS could involve lesions or dysfunction in one or more brain structures that, in turn, are responsible for the instantiation of specific cognitive processes. Chronic fatigue syndrome as a prolonged illness, could lead to a reactive depression, which would then affect effortful cognitive performance. The cognitive deficits in CFS could also represent an exaggerated behavioral response in certain personalities to a normally occurring fluctuation in immune system regulation [13,30–35]. In all these cases, there is much to be learned from relating the clinical neurobehavioral performance of the patient to the type of medical disorder. Because of the diagnostic dilemma posed by CFS patients, they are an interesting challenge for the neuropsychologist. Furthermore, studying patients whose illness results in a persistent fatigue can help neuropsychologists tease apart the effects of peripheral and central fatigue from specific cognitive deficits, an as yet unresolved quagmire in interpreting the results of the neuropsychological evaluation that can often last several hours.

CONCLUSIONS

Chronic fatigue syndrome is a diagnostic category that eludes a single etiological description [6,7,17,36–38]. Studies to date, in general, have revealed only relatively minor cognitive problems in patients. These problems lie in the domains of memory and attention and, yet, are related to the degree of mood state changes, as reported by the patient. Clearly, the severity of impairment in these areas of cognition, as reported by the CFS patient, exceeds their objective performance. Neuropsychological testing should be done in conjunction with a medical assessment. The diagnostic workup is targeted to evaluate whether the patient meets the CDC CFS criteria, which, unfortunately, are not strictly adhered to, but instead depends on the hospital, region, or country where the diagnosis is made [6,17].

Regardless of comparisons of CFS to neurasthenia or the words of pundits who dismiss CFS as nothing more than depression or a related psychiatric diagnosis, these patients present with veritable problems that require the involvement of trained neuropsychologists for assessment (and research purposes). The inclusion of a neuropsychological evaluation in the medical workup for CFS will surely lead to improved characterization of the disabling neurological and behavioral symptoms so often reported by patients with this disorder.

REFERENCES

1. Komaroff AL. Clinical presentation of chronic fatigue syndrome. In: Bock GR, Whelan J, eds. Chronic fatigue syndrome. Ciba Found Symp 1993, 173:43–61.
2. Grafman J, Johnson RJ, Scheffers M. Cognitive and mood-state changes in patients with chronic fatigue syndrome. Rev Infect Dis 1991; 13 (Suppl 1):S45–S52.
3. Gow JW, Behan WM, Clements GB, Woodall C, Riding M, Behan PO. Enteroviral RNA sequences detected by polymerase chain reaction in muscle of patients with postviral fatigue syndrome [see comments]. Br Med J 1991; 302:692–6.
4. Buchwald D, Cheney PR, Peterson DL, et al. A chronic illness characterized by fatigue, neurologic and immunologic disorders, and active human herpesvirus type 6 infection. Ann Intern Med 1992; 116:103–13.
5. Wessley S. The neuropsychiatry of chronic fatigue syndrome. In: Chronic fatigue syndrome. Ciba Found Symp 1993, 173:212–37.
6. Schluederberg A, Straus SE, Peterson P, et al. Chronic fatigue syndrome research: definition and medical outcome assessment. Ann Intern Med 1992; 117:325–31.
7. Schluederberg A, Straus SE, Grufferman S. Considerations in the design of studies of chronic fatigue syndrome. Rev Infect Dis 1991;13(suppl 1):S1–S140.
8. Imboden JB, Canter A, Cluff LB, Trever RW. Brucellosis: III. Psychological aspects of delayed convalescence. Arch Intern Med 1959; 103:406–14.
9. Grafman J, Schwartz V, Dale JK, Scheffers M, Houser C, Straus SE. Analysis of neuropsychological functioning in patients with chronic fatigue syndrome. J Neurol Neurosurg Psychiatry 1993; 56:684–89.
10. Abbey SE, Garfinkel PE. Chronic fatigue syndrome and depression: cause, effect, or covariate. Rev Infect Dis 1991; 13 (Suppl 1):S73–S83.
11. Weingartner H, Silberman E. Cognitive changes in depression. In: Post R, Ballenger J, eds. Neurobiology of mood disorders. Baltimore: Williams & Wilkins, 1987.
12. Ray C, Weir WRC, Cullen S, Phillips S. Illness perception and symptom components in chronic fatigue syndrome. J Psychosom Res 1992; 36:243–56.
13. Baumann LJ, Cameron LD, Zimmerman RS, Leventhal H. Illness representations and matching labels with symptoms. Health Psychol 1989; 8:449–69.
14. DeFreitas E, Hilliard B, Cheney PR, et al. Retroviral sequences related to human T-lymphotropic virus type II in patients with chronic fatigue immune dysfunction syndrome. Proc Natl Acad Sci USA 1991; 88:2922–6.
15. Behan PO, Bakheit AM. Clinical spectrum of postviral fatigue syndrome. Br Med Bull 1991; 47:793–808.
16. Lynch S, Seth R. Postviral fatigue syndrome and the VP-1 antigen [letter; comment]. Lancet 1989; 2:1160–1.
17. Levine PH, Jacobson S, Pocinki AG, et al. Clinical, epidemiologic, and virologic studies in four clusters of the chronic fatigue syndrome. Arch Intern Med 1992; 152:1611–6.
18. Altay HT, Toner BB, Brooker H, Abbey SE, Salit IE, Garfinkel PE. The neuropsychological dimensions of postinfectious neuromyasthenia (chronic fatigue syndrome): a preliminary report. Int J Psychiatry Med 1990; 20:141–9.
19. Riccio M, Thompson C, Wilson B, Morgan DJ, Lant AF. Neuropsychological and psychiatric abnormalities in myalgic encephalomyelitis: a preliminary report. Br J Clin Psychol 1992; 31:111–20.

20. Smith A. Cognitive changes in myalgic encephalomyelitis. In: Jenkins R, Mowbray JF, eds. Post-viral fatigue syndrome. Chichester: John Wiley & Sons, 1992:179–94.

21. Smith AP. Chronic fatigue syndrome and performance. In: Smith AP, Jones DM, eds. Handbook of human performance. vol 2. London: Academic Press, 1992:261–78.

22. Smith AP, Behan PO, Bell W, Millar K, Bakheit M. Behavioral problems associated with the chronic fatigue syndrome. Br J. Psychol 1993; 84:411–23.

23. Krupp L, Sliwinski MJ, Doscher C, Jandorf L, Burns L, Coyle PK. Fatigue, mood, and cognitive functions in chronic fatigue syndrome (CFS) and multiple sclerosis (MS). Albany Conference on Chronic Fatigue Syndrome. Albany, NY: 1992.

24. DeLuca J, Johnson SK, Natelson BH. Information processing efficiency in chronic fatigue syndrome and multiple sclerosis. Arch Neurol 1993; 50:301–4.

25. Katon W, Russo J. Chronic fatigue syndrome criteria: a critique of the requirement for multiple physical complaints. Arch Intern Med 1992; 152:1604–9.

26. Scheffers MK, Johnson RJ, Grafman J, Dale JK, Straus SE. Attention and short-term memory in chronic fatigue syndrome patients: an event-related potential analysis. Neurology 1992; 42:1667–75.

27. Prasher D, Smith A, Findley L. Sensory and cognitive event-related potentials in myalgic encephalomyelitis. J Neurol Neurosurg Psychiatry 1990; 53:247–53.

28. Lezak M. Neuropsychological assessment. 2nd ed. New York: Oxford University Press, 1983.

29. Wood C, Magnello ME, Sharpe MC. Fluctuations in perceived energy and mood among patients with chronic fatigue syndrome. J R Soc Med 1992; 85:195–98.

30. Abbey SE, Garfinkel PE. Neurasthenia and chronic fatigue syndrome: the role of culture in the making of a diagnosis. Am J Psychiatry 1991; 148:1638–46.

31. Franzen MD, Iverson GL, McCracken LM. The detection of malingering in neuropsychological assessment. Neuropsychol Rev 1990; 1:247–79.

32. Lane TJ, Manu P, Matthews DA. Depression and somatization in the chronic fatigue syndrome. Am J Med 1991; 91:335–44.

33. Othmer E, DeSouza C. A screening test for somatization disorder (hysteria). Am J Psychiatry 1985; 142:1146–9.

34. Wessely S. Old Wine in new bottles: neurasthenia and "ME." Psychol Med 1990; 20:35–53.

35. White PD. Fatigue and chronic fatigue syndromes. In: Bass CM, ed. Somatization: physical symptoms and psychological illness. London: Blackwell Scientific, 1990:104–40.

36. Durack DT, Street AC. Fever of unknown origin—reexamined and redefined. Curr Clin Top Infect Dis 1991; 11:35–51.

37. Holmes GP, Kaplan JE, Gantz NM, et al. Chronic fatigue syndrome: a working case definition. Ann Intern Med 1988; 108:387–9.

38. Peterson PK, Schenck CH, Sherman R. Chronic fatigue syndrome in Minnesota [see comments]. Minn Med 1991; 74:21–26.

11

Neuroendocrine Aspects of Chronic Fatigue Syndrome: Implications for Diagnosis and Research

Mark A. Demitrack

University of Michigan Medical Center,
Ann Arbor, Michigan

> Neurasthenia, indeed, has been the Central Africa of medicine—an unexplored territory into which few men enter, and those few have been compelled to bring reports that have been neither credited nor comprehended.
>
> George Beard, 1880

It is the premise of this chapter that chronic fatigue syndrome (CFS) is best understood as a clinical condition emerging from the complex interaction of a heterogeneous array of infectious and noninfectious antecedents, and perpetuated by specific pathological responses to these events, rather than representing a discrete disease with a singular cause. In this chapter I develop an analytic framework that suggests that a variety of apparently disparate antecedent factors, such as physical or emotional stress, psychiatric illness, or infection, may ultimately converge at the level of the central nervous system (CNS) in a final common pathway, resulting in the clinical syndrome of chronic fatigue. Although the precise components composing this pathway are not completely clear, I present a rationale and data to support the hypothesis that a specific disturbance in neuroendocrine function, especially of the hypothalamic–pituitary–adrenal (HPA) axis, serves as an important element in this final pathway, and may function as a biological mediator of several of the manifest signs and symptoms associated with this syndrome.

RATIONALE FOR A NEUROENDOCRINE APPROACH TO CHRONIC FATIGUE SYNDROME

In this chapter I assume that the currently termed CFS is not a new entity, but rather, has had many previous incarnations in the medical literature. A full discussion justifying this assumption is beyond the scope of this chapter and is dealt with in a more complete fashion elsewhere in this volume, and in other references [1]. One of the earliest and most persistent names for this clinical syndrome, neurasthenia, was coined by George Beard [2], and exists to the current day in certain illness classifications. The preeminent role of stress in the onset and perpetuation of this syndrome was alluded to, in general, by the choice of name (i.e., nervous exhaustion). More specifically, though, Beard observed, "Among the special exciting causes of neurasthenia may be mentioned the pressure of bereavement, business and family cares, parturition and abortion, sexual excesses, the abuse of stimulants and narcotics, and civilized starvation, such as is sometimes observed even among the wealthy order of society, and sudden retirement from business. . . ."

The repeated observation of the stress-responsive nature of this syndrome has led some to suggest that the prominence of neuropsychiatric symptoms in the clinical presentation is, in and of itself, a sufficient explanation of its etiology. In this view, CFS represents the behavioral aftermath of an acute, often infectious, stress in emotionally susceptible individuals (i.e., the psychiatric symptoms are synonymous with the illness itself). Indeed, such a framework is reflected quite bluntly by the exasperated conclusions articulated by Paul Wood in 1941, "patients should be informed of the nature of their illness and be treated as psychoneurotics; their distaste for this label may prove quite helpful. . . . The patient must be induced to believe that he is suffering from the effects of emotional disturbance and not from any disease or alteration of visceral function" [3].

In recent years, such a model would seem to be further bolstered by the results of studies using structured psychiatric interview techniques, which have suggested that the prevalence of psychiatric illness is higher in patients with CFS than in the general population, or even in other comparable somatically ill patients, and often precedes the onset of the fatigue syndrome by months or years [4–10]. To date, only one study refutes this position, showing a prevalence of psychiatric illness comparable with that of the general population, and a temporal relation suggesting that the psychiatric morbidity more often follows, rather than precedes, the development of the chronic fatigue [9]. Despite these data, a descriptive algorithm for the differentiation of primary psychiatric illnesses from

CFS remains elusive. Most investigators would agree that formally diagnosable psychiatric illnesses are present in well over half of all cases [4–10]. Indeed, it has been suggested that the specific requirement in the Centers for Disease Control (CDC) case definition of CFS for multiple somatic symptoms leads to an artifactual bias toward the overrepresentation of psychiatric illness in formal research studies of the illness [11]. A cautious conclusion from these studies would suggest that, in the absence of objective biological criteria, the use of descriptive criteria alone makes it difficult, if not impossible, to determine whether a psychiatric disorder is fully explanatory of the clinical presentation, a secondary manifestation of a primary disease process, or a coincident disease that modulates the presentation and course of the fatigue state.

Concurrent with the evolution of the preceding ideas, a competing pathophysiological model has maintained the primary importance of the infectious onset in the etiology of this syndrome. In this view, the constitutional symptoms associated with CFS emerge directly from persistent immune activation or other lasting pathophysiological changes caused by the initial infectious event. Such a "physiological" model has an equally lengthy history to its "psychological" counterpart. More recently, evidence supporting an infectious or persistent immune dysregulation hypothesis emerged largely from a series of reports that appeared between 1982 and 1985. These studies noted a spectrum of subtle abnormalities in cell-mediated and humoral immunity in these patients, along with Epstein–Barr virus and other viral antigens [12–14]. These immunological disturbances, coupled with the clinical observation that many of these patients developed the syndrome following an episode of acute infectious mononucleosis, led to the specific hypothesis that the illness was a manifestation of chronic Epstein–Barr viral infection. However, subsequent observations have challenged this idea [15–18] and suggest that, whereas immune stimulation may be present in a large proportion of these patients, persistent Epstein–Barr viral infection is almost certainly not a tenable explanation for most cases of the syndrome. Although no clear and convincing evidence has yet emerged to demonstrate a causal relation between infection with any specific viral or other microbial agent and the subsequent development of CFS, several viruses continue to receive attention and are dealt with more thoroughly in other chapters in this volume. Specific interest has focused on the herpesviruses (e.g., Epstein–Barr virus, herpes simplex viruses, cytomegalovirus, and human herpesvirus type-6), and the enteroviruses (e.g., Coxsackie B virus). A recent report has added a putative novel retroviral agent to this list [19]. Even though intriguing, these latter results have not been replicable using similar sequence probes in polymerase chain reaction (PCL) studies [20].

The mutually exclusive distinction between the strictly psychological or physiological etiologies summarized in the previous paragraphs may be more apparent than real. Indeed, we have argued elsewhere [21] that the phenomenologic overlap between CFS and a variety of primary psychiatric illnesses reflects the involvement of a shared psychobiological pathway that may be similarly dysregulated by a disparate variety of infectious or noninfectious pathophysiological antecedents. Considered in this light, several considerations would suggest that a focus on neuroendocrine function may be a particularly useful domain of study and help in establishing a more integrative view of this syndrome (Table 1). Several observations justify such a view.

First, a tremendous body of work has established the intimate relation between stress and the development of a variety of psychiatric disorders. As will be elaborated in the next section, there are several well-established neurobiological abnormalities that accompany these stress-related illnesses and are thought to play important roles in mediating the overall functional abnormalities of these disorders. The stress-responsive character of CFS is also an accepted clinical observation, and the presence of psychiatric symptoms and syndromes before and during the course of the illness is clearly known. What is less clearly known, however, is whether these specific psychiatric disorders in patients with CFS share the same pathophysiological mechanisms as in patients with primary psychiatric illnesses who do not also report the specific symptoms of CFS. Therefore, a detailed examination of the neuroendocrine correlates of CFS may be compared with similar findings in patients with primary psychiatric illnesses. Similarities of differences in biological phenotype may consequently refine our understanding of the relation between these two illness types and move our knowledge base beyond the limitations of the purely descriptive approaches detailed in the foregoing.

Second, it remains possible that an acute infectious illness serves as the precipitating event in many, but not all, patients with CFS. Acute infections are a profound physiological stress that results in substantial disturbances in neuroendocrine function. That these biological events may, in turn, have important consequences for the individual, and account for a major portion of the morbidity of the acute illness itself, is well established. For instance, various acute viral infections activate the HPA axis [22–24]. It has been suggested that this is an adaptive response, acting to contain the inflammatory process, and is presumed to occur as a result of the secretion of cytokines (e.g., interleukin-1),

Table 1 Reasons for an Interest in the Neuroendocrinology of Chronic Fatigue Syndrome

- Stress-responsive nature of chronic fatigue syndrome; comparison of biological phenotype with other stress-related illnesses
- Interrelated nature of central nervous system, immune system, and endocrine system
- Potential for acute viral infections to produce long-lasting changes in important homeostatic events

which directly stimulate central components of the axis [25]. Conversely, lack of an adequate glucocorticoid response in acute viral illness has been suggested to predict poor outcome and the need for supplemental glucocorticoid therapy. Neuroendocrine consequences of infectious events are not limited to pituitary–adrenal disturbances. For example, diabetes insipidus, due to either destructive lesions of the anterior hypothalamus or a functional inhibition of vasopressin secretion, has been described [26,27], as well as the inappropriate secretion of vasopressin [28], or more extensive patterns of hypothalamic–pituitary insufficiency [29]. In contrast to these observations in acute infections, chronic infectious states, such as viral hepatitis or infection with the human immunodeficiency virus (HIV), may also display more subtle derangements in neuroendocrine function, including mild grades of adrenal or gonadal failure [30–34]. Alternatively, and arguably of more relevance to a consideration of the role of infections in the development of CFS, it has been proposed that certain acute viral infections may result in long-lasting physiological changes. For example, Oldstone and colleagues have provided compelling evidence in animals demonstrating that viral infections may lead to persistent pathological changes in differentiated cellular functions, long after the infection itself has resolved [35]. With use of a poorly cytocidal murine RNA virus, the lymphocytic choriomeningitis virus, they showed that persistent infection alters levels of acetylcholine synthesis in neuroblastoma cells in vitro [36]. Furthermore, in mice, this virus displays a specific tropism for anterior pituitary somatotrophs, leading to a syndrome of retarded growth and abnormal glucose regulation caused by a specific impairment in the synthesis and secretion of growth hormone [37]. Similarly, others have shown that young mice infected with canine distemper virus later develop an obesity syndrome associated with specific alterations in brain catecholamine synthesis [38]. These syndromes develop in the absence of overt cellular lesions in brain tissue and no demonstrable viral antigen expression by immunofluorescent staining. In other words, it is possible that an infectious event early in the life of the individual may result in substantial and long-lasting changes in organismic homeostasis, without damaging the morphological appearance of the infected cells.

Finally, as has been alluded to in the preceding paragraphs, there are important bidirectional paths of communication between the central nervous system, the endocrine system, and the immunological cells of the body. Disturbance in the integrity of the system at any level may have important, and not readily predictable, implications for the outcome of the illness. Hence, a thorough understanding of the pathophysiology of CFS will most likely be enhanced by integrative, rather than strictly linear, models of illness development. For instance, in the historical work noted earlier, psychological vulnerability was appreciated essentially as a behavioral modifier, distorting the normal recuperative course from an acute infectious illness. Considered in light of the physiological connectivity among central nervous, endocrine, and immune systems, the psychological state of the individual takes on an additional dimension as an antecedent variable. Namely, psychological stress may alter immune responsiveness by modulation of autonomic nervous system reactivity [39] or by hormone-mediated effects on lymphoid tissue, or by a combination thereof [40]. In other words, psychological stress could directly alter host resistance to infection. Although the literature supporting this view is inconsistent [41], this additional avenue for psychological stress highlights the complex effects even a single factor may have in the overall development of CFS. Hence, an increased burden of psychological stress may both enhance susceptibility to the infectious agents involved in the pathophysiology of CFS and, at the same time, aggravate the longitudinal course of the illness by increasing the likelihood of abnormal illness behaviors during the recuperative process.

RELEVANT PREVIOUS STUDIES OF HYPOTHALAMIC–PITUITARY–ADRENAL FUNCTION

In the coordinated physiological response to physical and emotional stress, the HPA axis is generally considered to play a pivotal role. In this section I will highlight some of the important neurochemical and neuroanatomical features of this axis, and summarize basic observations in major depression and related psychiatric illnesses that bear on our work in CFS. Regulation of the HPA axis involves a complex array of biochemical events occurring principally among the hypothalamus, pituitary, and the cortex of the adrenal gland [42]. Key among these biochemical signals is corticotropin-releasing hormone (CRH), a 41-amino acid peptide hormone for which the major concentrations in brain are localized in discrete areas of the parvocellular subdivisions of the paraventricular nucleus (PVN) of the hypothalamus. Corticotropin-releasing hormone is also widely distributed in other, extrahypothalamic locations, including the limbic system, cerebral cortex, midbrain areas, pons, and medulla. Acute and chronic stress results in activation of hypothalamic CRH neurons as a final common event; CRH is then transported by nerve terminals in the median eminence of the hypothalamus into the portal plexus bathing the hormone-secreting cells of the anterior pituitary. Corticotropin (adrenocorticotropic hormone; ACTH) is then released into the systemic circulation, primarily to effect glucocorticoid release from the adrenal cortex. Complex short and long negative-feedback circuits among these three principal biochemical signals then converge to terminate activation of the axis. The specific suprahypothalamic biochemical signals that effect the activation of hypothalamic CRH in response to stress are complex, involving both peptide- as well as catecholamine-containing neural pathways [43]. Such pathways are usually redundant circuits, and are often composed of neuronal terminals that colocalize several peptide and nonpeptide elements. Less well studied than these biochemical signals, but of equal importance, are several specific neural circuits that have regulatory effects on the HPA axis. These areas include the amygdala, hippocampus, septal area, cingulate cortex, and certain brain stem regions. In addition to the stress-dependent activation of the HPA axis, it appears that intrinsic rhythmic elements in the suprachiasmatic nucleus drive the basal activity of the HPA axis in its characteristic circadian fashion. In humans, this circadian rhythm in ACTH and cortisol secretion is entrained to the sleep–wake cycle [44], with the trough of activity occurring in the evening and early night, and the peak in activity occurring just before waking.

Although a full review of the neuroendocrine correlates of the major psychiatric illnesses is beyond the scope of this chapter, several considerations pertinent to our findings in patients with CFS will be discussed here. A seminal observation that heralded the modern era of biological psychiatry was that patients with major depression demonstrated a characteristic disruption of the normal diurnal rhythmicity of the pituitary–adrenal axis [45]. This disturbance involved an elevation of adrenal glucocorticoid output, usually seen as an earlier onset of the morning surge of the axis, in conjunction with enhanced cortisol secretion in the late afternoon. Aberrant feedback regulation of the axis was suggested by studies employing the synthetic glucocorticoid, dexamethasone [46,47]. In normal individuals, administration of 1 mg of dexamethasone in the late evening results in a sustained suppression of endogenous glucocorticoid production over the next 24 hr. In contrast, approximately two-thirds of hospitalized patients with major depression "escape" from the suppressive effects of dexamethasone earlier than normal, with a return of supranormal endogenous glucocorticoid secretion [47]. Over the past decade, detailed studies of the HPA axis have further refined an understanding of the biochemical events responsible for this finding. A model of HPA axis dysregulation has been developed on the basis of this work, which suggests that, in major depression, there is an excessive central release of corticotropin-releasing hormone, with the subsequent development of adrenal gland hypertrophy from chronic overstimulation of the target organ itself. The specific mechanism underlying this central activation, however, remains elusive. For instance, the relative contribution of absent feedback inhibition, intrinsic overproduction, or impaired degradation of CRH, or sustained activation of the feed-forward biochemical and neural circuits driving the circadian rhythm of the axis are incompletely understood.

Although it was initially hoped that this line of investigation would result in a more specific, standardized laboratory diagnosis for major depression, this goal has not been realized. Indeed, although more recent investigations reinforce the idea that centrally mediated hypercortisolism is present in nearly two-thirds of inpatients with formally defined major depression, similar evidence of centrally mediated hypercortisolism has been described in other major psychiatric illnesses. Examples of this include anorexia nervosa [48], panic disorder [49], and alcoholism [50]. Nevertheless, these data have provided the fundamental groundwork informing our understanding of the neurobiological disturbances associated with acute and chronic stress.

The close phenomenologic similarity of CFS with major depression would suggest that a comparison of the specific neuroendocrine characteristics of these two clinical entities would be a fruitful line of inquiry. Several early reports are of particular interest relative to this point. In a study of benign myalgic encephalomyelitis employing the dexamethasone suppression test, only 1 of 16 subjects showed evidence of glucocorticoid nonsuppression, a remarkably low percentage [4]. Furthermore, in fibromyalgia, a syndrome that shares many of the clinical features of CFS, fewer than 5% of patients showed abnormal suppression to dexamethasone [51]. Patients with this latter syndrome also have reduced diurnal glucocorticoid levels [52] and impaired reactivity of the HPA axis to a variety of endocrine challenge strategies [53]. Interestingly, Poteliakhoff reported, in 1981, that subjects with both acute and chronic fatigue states showed reductions in plasma cortisol, when compared with nonfatigued individuals, along with altered circadian variation in capillary resistance and eosinophil counts [54]. These latter results suggested that even quite mild decrements in circulating glucocorticoids may be associated with measurable physiological changes.

In recent years, it has become increasingly apparent that depression is a heterogeneous condition from a psychological and from a physiological perspective. The initial investigations of the neuroendocrine correlates of depression, cited earlier, largely concerned the more classic, melancholic form of depression, namely that characterized by increased agitation, loss of sleep, loss of interest in all activities, persistent suicidal thoughts, and reduced appetite and libido. More recently, several alternative forms of depressive illness have been characterized, more often described as "atypical" or "anergic" depression owing to the absence of the features characteristic of the more classic, melancholic depression. These depressive subtypes are usually dominated by reduced energy, a reactive mood, a reversal of the typical pattern of vegetative features seen in classic depression. Examples of these depressive syndromes include the depressive phase of manic–depressive illness and the so-called seasonal affective disorder [55], atypical major depression [56], and the depressive syndromes seen in the context of certain endocrinopathies, such as primary hypothyroidism and the postoperative state of Cushing's disease. Interestingly, recent evidence suggests a pattern of HPA function in some of these syndromes reflecting inappropriately normal or frankly reduced activation of the axis [57–60]. Finally, it is also worth noting a recent series of studies of HPA function in patients with posttraumatic stress disorder, a paradigmatic stress-related illness. These patients show a reduced 24-hr urinary output of adrenal glucocorticoids, in conjunction with low rates of suppression after dexamethasone administration [61].

Taken together, these results we have briefly reviewed here suggest that the response to acute or chronic stress is heterogeneous, and not easily predictable. Many possible stable regulatory outcomes may exist, each of which may depend in critical ways on the constitutional endowment of the individual and the context and temporal sequence of the delivery of the stressful stimuli. In other words, factors such as the premorbid stress experience of the individual, the contextual nature of the delivery of the past and concurrent stressors, as well as the nature of concurrent physiological events (i.e., infectious episodes) may be important determinants of the long-term physiological response to stress.

STUDIES OF THE HYPOTHALAMIC–PITUITARY– ADRENAL AXIS IN CHRONIC FATIGUE SYNDROME

In light of these considerations, my colleagues and I have proposed a reconceptualization of the functional meaning of the symptoms seen in patients with CFS as an orienting context for our neuroendocrine studies. Specifically, a review of the clinical features of CFS shows considerable overlap with that seen in patients with glucocorticoid deficiency (Table 2). Indeed, one of the principal symptoms of glucocorticoid deficiency is debilitating fatigue. An abrupt onset precipitated by a stressor, feverishness, arthralgias, myalgias, adenopathy, postexertional fatigue, exacerbation of allergic responses, and disturbances in mood and sleep are also characteristic of glucocorticoid insufficiency [62]. Notably, these symptoms are often seen in the relatively rare syndrome of partial or subclinical adrenal insufficiency, which may be detectable only by ACTH stimulation or other endocrine testing in patients who fail to show the symptoms of classic Addison's disease, such as hypotension and abnormal fluid and electrolyte

Table 2 Similarity in Symptomatology of Chronic Fatigue Syndrome and Secondary Glucocorticoid-Deficient States

Secondary glucocorticoid deficiency	Chronic fatigue syndrome
Fatigue	Fatigue
Anorexia, nausea	Low-grade fever
Myalgias	Myalgias
Sleep disorder	Sleep disorder
Impaired cognition	Impaired cognition
Depression	Depression
Anxiety	Anxiety
Muscle weakness	Muscle weakness
Arthralgias	Arthralgias
Allergic responses	Allergic responses
	Headaches
	Pharyngitis

balance. Since glucocorticoids represent the most potent endogenous immunosuppressive compounds, we have further suggested that some of the
reported immunological disturbances in patients with CFS (e.g., exacerbation of
allergic responses, the profile of enhanced antibody titers to a variety of viral·
antigens, and elevations in cytokine levels) could also reflect a mild or relative
glucocorticoid deficiency. It has recently been shown, in animals, that a defect
in the responsiveness of the HPA axis to immune mediators confers a risk for
the development of inflammatory disease [63,64]. Furthermore, in humans,
withdrawal from hypercortisolemic states has been associated with the exacerbation of autoimmune thyroiditis [65], as well as the development of myalgias,
arthralgias, muscle weakness [66], and even severe fibromyalgia [67].

We have now completed a series of studies assessing the integrity of the HPA
axis in 30 patients with CFS and in 72 normal healthy volunteers [68]. These
studies comprised several different experimental procedures. The basal functional
activity of the axis was assessed by obtaining multiple evening baseline samples
for the measurement of total and free plasma cortisol concentrations, serial 24-hr
urine collections to assess urinary free cortisol excretion, and basal evening
measurement of plasma cortisol-binding globulin (CBG) binding capacity (Figs.
1 and 2). The latter measure was of interest, since levels of CBG are sensitive
to the negative-feedback effect of circulating glucocorticoids [69]. The results
of this basal assessment suggested a pattern of neuroendocrine dysfunction
characterized by a significant reduction in plasma and urinary glucocorticoid

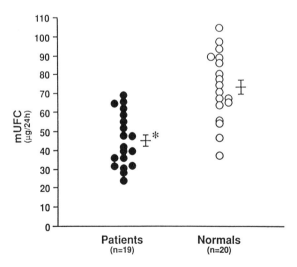

Figure 1   Urinary free cortisol (UFC) levels in patients with chronic fatigue syndrome
compared with healthy normal individuals (patients are represented by the filled circles,
normals by the open circles, *$p < 0.0002$). (From Ref. 68.)

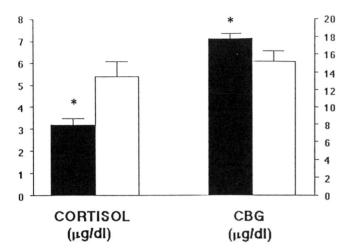

Figure 2   Basal evening plasma cortisol levels and CBG levels in patients with chronic fatigue syndrome compared with healthy normal individuals (patients are represented by the solid bars, normals by the open bars; $*p < 0.01$ for cortisol, $*p < 0.03$ for CBG).

levels. These findings contrast sharply with the sustained glucocorticoid excess seen in many patients with classic major depressive illness. Of particular interest, they are compatible with the observations noted in the previous section, including the reduced cortisol levels in chronic and acute fatigue states reported by Poteliakhoff [54], the low incidence of dexamethasone nonsuppression in patients with neuromyasthenia [4] and fibromyalgia [51], and the reduced diurnal glucocorticoid levels [52] and impaired HPA axis reactivity to neuroendocrine challenge [53] seen in primary fibromyalgia.

To more specifically characterize the locus of the disturbance in adrenal glucocorticoid secretion, we followed these studies of basal HPA axis activity with several specific challenge strategies. The plasma ACTH response to ovine CRH was used as a direct measure of corticotroph function, whereas adrenal functional activity was evaluated both indirectly by examining cortisol response to ovine CRH, and directly by measuring cortisol response to graded, submaximal stimulatory doses of ACTH. We also assessed gross central nervous system activity of the hypothalamic–pituitary–adrenal axis by measuring the levels of CRH and ACTH in cerebrospinal fluid (CSF) samples obtained by lumbar puncture. On the basis of the pattern of neuroendocrine response to these studies, we advanced the hypothesis that a primary adrenal deficit is an unlikely explanation for these results, rather, we have proposed that a failure in the central activation of the HPA axis may be a more likely and attractive hypothesis. It should be cautioned that this hypothesis is *inferential*, based on our interpretation of the observed data and with the following considerations in mind.

First, a primary disturbance in adrenal function would be expected to demonstrate reduced responsiveness of the adrenal cortex to all dose ranges of ACTH [57], and an exaggerated pituitary response to CRH administration [70]. In fact, CFS patients clearly did not demonstrate the latter response (as will be elaborated later) and, indeed, appeared to hyperrespond to low doses of ACTH in three different instances: (1) patients with CFS showed significantly higher net integrated cortisol responses at the two lowest doses of ACTH employed (Fig. 3), (2) compared with controls, patients with CFS showed a half-maximal cortisol response to a lower dose of ACTH (see Fig. 3), and (3) during evening challenge with ovine CRH, patients with CFS showed an exaggerated plasma cortisol response relative to the amount of ACTH released following ovine CRH administration (Fig. 4). The peak levels of plasma ACTH during CRH stimulation testing were comparable with those obtained after the administration of the lowest doses of exogenous ACTH we used.

Second, the net integrated pituitary ACTH response to ovine CRH was

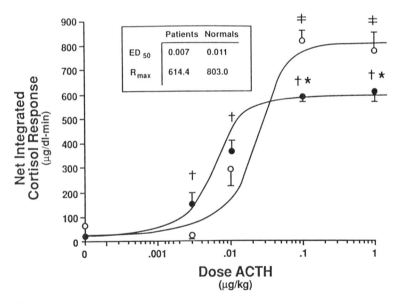

Figure 3 ACTH dose–response study in patients with chronic fatigue syndrome compared with healthy normal individuals (patients are represented by the filled circles, normals by the open circles; subject $\times$ dose interaction effect: $p = 0.0015$; post hoc comparisons: $*p < 0.05$ and $*p < 0.08$ for 0.1 and 1.0 μg/kg ACTH doses, respectively; within group effects: $\dagger p < 0.05$ for patients, all doses greater than placebo response; $\ddagger p < 0.05$ for normals, only 0.1 and 1.0 μg/kg doses greater than placebo). (From Ref. 68.)

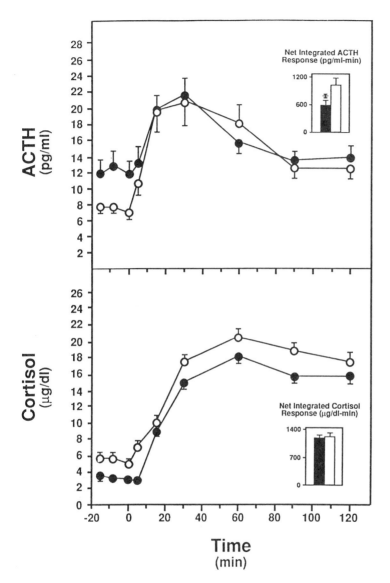

Figure 4   ACTH and cortisol response to evening administration of ovine CRH in patients with chronic fatigue syndrome compared with healthy normal individuals (patients are represented by the filled circles, normals by the open circles; insets show net integrated responses; *$p < 0.05$). (From Ref. 68.)

reduced (see Fig. 4), a finding that is the antithesis of that expected in primary adrenal failure, as noted earlier. Such a reduction in net pituitary responsiveness has been reported in several other clinical conditions, including major depression [71,72] and the underweight phase of anorexia nervosa [48]. Both of these illnesses are associated with hypercortisolism, and it has been postulated that the attenuated ACTH response to CRH reflects a pituitary corticotroph cell appropriately restrained in its responsiveness by high levels of circulating glucocorticoids. In support of this hypothesis is the finding of a significant negative correlation between bassl total cortisol levels and the net ACTH response to CRH in those patients [48]. It is clear that the blunted ACTH response to exogenous CRH in patients with CFS is not analogous to what has previously been reported in major depression or anorexia nervosa, since patients with CFS show *reduced*, rather than *increased*, glucocorticoid levels. However, a third context in which an attenuated net integrated ACTH response to CRH has been noted is in the hypothalamic CRH-deficient state described during the early postoperative period after curative surgery in patients with Cushing's syndrome [73,74]. Several lines of evidence suggest that this postoperative adrenal insufficiency reflects, in large part, a state of prolonged suppression of hypothalamic CRH. These patients will demonstrate measurable levels of plasma ACTH after the administration of CRH, indicating that if the patients' own hypothalamic CRH neurons were not suppressed by the long-standing hypercortisolism, one would expect to observe somewhat higher levels of basal plasma ACTH and cortisol. Furthermore, patients with Cushing's syndrome show a marked reduction in cerebrospinal fluid levels of CRH [57,58]. Finally, although these postoperative subjects show an attenuated ACTH response to exogenous CRH, it can be normalized rapidly with repeated administration of CRH, but this response cannot be sustained after the withdrawal of CRH [74]. These data suggest that, in the postoperative period, the pituitary corticotroph of patients with Cushing's syndrome becomes hyporesponsive to exogenous CRH owing to insufficient central priming by the long-standing, glucocorticoid- induced suppression of endogenous hypothalamic CRH. From these data we infer that the blunted ACTH response to CRH in patients with CFS, therefore, is more closely analogous to that seen in the context of postoperative Cushing's syndrome, rather than to that of hyper-cortisolemic major depression or the underweight phase of anorexia nervosa.

Third, the levels of cerebrospinal fluid CRH and ACTH in patients with CFS were normal, and not elevated. Although these findings are difficult to interpret with confidence, we consider such results to be *inappropriately* normal, given the magnitude of the putative reduction in glucocorticoid secretion in the periphery. Both CRH and ACTH in the CSF are responsive to the negative-feedback effects of circulating glucocorticoids [75,76]; hence, a reduction in peripheral glucocorticoid levels might be expected to result in increased levels of cerebrospinal fluid CRH and ACTH owing to a loss of this normal feedback inhibition, not the normal levels described here.

Although we argue that a centrally mediated failure in the regulation of the HPA axis exists in patients with CFS, several alternative hypotheses are also plausible and cannot be conclusively supported or refuted by the data we have now assembled. For instance, it has been suggested that adrenocortical sensitivity to ACTH, in both animals [77] and in humans [78], shows a diurnal variation. Shifts in circadian architecture as a result of sleep disturbances may then be reflected in a subtle loss of the synchronous activity of normal pituitary–adrenal communication. This may be compounded by disturbances in other pituitary or adrenal secretogogues such as AVP or angiotensin II, or circulating catecholamines [79]. Furthermore, variations in ACTH bioactivity, or the presence of increased circulating levels of ACTH from sources extrinsic to the HPA axis itself (i.e., from peripheral immunocytes [80]) may lead to apparent distortions in HPA axis function. There may also be multiple levels of dysregulation in the HPA axis (e.g., a disturbance in feedback regulation) with an enhancement of receptor-mediated counterregulation of hypothalamic–pituitary activity.

Nevertheless, we feel that the fundamental observation of a reduction in adrenal glucocorticoid output is consistent with previous observations in this and related syndromes, and provides a coherent theoretical framework on which to integrate some of the putative biological correlates that have been described in CFS patients. For example, CFS often follows in the aftermath of an acute infectious illness. Indeed, the diverse clinical and immunological features of patients with the syndrome have been argued to reflect a state of immune activation, with persistent release of cytokines and inflammatory mediators [81–84]. Evidence supporting such a model of immune activation is suggested by observations of lymphocyte phenotyping by Landay and colleagues and in CFS patients studied by Straus and colleagues [83,84]. These latter studies demonstrate a shift away from naive T-cells [CD45RA (2H4)-positive T cells] toward more differentiated, memory T-cells (CD45RO-positive T cells). Furthermore, our group has demonstrated an increase in cerebrospinal fluid levels of several key kynurenine metabolites and neopterin levels in patients with CFS [85], and an elevation in plasma levels of the serotonin metabolite 5-hydroxyindoleacetic acid (5-HIAA) [86], all of which represent biochemical correlates consistent with a state of persistent immune activation. Whether these immunological features actually cause the symptomatology of the syndrome or are merely epiphenomena is unclear. Glucocorticoids are the most potent endogenous anti-inflammatory compounds, and normally act to restrain the immune or inflammatory responses to infections [40]. A specific link between the hormonal abnormalities and immune disturbances is tenuous and remains unexplored. However, a number of recent human and animal studies speak to the potential clinical importance of such a link.

Although more speculative in nature, it is intriguing to speculate on the possible functional consequences of reduction in central CRH activation and its role in the specific symptom profile associated with CFS. Corticotropin-releasing hormone serves not only as the principal stimulus to the pituitary–adrenal axis, but it is also a behaviorally active neurohormone by which the central administration to animals and nonhuman primates induces signs of physiological and behavioral arousal, including activation of the sympathetic nervous system [87], hyperresponsiveness to sensory stimuli [88], and increased locomotion [89]. Hence, a relative or absolute deficiency of central nervous system sources of CRH could contribute to the profound lethargy and fatigue that are inherent characteristics of chronic fatigue syndrome, either through direct effects on the central nervous system or, indirectly, by causing a relative glucocorticoid deficiency. Although this is an attractive model, it should be emphasized that the assessment of CRH activity that we have established is as yet inferential, based primarily on peripheral pituitary–adrenal responses to hormonal challenge. Furthermore, the direct measurement of CRH in these patients has involved lumbar cerebrospinal fluid determinations, which may merely reflect cortical or spinal sources of CRH, and not direct functional CRH activity in the paraventricular nucleus (PVN). Finally, the relation between extrahypothalamic and hypothalamic sources of CRH in the mediation of the specific behavioral effects of CRH is not completely clear. Hence, there is no reason to presume that a functional deficit of CRH in the PVN is associated with similar reductions of CRH activity in limbic or cortical locations.

Taken together, these findings suggest that the interaction of neuroimmune and neuroendocrine signals may have important biochemical and behavioral consequences that may shape the clinical and biological presentation of patients with CFS.

WHAT DO THE FINDINGS TELL US? SUMMARY AND FORMULATION OF A MODEL

In summary, our own clinical observations and the studies we have performed have persuaded us that patients with CFS cannot be easily absorbed into any one preexisting diagnostic category. Rather, these data suggest that chronically fatigued patients, including those who meet the CDC case definition, are more properly regarded as manifesting a heterogeneous syndrome arising from the interplay of a variety of infectious and noninfectious events (Fig. 5). We feel it is unreasonable to presume that patients with CFS represent a discrete disease with a singular cause. Instead, a more useful formulation would characterize CFS as a *clinical condition*, rather than a diagnosis. In this sense, CFS is more analogous to a number of complex medical conditions, such as anemia or hypertension, in which several direct and indirect factors (some of which may

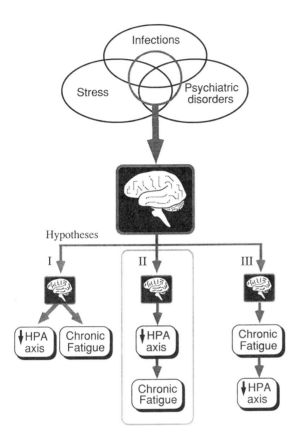

Figure 5   Schematic representation of important contributing factors in the development of chronic fatigue syndrome and hypothetical models suggesting a role for HPA axis dysfunction.

be psychological) lead to the development of the observable clinical syndrome. Such a model rejects a unitary etiologic event to explain the condition, but nevertheless allows the presence of shared pathophysiological processes, and emphasizes the interactive relation between these many disparate factors.

With these considerations in mind, we hypothesize that, in CFS, specific pathophysiological antecedents (e.g., acute infection, stress, preexisting or concurrent psychiatric illness) may ultimately converge in a final common biological pathway, coordinated at the level of the central nervous system, resulting in the clinical syndrome of chronic fatigue. Such a formulation provides a more congenial theoretical framework on which to integrate the varied biological and behavioral manifestations of the syndrome. Although the precise elements composing this final common pathway are not readily apparent, we believe the neuroendocrine data we have described in this chapter support the notion that, in part, a reduction in adrenal glucocorticoid secretion, caused by a central nervous system-mediated failure in the activation of the HPA axis, serves an important pathophysiological role in the development of many of the biological and behavioral features of the syndrome.

The relative contribution of each of the antecedent factors toward increasing the morbid risk for the development of CFS in an individual patient is difficult to specify with certitude. Indeed, it is difficult, if not impossible, for a single experimental paradigm to elucidate all of the causal interactions among these antecedent factors, and the consequent sequence of pathophysiological events, with complete surety. However, the phenomenologic considerations discussed earlier, taken together with the biological data now reported in this syndrome, favor the conceptual paradigm of illness suggested in model II of Figure 5. In this model, acquired factors as cumulative life stress, or psychiatric illness, or an intrinsic deficit in HPA axis reactivity render the individual incapable of mounting an adequate response to an acute stress, such as an infection. As a consequence, a relative or absolute reduction of adrenal glucocorticoids ensues, resulting in the loss of some or all of the normal counterregulatory effects of the HPA axis called into play in response to the stress. In this model, some of the clinical features of CFS, such as the putative mild immune system activation, may theoretically be considered as epiphenomena of the reduction in adrenocortical activity. Although increased immune system activity would be expected to activate HPA axis function, the previously established functional loss of HPA axis reactivity prevents this normative response, a new homeostatic set-point is achieved, and the syndromal illness emerges.

Studies of the pathophysiological mechanisms involved in the development of CFS are in their infancy. Unfortunately, most, if not all, prior studies have been plagued by substantial methodologic inadequacies reflecting an initial absence of appreciation of the interdisciplinary approach necessary for study of this syndrome. For example, the now obvious presence of substantial behavioral symptoms in chronic fatigue patients has called for a renewed emphasis on the systematic use of appropriately chosen clinically ill comparison groups. The observation of immunological and neuroendocrine dysregulation in patients with various psychiatric illnesses, which in some instances is quite similar to the patterns seen in patients with chronic fatigue, makes this fundamental step all the more important if the findings are to be placed in proper perspective. With these considerations in mind, it is important to note that several alternative models of the biological findings of CFS need to be addressed in any studies of this illness. In reference to our own work, for example, the disruption in sleep–wake and activity–rest cycles in patients with CFS may produce an alteration in the circadian rhythm of the HPA axis. In such a scheme, disturbances in HPA axis function may be a concurrent effect of this disruption, but may be causally unrelated to the symptomatic presentation of CFS itself (i.e., the sequence of events in hypothetical model I). Alternatively, as noted by ourselves and others, the pathophysiology of CFS may result in certain behavioral characteristics, such as prolonged physical inactivity. In this latter formulation, the disturbances in HPA axis function emerge as a nonspecific corollary of the illness itself (i.e., the sequence of events depicted in model III). Critical appraisal of these methodologic issues should be a requisite feature of all future work in this field if genuinely new ground is to be broken.

REFERENCES

1. Abbey SE, Garfinkel PE. Neurasthenia and chronic fatigue syndrome: the role of culture in the making of a diagnosis. Am J Psychiatry 1991; 148:1638–46.
2. Beard G. Neurasthenia, or nervous exhaustion. Boston Med Surg J 1869; 3:217–21.
3. Wood P. Aetiology of Da Costa's syndrome. Br Med J, 1941; 92:849.
4. Taerk GS, Toner BB, Salit IE, Garfinkel PE, Ozersky S. Depression in patients with neuromyasthenia (benign myalgic encephalomyelitis). Int J Psychiatry Med 1987; 17:49–56.
5. Manu P, Lane TJ, Matthews DA. The frequency of the chronic fatigue syndrome in patients with symptoms of persistent fatigue. Ann Intern Med 1988; 109:554–6.
6. Manu P, Matthews DA, Lane TJ, Tennen H, Hesselbrock V, Mendola R, Affleck G. Depression among patients with a chief complaint of chronic fatigue. J Affect Dis 1989; 17:165–72.
7. Kruesi MJP, Dale JK, Straus SE. Psychiatric diagnoses in patients with the chronic fatigue syndrome. J Clin Psychiatry 1989; 50:53–6.
8. Gold D, Bowden R, Sixbey J, et al. Chronic fatigue: a prospective clinical and virologic study. JAMA 1990; 264:48–53.
9. Hickie I, Lloyd A, Wakefield D, Parker G. The psychiatric status of patients with chronic fatigue. Br J Psychiatry 1990; 156:534–40.
10. Katon WJ, Buchwald DS, Simon GE, Russo JE, Mease PJ. Psychiatric illness in patients with chronic fatigue and those with rheumatoid arthritis. J Gen Intern Med 1991; 6:277–85.
11. Katon W, Russo J, Chronic fatigue syndrome: a critique of the requirement for multiple physical complaints. Arch Intern Med 1992; 152:1604–9.
12. Tobi M, Ravid Z, Feldman-Weiss V, et al. Prolonged atypical illness associated with serological evidence of persistent Epstein–Barr virus infection. Lancet 1982; 1:61–4.
13. Jones JF, Ray G, Minnich LL, Hicks MJ, Kibler R, Lucas DO. Evidence for active Epstein–Barr virus infection in patients with persistent, unexplained illnesses: elevated anti-early antigen antibodies. Ann Intern Med 1985; 102:1–7.
14. Straus SE, Tosato G, Armstrong G, et al. Persisting illness and fatigue in adults with evidence of Epstein–Barr virus infection. Ann Intern Med 1985; 102:7–16.

15. Horowitz CA, Henle W, Henle G, Rudnick H, Latts E. Long-term serological follow-up of patients for Epstein–Barr virus after recovery from infectious mononucleosis. J Infect Dis 1985; 151:1150–3.

16. Holmes GP, Kaplan JE, Stewart JA, Hunt B, Pinsky PF, Schonberger LB. A cluster of patients with a chronic mononucleosis-like syndrome: is Epstein–Barr virus the cause? JAMA 1987; 257:2297–302.

17. Buchwald D, Sullivan JL, Komaroff AL. Frequency of "chronic active Epstein–Barr virus infection" in a general medical practice. JAMA 1987; 257:2303–7.

18. Straus SE, Dale JK, Tobi M, et al. Acyclovir treatment of the chronic fatigue syndrome: lack of efficacy in a placebo-controlled trial. N Engl J Med 1988; 319:1692–8.

19. DeFreitas E, Hilliard B, Cheney PR, Bell DS, Kiggundu E, Sankey D, Wroblewska Z, Palladino M, Woodward JP, Koprowski H. Retroviral sequences related to human T-lymphotropic virus type II in patients with chronic fatigue immune dysfunction syndrome. Proc Natl Acad Sci USA 1991; 88:2922–6.

20. Khan A, Heneine W, Chapman L, Gary H, Folks T, Schonberger L. Assessment of retroviral sequences and risk factors in adults with chronic fatigue syndrome. Progr Abstr 32nd Ann Intersci Conf Antimicrob Agents Chemother p. 221, no. 665.

21. Demitrack MA, Greden JF. Chronic fatigue syndrome: the need for an integrative approach. Biol Psychiatry 1991; 30:747–52.

22. Preeyasombat C, Richards C, Silverman M, Kenny FM. Cortisol production III. Rubella and varicella encephalopathy, with a note on their treatment with steroids. Am J Dis Child 1965; 110:370–3.

23. White MG, Carter NW, Rector FC, et al. Pathophysiology of epidemic St Louis encephalitis I. Inappropriate secretion of antidiuretic hormone II. Pituitary–adrenal function III. Cerebral blood flow and metabolism. Ann Intern Med 1969; 71:691–702.

24. Zeitoun MM, Hassan AI, Hussein ZM, Fahmy MS, Ragab M, Hussein M. Adrenal glucocorticoid function in acute viral infections in children. Acta Paediatr Scand 1973; 62:608–14.

25. Besedovsky HO, Del Rey A. Mechanism of virus-induced stimulation of the hypothalamus–pituitary–adrenal axis. J Steroid Biochem 1989; 34:235–9.

26. Jones GM. Diabetes insipidus. Clinical observations in forty-two cases. Arch Intern Med 1944; 74:81.

27. McReynolds EW, Roy S. Diabetes insipidus secondary to group B beta streptococcal meningitis. J Tenn Med Assoc 1974; 117:117–20.

28. Hagg E, Astrom L, Steen L. Persistent hypothalamic–pituitary insufficiency following acute meningoencephalitis. Acta Med Scand 1978; 203:231–5.

29. Kupari M, Pelkonen R, Valtonen V. Post-encephalitic hypothalamic–pituitary insufficiency. Acta Endocrinol 1980; 94:433–8.

30. Kedrowa S. Assessment of adrenocortical function in the course of viral hepatitis. Pol Med J 1965; 5:44–51.

31. Membreno L, Irony I, Dere W, Klein R, Biglieri EG, Cobb E. Adrenocortical function in acquired immunodeficiency syndrome. J Clin Endocrinol Metab 1987; 65:482–7.

32. Croxson TS, Chapman WE, Miller KL, Levit CD, Senie R, Zumoff B. Changes in the hypothalamic–pituitary–gonadal axis in human immunodeficiency virus-infected homosexual men. J Clin Endocrinol Metab 1989; 68:317–21.

33. Schlienger JL, Lang JM. Endocrine consequences of HIV infection [in French]. Pathol Biol 1989; 37:921–6.

34. Merenich JA, McDermott MT, Asp AA, Harrison SM, Kidd GS. Evidence of endocrine involvement early in the course of human immunodeficiency virus infection. J Clin Endocrinol Metab 1990; 70:566–71.

35. Southern P, Oldstone MBA. Medical consequences of persistent viral infection. N Engl J Med 1986; 314:359–67.

36. Oldstone MBA, Holmstoen J, Welsh RM Jr. Alterations of acetylcholine enzymes in neuroblastoma cells persistently infected with lymphocytic choriomeningitis virus. J Cell Physiol 1977; 91:459–72.

37. Oldstone MBA, Sinha YN, Blount P, et al. Virus-induced alterations in homeostasis: alterations in differentiated functions of infected cells in vivo. Science 1982; 218:1125–7.

38. Lyons MJ, Faust IM, Hemmes RB, Buskirk DR, Hirsch J, Zabriskie JB. A virally induced obesity syndrome in mice. Science 1982; 216:82–5.

39. Livnat S, Felten SY, Carlson SL, Bellinger DL, Felten DL. Involvement of peripheral and central catecholamine systems in neural–immune interactions. J Neuroimmunol 1985; 10:5–30.

40. Munck A, Guyre PM, Holbrook NJ. Physiological functions of glucocorticoids in stress and their relation to pharmacological actions. Endocr Rev 1984; 5:25–44.

41. Cohen S, Williamson G. Stress and infectious disease in humans. Psychol Bull 1991; 109:5–24.

42. Swanson LW, Sawchenko PE, Rivier J, Vale WW. Organization of ovine corticotropin-releasing factor immunoreactive cells and fibers in the rat brain. An immunohistochemical study. Neuroendocrinology 1983; 36:165–86.

43. Herman JP, Wiegand S, Watson SJ. Regulation of basal corticotropin releasing hormone and arginine vasopressin mRNA expression in the paraventricular nucleus: effects of selective hypothalamic deafferentation. Endocrinology 1990; 127:2408–17.

44. Krieger DT. Rhythms in CRH, ACTH and corticosteroids. Endocr Rev 1979; 1:123.

45. Sachar EJ, Hellman L, Roffwarg HP, Halpern FS, Fukush DK, Gallagher TF. Disrupted 24 hour patterns of cortisol secretion in psychotic depressives. Arch Gen Psychiatry 1973; 28:19–24.

46. Carroll BJ, Curtis GC, Mendels J. Neuroendocrine regulation in depression I. Limbic system–adrenocortical dysfunction. Arch Gen Psychiatry 1976; 33:1039–44.

47. Carroll BJ, Feinberg M, Greden JF, Tarika J, Albala AA, Hasket RF, James NM, Kronfol Z, Lohr N, Steiner M, de Vigne JP, Young E. A specific laboratory test for the diagnosis of melancholia: standardization, validation, and clinical utility. Arch Gen Psychiatry 1981; 38:15–22.

48. Gold PW, Gwirtsman H, Avgerinos PC, et al. Abnormal hypothalamic–pituitary–adrenal function in anorexia nervosa: pathophysiologic mechanisms in underweight and weight-corrected patients. N Engl J Med 1986; 314:1335–42.

49. Roy-Byrne PP, Uhde TW, Post RM, Gallucci W, Chrousos GP, Gold PW. The

corticotropin-releasing hormone stimulation test in patients with panic disorder. Am J Psychiatry 1986; 143:896–9.

50. Adinoff B, Martin PR, Bone GH, Eckardt MJ, Roehrich L, George DT, Moss HB, Eskay R, Linnoila M, Gold PW. Hypothalamic–pituitary–adrenal axis functioning and cerebrospinal fluid levels in alcoholics after recent and long-term abstinence. Arch Gen Psychiatry 1990; 47:325–30.

51. Hudson JI, Pliner LF, Hudson MS, Goldenberg DL, Melby JC. The dexamethasone suppression test in fibrositis. Biol Psychiatry 1984; 19:1489–93.

52. McCain GA, Tilbe KS. Diurnal hormone variation in fibromyalgia syndrome: a comparison with rheumatoid arthritis. J Rheumatol Suppl 1989; 16:154–7.

53. Griep EN, Boersma JW, DeKloet ER. Disturbed neuroendocrine reactivity in the primary fibromyalgia syndrome (PFS): a stress-related disorder? Presented at the Annual Meeting of the International Society for Psychoneuroendocrinology, Siena, Italy, June 1991.

54. Poteliakhoff A. Adrenocortical activity and some clinical findings in acute and chronic fatigue. J Psychosom Res 1981; 25:91–5.

55. Rosenthal NE, Sack DA, Gillin JC, Lewy AJ, Goodwin FK, Davenport Y, Mueller PS, Newsome DA, Wehr TA. Seasonal affective disorder: a description of the syndrome and preliminary findings with light therapy. Arch Gen Psychiatry 1984; 41:72–80.

56. Quitkin FM, McGrath PJ, Stewart JW, Harrison W, Wager SG, Nunes E, Rabkin JG, Tricamo E, Markowitz J, Klein DF. Phenelzine and imipramine in mood reactive depressives: further delineation of the syndrome of atypical depression. Arch Gen Psychiatry 1989; 46:787–93.

57. Kling MA, Roy A, Doran AR, et al. Cerebrospinal fluid immunoreactive CRH and ACTH secretion in Cushing's disease and major depression: potential clinical implications. J Clin Endocrinol Metab 1991; 72:260–71.

58. Tomori N, Suda S, Tozawa F, Demura H, Shizume K, Mouri T. Immunoreactive corticotropin-releasing factor concentrations in cerebrospinal fluid from patients with hypothalamic–pituitary–adrenal disorders. J. Clin Endocrinol Metab 1983; 56:1305–7.

59. Kamilaris TC, DeBold CR, Pavlou SN, Island DP, Hoursandis A, Orth DN. Effect of altered thyroid hormone levels on hypothalamic–pituitary–adrenal function. J Clin Endocrinol Metab 1987; 65:994–9.

60. Joseph-Vanderpool JR, Rosenthal NE, Chrousos GP, Wehr TA, Skwerer R, Kasper S, Gold PW. Abnormal pituitary–adrenal responses to CRH in patients with seasonal affective disorder: clinical and pathophysiological implications. J Clin Endocrinol Metab 1991; 72:1382–7.

61. Yehuda R, Southwick SM, Krystal JH, Bremner D, Charney DS, Mason JW. Enhanced suppression of cortisol following dexamethasone administration in posttraumatic stress disorder. Am J Psychiatry 1993; 150:83–6.

62. Baxter JD, Tyrell JB. The adrenal cortex. In: Felig P, Baxter JD, Broadus AE, Frohman LA, eds. Endocrinology and metabolism. New York: McGraw-Hill, 1981:385–510.

63. Sternberg EM, Hill JM, Chrousos GP, et al. Inflammatory mediator-induced hypothalamic–pituitary–adrenal activation is defective in streptococcal cell wall arthritis-susceptible rats. Proc Natl Acad Sci USA 1989; 86:2374–8.

64. Sternberg EM, Young WS III, Bernardini R, et al. A central nervous system defect in biosynthesis of corticotropin-releasing hormone is associated with susceptibility to streptococcal cell wall-induced arthritis in Lewis rats. Proc Natl Acad Sci USA 1989; 86:4771–5.

65. Takasu N, Komiya I, Nagasawa Y, Asawa T, Yamada T. Exacerbation of autoimmune thyroid dysfunction after unilateral adrenalectomy in patients with Cushing's syndrome due to an adrenocortical adenoma. N Engl J Med 1990; 322:1708–12.

66. Dixon RB, Christy NP. On the various forms of corticosteroid withdrawal syndrome. Am J Med 1980; 68:224–30.

67. Disdier P, Harle J-R, Brue T, Jaquet P, Chambourlier P, Griscoll F, Weiller P-J. Severe fibromyalgia after hypophysectomy for Cushing's disease. Arthritis Rheum 1991; 34:493–5.

68. Demitrack MA, Dale JK, Straus SE, Laue L, Listwak SJ, Kruesi MJP, Chrousos GP, Gold PW. Evidence for impaired activation of the hypothalamic–pituitary–adrenal axis in patients with chronic fatigue syndrome. J Clin Endocrinol Metab 1991; 73:1224–34.

69. Nieman LK, Chrousos GP, Schulte HM, Loriaux DL, Nisula BC. Adrenal regulation of corticosteroid binding globulin. In: Int Congr Ser 1984; 652:1096, abstract 1672A.

70. Schulte HM, Chrousos GP, Avgerinos PC, et al. The corticotropin-releasing hormone stimulation test: a possible aid in the evaluation of patients with adrenal insufficiency. J Clin Endocrinol Metab 1984; 58:1064–7.

71. Gold PW, Loriaux DL, Roy A, et al. Responses to corticotropin-releasing hormone in the hypercortisolism of depression and Cushing's disease: pathophysiologic and diagnostic implications. N Engl J Med 1986; 314:1329–34.

72. Holsboer F, VonBardeleben U, Gerken A, Staller GK, Muller OA. Blunted corticotropin and normal cortisol response to human corticotropin-releasing factor in depression. N Engl J Med 1984; 31:1127.

73. Avgerinos PC, Chrousos GP, Nieman LK, Oldfield EH, Loriaux DL, Cutler GB. The corticotropin-releasing hormone test in the postoperative evaluation of patients with Cushing's syndrome. J Clin Endocrinol Metab 1987; 65:906–13.

74. Muller OA, Staller GK, von Werder K. Corticotropin-releasing factor in humans II. CRF stimulation in patients with diseases of the hypothalamic–pituitary–adrenal axis. Horm Res 1987; 25:185–98.

75. Garrick NA, Hill JL, Szele FG, Tomai TP, Gold PW. Corticotropin-releasing factor: a marked circadian rhythm in primate cerebrospinal fluid peaks in the evening and is inversely related to the cortisol circadian rhythm. Endocrinology 1987; 121:1329–34.

76. Carnes M, Barksdale CM, Kalin NH, Brownfield MS, Lent SJ. Effect of dexamethasone on central and peripheral ACTH systems in the rat. Neuroendocrinology 1987; 45:160–4.

77. Kaneko M, Kaneko K, Shinsako J, Dallman M. Adrenal sensitivity to adrenocorticotropin varies diurnally. Endocrinology 1981; 109:70–5.

78. DeCherney GS, DeBold CR, Jackson RV, Sheldon WR, Island DP, Orth DN. Diurnal variation in the response of plasma adrenocorticotropin and cortisol to

intravenous ovine corticotropin-releasing hormone. J Clin Endocrinol Metab 1985; 61:273–9.

79. Vale W, Vaughan J, Smith M, Yamamoto G, Rivier J, Rivier C. Effects of synthetic ovine corticotropin-releasing factor, glucocorticoids, catecholamines, neurohypophysial peptides, and other substances on cultured corticotropic cells. Endocrinology 1983; 113:1121–31.

80. Blalock JE. Molecular mechanisms of bidirectional communication between the immune and neuroendocrine systems. Int J Neurosci 1990; 51:363–4.

81. Cheney PR, Dorman SE, Bell DS. Interleukin-2 and the chronic fatigue syndrome. Ann Intern Med 1989; 110:321.

82. Chao CC, Gallagher M, Phair J, Peterson PK. Serum neopterin and interleukin-6 levels in chronic fatigue syndrome. J Infect Dis 1990; 162:1412–3.

83. Landay AL, Jessop C, Lennette ET, Levy JA. Chronic fatigue syndrome: clinical condition associated with immune activation. Lancet 1991; 338:707–12.

84. Straus SE, Fritz S, Dale J, Gould B, Strober W. Lymphocyte phenotype analysis suggests chronic immune stimulation in patients with chronic fatigue syndrome. J Clin Immunol 1993; 13:30–40.

85. Heyes MP, Saito K, Crowley J, Davis LE, Demitrack MA, Der M, Kruesi MJP, Lackner A, Larsen SA, Lee K, Leonard H, Martin A, Markey SP, Milstein S, Mouradian MM, Pranzanelli MR, Quearry BJ, Rapoport JL, Salazar A, Smith M, Straus SE, Sunderland T, Swedo S, Toutellotte WW. Neuroactive kynuerines in cerebral and meningeal infections, sepsis, neuropsychiatric disorders and chronic neurodegenerative diseases of man. Brain 1992; (in press).

86. Demitrack MA, Gold PW, Dale JK, Krahn DD, Kling MA, Straus SE. Plasma and cerebrospinal fluid monoamine metabolites in patients with chronic fatigue syndrome: preliminary findings. Biol Psychiatry 1992; 32:1065–77.

87. Brown MR, Fisher LA, Spiess J, Rivier C, Rivier J, Vale W. Corticotropin-releasing factor: actions on the sympathetic nervous system and metabolism. Endocrinology 1982; 111:928–31.

88. Swerdlow NR, Geyer MA, Vale WW, Koob GF. Corticotropin-releasing factor potentiates acoustic startle in rats: blockade by chlordiazepoxide. Psychopharmacology 1986; 88:147–52.

89. Sutton RE, Koob GF, LeMoal M, Rivier J, Vale W. Corticotropin-releasing factor produces behavioural activation in rats. Nature 1982; 297:331–3.

IV

RELATION TO OTHER DISORDERS

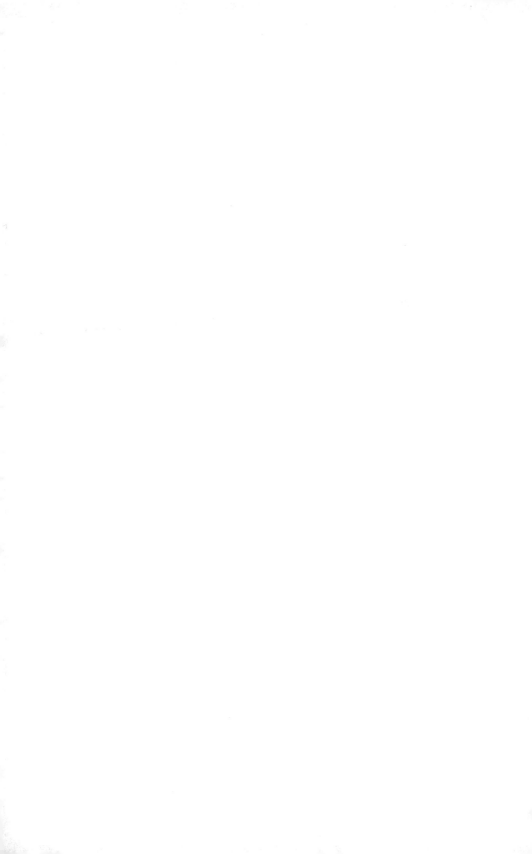

12

The Fibromyalgia Syndrome and Chronic Fatigue Syndrome

Don L. Goldenberg
Newton–Wellesley Hospital,
Newton, Massachusetts,
and Tufts University School of Medicine,
Boston, Massachusetts

EVOLUTION OF FIBROMYALGIA AS A DISCRETE DISORDER

The historical evolution of fibromyalgia was strikingly similar to that of chronic fatigue syndrome (CFS). Both disorders became popular in the late 1800s, CFS under the term neurasthenia, whereas fibromyalgia was most often called fibrositis. Early clinical descriptions of both disorders were nearly identical. Mitchell et al. described the constitutional aspects of this syndrome: "The sleep is restless, the temper changes and becomes irritable" [1]. Gowers emphasized the heightened pain sensitivity and localized soft-tissue tenderness in fibrositis [2]. Similarly, Beard reported in neurasthenia, "heaviness and vague aching of loins and limbs and sometimes of the whole body . . . quite apt to follow over physical exertion, as in walking or standing, but may come on without any apparent or special exciting causes. Neurasthenia may also simulate rheumatism and is frequently mistaken for it" [3].

Whereas the focus of research in CFS during the past century has been a search for an infectious etiology, the focus in fibromyalgia has been to define muscle pathophysiology. Unfortunately, most studies of muscle pain disorders did not differentiate localized or generalized, acute or chronic, or inflammatory versus noninflammatory conditions. Fibrositis was often used as a wastebasket diagnosis for any form of unexplained muscular rheumatism. The initial pathological description of muscle inflammation in fibrositis could not be verified, although the term fibrositis continued to be used, until recently. Kellgren and Lewis described reproducible patterns of referred pain and tenderness following hypertonic saline injections into muscle [4]. Travell and co-workers suggested that "trigger points" in muscle were the source of many forms of regional pain [5]. However, the current concept of fibromyalgia can be traced to studies by Smythe and Moldofsky in the mid-1970s. Smythe demonstrated that patients with fibromyalgia were excessively tender at discrete anatomical locations [6], and Moldofsky described specific sleep disturbances in patients with fibromyalgia [7].

The demonstration of a physical finding, the tender points, and a potential laboratory abnormality, the polysomnographic demonstration of alpha-intrusion in slow wave, deep sleep, led to the first critical investigations of fibromyalgia in the early 1980s. These studies noted that characteristic symptoms, such as generalized pain, fatigue, and sleep disturbances, in combination with the presence of multiple tender points, and in the absence of synovitis or myositis, could differentiate fibromyalgia patients from healthy controls or from patients with rheumatic diseases [8–10]. These symptoms and signs were then field-tested in search of optimal diagnostic criteria, which culminated in the 1990 American College of Rheumatology (ACR) classification criteria for the diagnosis of fibromyalgia [11] (Table 1). This North American multicenter study enrolled 293 patients previously diagnosed with fibromyalgia and 265 patients with a rheumatic condition that would be most difficult to differentiate from fibromyalgia, such as chronic regional pain. If a patient with fibromyalgia also had a concomitant systemic rheumatic disease, such as rheumatoid arthritis (RA), that patient was matched to the next clinic patient with the same systemic connective tissue disease. Each patient was evaluated by a blinded assessor, with an extensive protocol including a detailed history, physical examination that included a manual and dolorimetry tender point examination, laboratory assessments, and radiological tests. Numerous possible combinations were evaluated to determine which symptoms and signs would provide optimal discriminating value. The criteria selected were (1) diffuse pain, present for at least 3 months, and involving right and left sides, above and below the waist, as well as axial; and (2) tenderness on moderate pressure palpation of at least 11 of 18 tender points (see Table 1). These criteria were 88% sensitive and 81% specific in distinguishing the fibromyalgia patients from the other patients with chronic pain. No laboratory or radiological tests were diagnostically informative. There were no clinical differences in fibromyalgia patients who had a concurrent rheumatic disease and, for purposes of the diagnosis of fibromyalgia, the concept of "primary" and "secondary" fibromyalgia was abandoned.

Recently, the prevalence of fibromyalgia has been evaluated using these validated diagnostic criteria. Estimates of fibromyalgia prevalence in random population studies have varied from 1 to 10.5% [12]. Other studies have reported

Table 1 The American College of Rheumatology 1990 Criteria for the Classification of Fibromyalgia[a]

1. History of widespread pain

   Definition. Pain is considered widespread when all of the following are present: pain in the left side of the body, pain in the right side of the body, pain above the waist, and pain below the waist. In addition, axial skeletal pain (cervical spine or anterior chest or thoracic spine or low back) must be present. In this definition, shoulder and buttock pain is considered as pain for each involved side. "Low-back pain is considered lower segment pain.

2. Pain in 11 of 18 tender point sites on digital palpation

   Definition. Pain, on digital palpation, must be present in at least 11 of the following 18 tender point sites:

   Occiput: bilateral, at the suboccipital muscle insertions.

   Low cervical: bilateral, at the anterior aspects of the intertransverse spaces at C5-7

   Trapezius: Bilateral, at the midpoint of the upper border

   Supraspinatus: bilateral, at origins, above the scapula spine near the medial border

   Second rib: bilateral, at the second costochondral junctions, just lateral to the junctions on upper surfaces

   Lateral epicondyle: bilateral, 2-cm distal to the epicondyles

   Gluteal: bilateral, in upper outer quadrants of buttocks in anterior fold of muscle

   Greater trochanter: bilateral, posterior to the trochanteric prominence

   Knee: bilateral, at the medial fat pad proximal to the joint line

   Digital palpation should be performed with an approximate force of 4 kg. For a tender point to be considered "positive" the subject must state that the palpation was painful. "Tender" is not to be considered "painful."

[a]For classification purposes, patients will be said to have fibromyalgia if both criteria are satisfied. Widespread pain must have been present for at least 3 months. The presence of a second clinical disorder does not exclude the diagnosis of fibromyalgia.
Source: Ref. 11.

that 2–6% of patients in primary care clinics and 5–20% of patients in rheumatology clinics have fibromyalgia [13]. After RA, fibromyalgia now occupies the most amount of time in rheumatology practices, 16%, compared with 24% for RA [14].

DEMOGRAPHIC AND CLINICAL CHARACTERISTICS

Fibromyalgia has been reported primarily in women aged 20–60 years [8–10]. In most studies, the female/male ratio has been about 10:1. The average age at diagnosis has been 40–45 years, but most patients have been symptomatic for at least 5 years before diagnosis. Although most early reports were from preponderantly white, middle-class patient populations, fibromyalgia has been reported in Hispanic, black, and Asian populations. Fibromyalgia has been described in children and the elderly, and the clinical manifestations have been identical with those in the more typical-aged range.

Approximately one-half of our patients report that their symptoms began coincident to or shortly after a precipitating event [10]. Physical trauma, such as an injury at work, a motor vehicle accident, or surgery, has been the most common precipitating factor. However, a flulike or viral illness has also been common, and one-third of our patients report such a precipitating factor. Other commonly reported precipitating factors include emotional trauma, steroid withdrawal, and specific infections such as Lyme disease and human immunodeficiency virus (HIV) infection. The other fibromyalgia patients report an indolent onset and are unable to identify any such triggering events.

The cardinal symptom of fibromyalgia is generalized musculoskeletal pain. Pain is often reported as a deep, persistent, aching, but may be sharp, radiating, burning, gnawing, "flulike," or a combination of these. Myalgias as well as arthralgias are reported. Although most patients describe neck, shoulder, and back pain, the pain is often migratory or additive in nature. The musculoskeletal symptoms often mimic other disorders. For example, fibromyalgia patients often describe arthralgias in small joints, including hands and wrists, and "feel swollen," suggesting the possibility of rheumatoid arthritis or another systemic arthritis. Many patients report muscle weakness, which may simulate a myopathy or myositis. The numbness, tingling, and burning of the extremities may mimic carpal tunnel syndrome, a radiculopathy, or multiple sclerosis.

Fatigue is reported in 70–90% of patients in most large studies. In general, the fatigue parallels the pain complaints. Our studies have documented that fatigue in fibromyalgia is similar to that in CFS, including approximately one-third of patients who became bedridden or markedly limited because of fatigue (Table 2). Sleep disturbances, best elicited by the question "do you feel rested on awakening?", have also been reported in 70–90% of patients. Although some patients described insomnia, most report light sleep with many nocturnal awakenings. Gastrointestinal symptoms suggestive of irritable bowel syndrome, chronic and recurrent headaches, most often muscular, but also migraine, and paresthesis, all have been reported in more than 50% of patients. Less common, but still prominent, symptoms include depression, anxiety, Raynaud's-like phenomenon, and bladder irritability.

The finding of multiple tender points on examination is the only reproducible physical finding in fibromyalgia. These tender points can discriminate patients with fibromyalgia from normal controls and from those with systemic rheumatic diseases. Whereas many healthy individuals will have a few "points" that are very tender, fibromyalgia patients have many such points. Since most physicians have not been trained to examine patients for muscle tenderness, some basic concepts are important. First, one should palpate predefined areas that have been most useful in diagnostic studies of fibromyalgia (Fig. 1). These locations are

Table 2 Fibromyalgia and CFS Patients

	Fibromyalgia $(n = 20)$	CFS $(n = 27)$	
		With pain $(n = 19)$	Without pain $(n = 8)$
Mean age	42 + 10.9	37 + 11.6	36 + 15.3
Duration of symptoms, mo	84 + 27.8	59 + 33.4	51 + 28.9
Fatigue, n(%)	18(90)	19(100)	8(100)
Sleep disturbance, n(100)	19(90)	18(95)	6(75)
Morning stiffness, n(%)	19(95)	12(63)	5(63)
Irritable bowel syndrome, n(%)	16(80)	10(53)	5(63)
Numbness and tingling, n(%)	17(85)	13(68)	4(50)
Raynaud's phenomenon, n(%)	2(10)[a]	7(37)	4(50)
Currently seeing mental health professional, n(%)	2(10)[a]	11(58)	4(50)
Past psychiatric disorder,[b] n(%)	5(25)	4(21)	2(25)
Current psychiatric disorder[b]	7(35)	6(32)	3(38)
Tender points (manual exam), n	19 ± 4.2	14 ± 6.7	6.4 ± 5.4
Mean dolorimeter tender point score, kg/cm^3	3.6 ± 1.4	3.8 ± 1.2	5.8 ± 1.6[c]

[a] $p < 0.05$, fibromyalgia versus CFS patients.
[b] Past and current psychiatric diagnosis according to patients self-account.
[c] $p < 0.05$, CFS patients without pain vs other two groups.
Source: Modified from Ref. 17.

often anatomically "vulnerable," and often correspond to sites of tendonitis, such as just below the lateral epicondyle where tenderness is present in "tennis elbow" or over the greater trochanter, a common site of bursitis. Second, the correct amount of pressure to apply should correspond to a dolorimeter pressure of 4 kg/cm^2, and be slowly applied waiting to see if the patient reports pain at that site. Each anatomical site should be palpated bilaterally and control sites, such as the thumbnail, forehead, or midforearm should be similarly palpated. Patients with fibromyalgia will be more tender in the predefined anatomical sites, although they do have a heightened pain sensitivity in many muscles and soft-tissue sites. This tender point examination can be learned quickly, takes less than 3 minutes to perform, and has been noted to be reliable and valid in intra- and interobserver error [9,15]. The physical examination is otherwise unremarkable in fibromyalgia patients. As in CFS, laboratory tests are not helpful diagnostically, other than to help exclude other conditions. Routine laboratory tests should be kept to a minimum and may include a complete blood count, thyroid function studies, and an erythrocyte sedimentation rate.

Fibromyalgia may also occur concurrently with other common rheumatic conditions, such as RA or osteoarthritis (OA), or with endocrine disorders, such as hypothyroidism, or during steroid withdrawal. Such situations were called

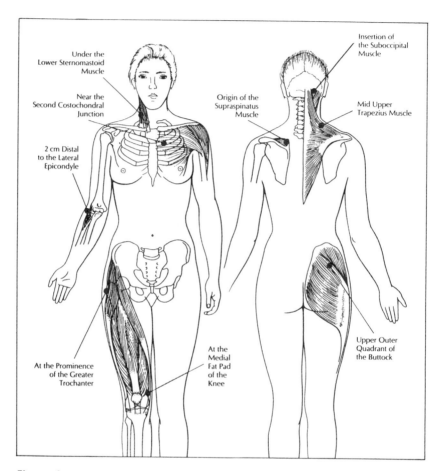

Figure 1 The nine pair of tender points used for the ACR diagnostic criteria study of fibromyalgia. Each site should be bilaterally tender on digital palpation. (From Ref. 78.)

secondary; however, there is no evidence that the concurrent illness is etiologically related to fibromyalgia. For example, fibromyalgia patients with a history of hypothyroidism are generally euthyroid when fibromyalgia develops, and giving more thyroid hormone does not help their symptoms.

CLINICAL OVERLAP WITH CHRONIC FATIGUE SYNDROME

The demographic and clinical manifestations of fibromyalgia and CFS are very similar [16,17] (see Table 2). Both are preponderant in younger women, and are associated with fatigue, myalgias, headaches, sleep disturbances, neurocognitive and neuropsychiatric symptoms. In view of these similarities, we performed two studies on the relation of CFS to fibromyalgia. In the first, we surveyed fibromyalgia patients for symptoms suggestive of CFS [16]. As expected, symptoms of myalgias, fatigue, and sleep disturbances were similar. Surprisingly, more than 50% of patients with fibromyalgia reported recurrent sore throats and often reported swollen glands. Patients were asked: "Do you feel that your symptoms began with a flu- or viral-like illness?" Fifty-five percent of these fibromyalgia patients surveyed felt that their symptoms began after a flulike illness. In the second study, we performed a manual and dolorimetry tender point examination on 27 patients followed in a primary care setting for chronic fatigue (see Table 2) [17]. Although the study was completed before the Centers for Disease Control (CDC) working case definition for CFS were published, most patients did meet the CDC criteria for CFS. Eight of the chronic fatigue patients did not have chronic musculoskeletal pain, and their tender point scores were similar to healthy controls. In contrast, the tender point scores of the other 19 chronic fatigue patients who did complain of pain were identical with those of fibromyalgia patients. Thus, most patients with chronic fatigue will have coexistent fibromyalgia. In recognition of this overlap, a recent National Institutes of Health (NIH) conference on revision of the working case definition for CFS suggested that fibromyalgia not be an exclusionary criteria in the diagnosis of CFS [18].

The potential role of infectious agents in fibromyalgia has also attracted more research interest. Fibromyalgia has been reported to follow well-documented viral illness, including HIV [19,20], coxsackievirus [21], and parvovirus [22] infections. The most interesting association of fibromyalgia has been with Lyme disease (Table 3). It would not be surprising that patients who are very anxious about contracting Lyme disease and who live in endemic areas may actually have fibromyalgia, rather than Lyme disease. Indeed, at Lyme disease clinics in the Northeast, fibromyalgia is diagnosed in approximately 25% of patients, and most

Table 3 The Association of Fibromyalgia and Lyme Disease

Author [Ref.]	Methodology	Results
Sigal [23]	Retrospective; all patients referred to Lyme clinic	Only 25% have Lyme disease; 25% have fibromyalgia; most with fibromyalgia did have prior Lyme disease. No response of fibromyalgia to antibiotics.
Dinerman [24]	Prospective; only patients with Lyme disease	Of the Lyme disease patients 8% had fibromyalgia that developed concurrently with Lyme disease. No response of fibromyalgia to antibiotics.

patients referred for chronic, treatment-resistant Lyme disease have fibromyalgia [23]. However, surprisingly, one-half of such patients did have prior Lyme disease that responded to antibiotics, but the patients then developed fibromyalgia symptoms. In a prospective study from another Lyme disease clinic, 8% of patients with new onset of Lyme disease concurrently reported fibromyalgia symptoms [24]. The symptoms of Lyme disease, but not those of fibromyalgia, responded to antibiotics.

The diagnosis of Lyme disease should be based on the clinical features of a characteristic dermatitis and typical later manifestations, including arthritis, central nervous system (CNS) and cardiovascular features. Appropriate seasonal and geographic exposure and serological studies are confirmatory, but are misleading without typical clinical features. The combination of an enzyme-linked immunosorbent assay (ELISA) to detect IgM and IgG anti–*Borrelia burgdorferi* antibodies, and a Western blot confirmation are currently the most sensitive and specific laboratory tests for the diagnosis of Lyme disease. However, the predictive value of these serological tests is dependent on the likelihood of an accurate clinical diagnosis. Indiscriminately obtaining serological tests for Lyme disease in patients with nonspecific symptoms of fibromyalgia or chronic fatigue will yield a high proportion of false-positive tests or may just indicate prior exposure.

PATHOPHYSIOLOGY

Most of the pathophysiological studies on fibromyalgia during the past century have focused on muscle and soft tissue. However, at present, one cannot clearly discern whether lesions are present in fibromyalgia muscle, skin, nerve, or other peripheral tissue. Histopathologic examination of fibromyalgia muscle demonstrates type II fiber atrophy, ragged red fibers, and variable ultrastructural changes [25]. However, when matched with appropriate controls, no significant differences have been found [26]. The most exciting muscle studies, using techniques such as oxygen probe analysis and chemical or spectral analysis, have suggested a relative hypoxia, with elevated intracellular acidosis [27,28]. In one report, the trapezius muscle of fibromyalgia patients demonstrated reduced ATP and phosphocreatine values below 2 SD, or more, of that in normal controls [27]. However, many of these studies did not adequately control for levels of physical activity, and recent controlled studies have not found significant differences in fibromyalgia and appropriate controls [29]. Nevertheless, muscle microtrauma remains a viable explanation for the muscle pain characteristic of fibromyalgia.

In addition to muscle hyperalgesia, there is evidence of a more generalized peripheral nervous system hyperactivity in fibromyalgia. For example, 30–40% of patients with fibromyalgia have Raynaud's phenomenon and Bennett et al. demonstrated that the vasomotor instability may correlate with alterations in serotonin reuptake [30]. There is an exaggerated local skin response to pressure (dermatographism) or to application of chemical irritant, such as capsaisin in fibromyalgia patients [31]. Marked transient improvement in pain following a complete sympathetic block [32] suggests that the sympathetic nervous system plays a role in fibromyalgia.

There is also evidence to support a role of the central nervous system (CNS) in fibromyalgia. Sleep disturbances, present in most patients historically, and confirmed by overnight polysomnography, suggest central abnormalities [7,33]. However, the early-wave intrusion in slow-wave sleep initially thought to be characteristic of fibromyalgia is neither specific nor highly sensitive for the disorder. This sleep pattern is found in many chronic pain conditions, including most patients with rheumatoid arthritis [34], and is also prominent in CFS [35]. Patients with fibromyalgia may also have other sleep abnormalities, such as sleep apnea or nocturnal myoclonus [36].

Patients with fibromyalgia have levels of depression and anxiety that are in excess of community controls or of those found in RA [37] (Table 4). For example, by using structured psychiatric interviews, we found a 25% prevalence of current depression and a 70% lifetime history of depression in fibromyalgia, both significantly higher than in RA controls [38]. A family history of major depression was also greater than in RA. The levels of current and past depression are comparable with those in most reports of CFS (see Table 4). Excess anxiety, stress, helplessness, and inability to cope are also more common in fibromyalgia than in RA [37,39]. However, most fibromyalgia patients do not meet the *Diagnostic and Statistical Manual of Mental Disorders*, 3rd ed. (*DSM-III*) criteria for any active psychiatric diagnosis [39].

In attempting to integrate the clinical characteristics of abnormal pain perception, sleep disturbances, fatigue, and mood disturbances, investigators

Table 4 Current and Lifetime History of Psychiatric Illness (% of Patients) in Chronic Fatigue, Fibromyalgia, and Rheumatoid Arthritis

Psychiatric illness[a]	Chronic fatigue		Fibromyalgia		Rheum arthr	
	Now	Ever	Now	Ever	Now	Ever
Depression	15	77	24	64	3	42
Panic	11	29	15	33	3	4
Somatization	20	20	21	21	0	0
No illness	55	14	62	18	94	52

[a]All psychiatric diagnoses determined according to structured psychiatric interviews.
Source: Modified from Ref. 37 for chronic fatigue (*n* = 98) and RA (*n* = 31); and Ref. 38 for fibromyalgia (*n* = 33).

have recently been evaluating neurohormones and neurotransmitters in fibro-myalgia. The plasma and cerebrospinal fluid (CSF) concentrations of a number of amino acids, including metabolites of serotonin, such as 5-hydroxyindoleacetic acid (5-HIAA), were lower in fibromyalgia than in normal persons and than in RA [40,41]. Levels of CSF substance P were significantly higher than in healthy, pain-free controls [42]. In the periphery, substance P release provokes neurogenic inflammation. The heightened pain perception in fibromyalgia, therefore, might be explained by inappropriately low levels of serotonin, which would allow greater uninhibited release of substance P following a noxious stimulus [43]. Recent studies have also noted hypothalamic–pituitary–adrenal (HPA) axis abnormalities in a subset of fibromyalgia patients [44–46]. The HPA axis alterations are consistent with reports that fibromyalgia may be associated with steroid withdrawal, hypothyroidism, and following surgically induced panhypopituitarism [47]. Fibromyalgia patients had less variations between peak and trough cortisol when compared with RA patients [44]. A hyperprolactinemic response to thyrotropin-releasing hormone has been reported by two investigators [45,46]. Bennett et al. found significantly lower levels of somatomedin C in fibromyalgia patients, compared with healthy controls [48]. Somatomedin C is the major indicator of growth hormone's anabolic action and is produced by the liver in response to growth hormone. Eighty percent of growth hormone is produced during stage 4 sleep, and growth hormone has major effects on muscle mass and homeostasis [49]. Alterations in neurohormones have also been reported in patients with rheumatoid arthritis [50] and CFS [51]. Demitrack et al. suggested that patients with CFS may have a hypofunctioning corticotropin-releasing hormonal system. These studies all raise the exciting possibility that interactions of the immune and central nervous systems may account for the overlap of common conditions, such as rheumatoid arthritis, fibromyalgia, or CFS, and depression [52].

There have been fewer extensive microbiological studies in patients with fibromyalgia in comparison with those with CFS. Clearly, very few patients with fibromyalgia have evidence of active or recent infections, such as Lyme disease or parvovirus infection. Geometric mean antibody titers to Epstein–Barr virus (EBV) were not significantly different in fibromyalgia patients from those with chronic fatigue, and neither group differed significantly from normal, healthy controls [16]. However, elevated levels of antibody to human herpes virus-6 (HHV-6), comparable with the levels reported in CFS, have been described in fibromyalgia [53]. There is also little evidence to suggest major immune abnormalities in fibromyalgia. Standard serological tests, such as antinuclear antibodies and anti-smooth muscle antibodies do not differ from controls [54]. Most reports of cell-mediated immunity, including lymphocyte subsets and functional activity, have demonstrated no consistent abnormalities [55,56]. However, a defect in interleukin-2 (IL-2) secretion, possibly related to protein kinase C activation was found in one study [57]. Anecdotally, patients often report cognitive difficulties, but there have been no controlled studies of neuropsychological testing or CNS studies such as brain magnetic resonance imaging (MRI) in fibromyalgia patients.

TREATMENT AND OUTCOME

As with CFS, there is no satisfactory treatment for fibromyalgia. However, during the past decade there have been more than a dozen randomized, controlled, clinical trials employing both medicinal and nonmedicinal therapies in fibromyalgia [58–70] (Table 5).

Several trials have demonstrated that low doses of tricyclic antidepressants (TCA) are more effective than placebo or nonsteroidal anti-inflammatory drugs (NSAIDs) in fibromyalgia [58–62]. In contrast, NSAIDs alone, such as naproxen or ibuprofen [59,70], or modest doses of prednisone [71] have not been effective in clinical trials. The typical dose of the TCA has been low, such as 25–50 mg of amitriptyline, or 20–30 mg of cyclobenzaprine. Unpleasant side effects, such as dry mouth and constipation, have been common. Unfortunately, treatments

Table 5 Controlled Therapeutic Trials in Fibromyalgia

Author [Ref.]	Therapy	Medication dose (mg/day)
Medicinal therapy		
Carette [58]	Amitriptyline	25–50
Goldenberg [59]	Amitriptyline	25
	Naproxen[a]	1000
Bennett [60]	Cyclobenzaprine	10–40
Quimby [61]	Cyclobenzaprine	10–40
Caruso [62]	Dothiepin	75
Vaeroy [63]	Soma compd[b]	6 tabs
Caruso [64]	5-Hydroxytryptophan	300
Russell [65]	Alprazolam and ibuprofen[c]	0.5–3
		2400
Jacobsen [66]	*S*-Adenosylmethionine	800
Nonmedicinal therapy		
McCain [67]	Cardiovascular fitness training	
Ferraccioli [68]	EMG-biofeedback training	
Haanen [69]	Hypnotherapy	
Nielsen [72]	Cognitive–behavioral therapy	

[a]Amitriptyline alone, but not naproxen alone, better than placebo.
[b]Equivalent = 1200 mg carisoprodol, 960 mg acetaminophen, 192 mg caffeine.
[c]Combination better than placebo.

in most of the reports have been of 6- to 12-weeks duration, and there is evidence that over time these medications may lose some of their efficacy [70]. Other CNS-active medications noted to be effective in clinical trials include alprazolam [65] and *S*-adenosylmethionine [66].

In most of these trials, only about 25–35% of patients improved in a meaningful fashion [70]. Younger age, less severity of symptoms, and shorter duration may predict responsiveness to some degree [59]. The mechanisms of action of TCAs in fibromyalgia are unknown. It is unlikely that the TCAs are improving depression, since the doses have been "subtherapeutic" and the treatment response has been quicker than that usually noted in depression. We have also failed to find any correlation of response to TCAs with premorbid psychopathology. The TCAs may improve the sleep disturbances, although there is now no direct evidence for that. They have an analgesic effect that is independent of their antidepressant action, and this may be responsible for their efficacy in fibromyalgia, as well as in other chronic pain conditions. Serotonin-reuptake blockers, including fluoxetine, have not been studied in controlled trials, although, anecdotally, they have often helped associated mood disturbances, but they have not been particularly effective for sleep or pain. Some patients do respond best to combinations of CNS-active medications, such as a low dose of fluoxetine in the morning and a low dose of TCA at bedtime.

Nonmedicinal treatment noted to be effective in controlled trials include cardiovascular fitness exercise [67], electromyogram (EMG) biofeedback [68], hypnotherapy [69], and cognitive behavioral therapy [72]. Other treatments often used, but not adequately evaluated, include physical therapy, massage, flexibility exercises, biofeedback, manipulation, and acupuncture. The most effective treatment programs have also emphasized patient and family education. Once a diagnosis is established and a patient better understands the disorder, an attitude of wellness, rather than sickness and uncertainty, can be promoted. Often this requires active, cognitive behavioral therapy (CBT). The CBT programs that employ cognitive restructuring, relaxation strategies, imagery, and problem-solving have been described for fibromyalgia [72]. Patients can assume more independence relative to their illness. Physical therapists, physiatrists, psychologists, psychiatrists, and other health professionals form a team approach to patient care.

Unfortunately, despite improved recognition and therapy of fibromyalgia, most patients continue to have chronic pain and fatigue [73,74]. In contrast with what would be expected in exaggerated pain syndromes or somatization, the symptoms of most patients are stable over time, although they vary significantly from one patient to another. Most longitudinal reports have been from tertiary referral centers, and the severity and outcome of "community fibromyalgia" may be quite different. Nevertheless, these reports describe persistent, high levels of pain, fatigue, and sleep disturbances [74]. Patients' self-rating of pain severity is greater than in RA, and their perceived levels of disability are comparable with those of RA [75]. The functional ability to perform standardized work tasks was similar in fibromyalgia and RA [75]. Both patient groups performed about 60% of the work accomplished by healthy age- and sex-matched controls. Thus, it is not surprising that patients with fibromyalgia often apply for some form of work-related financial compensation. In Sweden, with liberal national health insurance compensation, most patients with fibromyalgia are receiving either partial or total disability payments. In the United States, although 25–35% of patients report that they are unable to adequately perform their prior job, only about 12% receive any form of disability compensation [76].

CONCLUSIONS AND FUTURE DIRECTION

It is obvious that fibromyalgia and CFS share similar historical, clinical, and laboratory features. Our own research has demonstrated that most patients with CFS do meet current criteria for fibromyalgia. Possibly the most important factor in the evolution of these two conditions as discrete from each other relates to preconceived notions about their etiologies. Thus, fibromyalgia has been thought of as a primary muscle disorder, whereas CFS has been considered to be related to an infectious agent. Nevertheless, the clinical descriptions of the course of these two syndromes, as well as much of the research on etiopathogenesis, have been strikingly similar.

In the future, we should better appreciate the overlapping nature of these syndromes and that they share features with other poorly understood common disorders, such as migraine, irritable bowel syndrome, and depression. To understand these relations, we recently used structured interview techniques to evaluate 33 women with fibromyalgia followed in a tertiary referral center [77]. We found that patients with fibromyalgia displayed high lifetime rates of migraine, irritable bowel syndrome, major depression, panic disorder, as well

Table 6 Current and Lifetime Medical and Psychiatric Diagnoses in 33 Women with Fibromyalgia[a]

Diagnosis	% Current diagnosis	% Lifetime diagnosis
CFS	70	70
Migraine	45	55
Irritable bowel syndrome	39	52
Depression	18	58
Panic disorder	15	33

[a]All diagnoses made with structured interviews, according to operational diagnostic criteria.
Source: Modified from Ref. 77.

as CFS (Table 6). Whereas the migraine, irritable bowel syndrome, and depression usually antedated symptoms of fibromyalgia, the onset of CFS and fibromyalgia were concurrent. Thus, either the current diagnostic criteria do not adequately distinguish fibromyalgia from CFS, or they are the same illness. Of note, some of the most interesting, current investigation in the areas of fibromyalgia and CFS involve the neuroendocrine system [44–52]. In the future, recognition that these conditions may have more similarities than differences should foster collaborative research and better our understanding of these perplexing problems.

REFERENCES

1. Mitchell SW, Moorehouse GR, Keen WW. Gunshot wounds and other injuries of nerves. Philadelphia: JB Lippincott, 1864.
2. Gowers WR. Lumbago: its lessons and analogues. Br Med J 1904; 1:117–21.
3. Beard GM. Neurasthenia, or nervous exhaustion. Boston Med Surg J 1869; 3:217–20.
4. Kellgren JH. On distribution of pain arising from deep somatic structures with charts of segmental pain areas. Clin Sci 1939; 4:35–46.
5. Travell J, Simons DG. Myofascial pain and dysfunction: the trigger point manual. Baltimore: Williams & Willkins, 1983.
6. Smythe HA, Moldofsky H. Two contributions to understanding of the "fibrositis" syndrome. Bull Rheum Dis 1977; 28:928–31.
7. Moldofsky H, Lue FA. The relationship of alpha and delta EEG frequencies to pain and mood in "fibrositis" patients treated with chlorpromazine and L-tryptophan. Electroencephalogr Clin Neurophysiol 1980; 50:71–80.
8. Yunus MB, Masi AT, Calabro JJ, Miller KA, and Feigenbaum SL. Primary fibromyalgia (fibrositis): clinical study of 50 patients with matched normal controls. Semin Arthritis Rheum 1981; 11:151–71.
9. Wolfe F, Cathey MA. The epidemiology of tender points: a prospective study of 1520 patients. J Rheumatol 1985; 12:1164–8.
10. Goldenberg DL. Fibromyalgia syndrome. An emerging but controversial conditon. JAMA 1987; 257:2782–7.
11. Wolfe F, Smythe HA, Yunus MB, Bennett RM, Bombardier, Goldenberg DL, Tugwell P, Abeles M, Campbell SM, Clark P, Fam AG, Farber SJ, Fiechtner JJ, Franklin CM, Gatter RA, Hamaty D, Lessard J, Lichtbroun AS, Masi AT, McCain GA, Reynolds WJ, Romano TJ, Russell IJ, Sheon R. The American College of Rheumatology 1990 criteria for the classification of fibromyalgia: report of the multicenter criteria committee. Arthritis Rheum 1990; 33:160–172.
12. Forseth KO, Gran JT. The prevalence of fibromyalgia among women aged 20–49 years in Arendal, Norway. Scand J Rheumatol 1992; 21:74–8.
13. Wolfe F, and Cathey MA. Prevalence of primary and secondary fibrositis. J Rheumatol 1983; 10:965–8.
14. Marder WD, Meenan RF, Felson DT, Reichlin M, Birnbaum NS, Croft JD, Dore RK, Kaplan H, Kaufman RL, Stobo JD. The present and future adequacy of rheumatology manpower. Arthritis Rheum 1991; 34:1209–17.

15. Simms RW, Goldenberg DL, Felson DT, Mason JH. Tenderness in 75 anatomic sites: distinguishing fibromyalgia patients from controls. Arthritis Rheum 1988; 31:182–7.

16. Buchwald D, Goldenberg DL, Sullivan JL, Komaroff AL. The "chronic, active Epstein–Barr virus infection" syndrome and primary fibromyalgia. Arthritis Rheum 1987; 30:1132–6.

17. Goldenberg DL, Simms RW, Geiger A, Komaroff AL. High frequency of fibromyalgia in patients with chronic fatigue seen in a primary care practice. Arthritis Rheum 1990; 33:381–7.

18. Schluederberg A, Straus SE, Peterson P, Blumenthal S, Komaroff AL, Spring SB, Landay A, Buchwald D. Chronic fatigue syndrome research. Ann Intern Med 1992; 117:325–31.

19. Buskila D, Gladman DD, Langevitz P, Urowitz S, Smythe HA. Fibromyalgia in human immunodeficiency virus infection. J Rheumatol 1990; 17:1202–6.

20. Simms RW, Zerbini CAF, Ferrante N, Anthony J, Felson D. Craven DE. Fibromyalgia syndrome in patients infected with human immunodeficiency virus. Am J Med 1992; 92:368–74.

21. Nash P, Chard M, Hazleman B. Chronic Coxsackie B infection mimicking primary fibromyalgia. J Rheumatol 1989; 16:1506–8.

22. Leventhal LJ, Naides SJ, Freundlich B. Fibromyalgia and parvovirus infection. Arthritis Rheum 1991; 34:1319–24.

23. Sigal LH. Summary of the first 100 patients seen at a Lyme disease referral center. Am J Med 1990; 88:577–81.

24. Dinerman H, Steere AC. Lyme disease associated with fibromyalgia. Ann Intern Med 1992; 117:281–5.

25. Henriksson KG, Bengtsson A. Fibromyalgia—a clinical entity? Can J Physiol Pharmacol 1991; 69:672–7.

26. Yunus MB, Kalyan-Raman UP, Masi AT, Aldag JC. Electron microscopic studies of muscle biopsy in primary fibromyalgia syndrome: a controlled and blinded study. J Rheumatol 1989; 16:97–101.

27. Bengtsson A, Henriksson KG, Larsson J. Reduced high-energy phosphate levels in the painful muscles of patients with primary fibromyalgia. Arthritis Rheum 1986; 29:817–21.

28. Lund N, Bengtsson A, Thorborg P. Muscle tissue oxygen pressure in primary fibromyalgia. Scand J Rheumatol 1986; 15:165–73.

29. de Blecourt AC, Wolf RF, van Rijswijk MH, Kamman RL, Knipping AA, Mooyaart EL. In vivo ^{31}P magnetic resonance spectroscopy (MRS) of tender points in patients with primary fibromyalgia syndrome. Rheumatol Int 1991; 11:51–4.

30. Bennett RM, Clark SR, Campbell SM, Ingram S, Burkhardt CS, Nelson DL, Porter JM. Symptoms of Raynaud's syndrome in patients with fibromyalgia—a study utilizing the Nielsen test, digital photoplethysmography, and measurements of platelet alpha adrenergic receptors. Arthritis Rheum 1991; 34:264–9.

31. Littlejohn GO, Weinstein C, Helme RD. Increased neurogenic inflammation in fibrositis syndrome. J Rheumatol 1987; 14:1022–5.

32. Bengtsson A, Bengtsson M. Regional sympathetic blockade in primary fibromyalgia. Pain 1988; 33:161–7.

33. Moldofsky H. Sleep and fibrositis syndrome. Rheum Dis Clin North Am 1989; 15:91–103.

34. Mahowald MW, Mahowald ML, Bundlie SR, et al. Sleep fragmentation and daytime sleepiness in rheumatoid arthritis. Sleep Res 1987; 16:487.

35. Moldofsky H. Nonrestorative sleep and symptoms after a febrile illness in patients with fibrositis and chronic fatigue syndromes. J Rheumatol Suppl 1989; 9:150–3.

36. Moldofsky H, Tullis C, Lue FA, Quance G, Davidson J. Sleep-related myoclonus in rheumatic pain modulation disorder (fibrositis syndrome) and in excessive daytime somnolence. Psychosom Med 1984; 46:145–51.

37. Katon WJ, Buchwald DS, Simon GE, Russo JE, Mease PJ. Psychiatric illness in patients with chronic fatigue and those with rheumatoid arthritis. J Gen Intern Med 1991; 6:277–85.

38. Hudson JI, Hudson MS, Pliner LF, Goldenberg DL, Pope HG Jr. Fibromyalgia and major affective disorder: a controlled phenomenology and family history study. Am J Psychiatry 1985; 142:441–6.

39. Goldenberg DL. An overview of psychologic studies in fibromyalgia. J Rheumatol Suppl 1989; 19:12–4.

40. Russell IJ, Michalek JE, Vipraio GA, Fletcher EM, Javors MA, Bowden CA. Platelet ^{3}H-imipramine uptake receptor density and serum serotonin levels in patients with fibromyalgia/fibrositis syndrome. J Rheumatol 1992; 19:104–9.

41. Russell IJ, Vaeroy H, Javors M, Nyberg F. Cerebrospinal fluid biogenic amine metabolites in fibromyalgia/fibrositis syndrome and rheumatoid arthritis. Arthritis Rheum 1992; 35:550–6.

42. Vaeroy H, Helle R, Frre O, Kass E, Terenius L. Elevated CSF levels of substance P and high incidence of Raynaud phenomenon in patients with fibromyalgia: new features for diagnosis. Pain 1988; 32:21–6.

43. Russell IJ. Neurohormonal aspects of the fibromyalgia syndrome. Rheum Dis Clin North Am 1989; 15:149–68.

44. McCain GA, Tilbe KS. Diurnal hormone variation in fibromyalgia syndrome: a comparison with rheumatoid arthritis. J Rheumatol [Suppl] 1989; 16:154–7.

45. Ferraccioli G, Cavalieri F, Salaffi F, Fontana S, Scita F, Nolli M, Maestri D. Neuroendocrinologic findings in primary fibromyalgia (soft tissue chronic pain syndrome) and in other chronic rheumatic conditions (rheumatoid arthritis, low back pain). J Rheumatol 1990; 17:869–73.

46. Neeck G, Riedel W. Thyroid function in patients with fibromyalgia syndrome. J Rheumatol 1992; 19:1120–2.

47. Disdier P, Harle J-R, Brue T, Jacuet P, Chambourlier P, Grisol F, Weiller P-J. Severe fibromyalgia after hypophysectomy for Cushing's disease. Arthritis Rheum 1991; 34:493–5.

48. Bennett RM, Clark SR, Campbell SM, Burckhardt CS. Low levels of somatomedin C in patients with the fibromyalgia syndrome: a possible link between sleep and muscle pain. Arthritis Rheum 1992; 35:1113–6.

49. Fryburg DA, Louard RJ, Gerow KE, Gelfand RA, Barrett EJ. Growth hormone stimulates skeletal muscle protein and antagonizes insulin's antiproteolytic action in humans. Diabetes 1992; 41:424–9.

50. Chikanza IC, Petrou P, Kingsley G, Chrousos G, Panayi GS. Defective hypothalamic response to immune and inflammatory stimuli in patients with rheumatoid arthritis. Arthritis Rheum 1992; 35:1281–8.

51. Demitrack M, Dale JK, Straus SE, Laue L, Listwak SJ, Kruesi MJ, Chrousos GP, Gold PW. Evidence for impaired activation of the hypothalamic–pituitary–adrenal axis in patients with chronic fatigue syndrome. J Clin Endocrinol Metab 1991; 73:1224–34.

52. Sternberg EW, Chrousos GP, Wilder RL, Gold PW. The stress response and the regulation of inflammatory disease. Ann Intern Med 1992; 117:854–66.

53. Buchwald D, Saxinger C, Goldenberg DL, Gallo RC, Komaroff Al. Primary fibromyalgia (fibrositis) and human herpes virus-6: a serologic association. Clin Res 1988; 36:332A.

54. Bengtsson A, Ernerudh J, Vrethem M, Skogh T. Absence of autoantibodies in primary fibromyalgia. J Rheumatol 1990; 17:1682–84.

55. Russell IJ, Vipraio GA, Michalek J, Fletcher E. Abnormal T cell subpopulations in fibrositis syndrome. Arthritis Rheum 1988; 31(suppl 4):S24.

56. Peter JB, Wallace DJ. Abnormal immune regulation in fibromyalgia. Arthritis Rheum 1988; 31:S24.

57. Hader N, Rimon D, Kinarty A, Lahat N. Altered interleukin-2 secretion in patients with primary fibromyalgia syndrome. Arthritis Rheum 1991; 34:866–72.

58. Carette S, McCain GA, Bell DA, Fam AG. Evaluation of amitriptyline in primary fibrositis. A double-blind, placebo-controlled study. Arthritis Rheum 1986; 29:655–9.

59. Goldenberg DL, Felson DT, Dinerman H. A randomized, controlled trial of amitriptyline and naproxen in the treatment of patients with fibromyalgia. Arthritis Rheum 1986; 29:1371–7.

60. Bennett RM, Gatter RA, Campbell SM, Andrews RP, Clark SR, Scarola JA. A comparison of cyclobenzaprine and placebo in the management of fibrositis. A double-blind controlled study. Arthritis Rheum 1988; 31:1535–42.

61. Quimby LG, Gratwick GM, Whitney CD, Block SR. A randomized trial of cyclobenzaprine for the treatment of fibromyalgia. J Rheumatol 1989; S19:140–3.

62. Caruso I, Sarzi Puttini PC, Boccassini L, Santandrea S, Locati M, Volpato R, Montrone F, Benvenuti C, Beretta A. Double-blind study of dothiepin versus placebo in the treatment of primary fibromyalgia syndrome. J Int Med Res 1987; 15:154–9.

63. Vaeroy H, Abrahamsen A, Frre O, Kass E. Treatment of fibromyalgia (fibrositis syndrome): a parallel double blind trial with carisoprodol, paracetamol and caffeine (Somadril comp) versus placebo. Clin Rheumatol 1989; 8:245–50.

64. Caruso I, Sarzi Puttini P, Cazzola M, Azzolini V. Double-blind study of 5-hydroxytryptophan versus placebo in the treatment of primary fibromyalgia syndrome. J Int Med Res 1990; 18:201–9.

65. Russell IJ, Fletcher EM, Michalek JE, Mcbroom PC, Hester GG. Treatment of primary fibrositis/fibromyalgia syndrome with ibuprofen and alprazolam—a double-blind, placebo-controlled study. Arthritis Rheum 1991; 34:552–60.

66. Jacobsen S, Danneskiold-Samsoe B, Andersen RB. Oral *S*-adenosylmethionine in primary fibromyalgia. Double blind clinical evaluation. Scand J Rheumatol 1991; 20:294–302.

67. McCain GA, Bell DA, Mai FM, Halliday PD. A controlled study of the effects of a supervised cardiovascular fitness training program on the manifestations of fibromyalgia. Arthritis Rheum 1988; 31:1135–41.

68. Ferraccioli G, Ghirelli L, Scita F, Nolli M, Mozzani M, Fontana S, Scorsonelli M, Tridenti A, De Risio C. EMG-biofeedback training in fibromyalgia syndrome. J Rheumatol 1987; 14:820–5.

69. Haanen HCM, Hoenderdos HTW, van Romunde LKJ, Hop WCJ, Mallee C, Terwiel JP, Hekster GB. Controlled trial of hypnotherapy in the treatment of refactory fibromyalgia. J Rheumatol 1991; 18:72–5.

70. Goldenberg DL. Treatment of fibromyalgia syndrome. Rheum Dis Clin North Am 1989; 15:61–71.

71. Clark S, Tindall E, Bennett RM. A double blind crossover trial of prednisone versus placebo in the treatment of fibrositis. J Rheumatol 1985; 12:980–3.

72. Nielson WR, Walker C, McCain GA. Cognitive behavioral treatment of fibromyalgia syndrome: preliminary findings. J Rheumatol 1992; 19:98–103.

73. Cathey MA, Wolfe F, Kleinheksel SM, Hawley DJ. Socioeconomic impact of fibrositis. A study of 81 patients with primary fibrositis. Am J Med 1986; 81:78–84.

74. Felson DT, Goldenberg DL. The natural history of fibromyalgia. Arthritis Rheum 1986; 29:1522–6.

75. Cathey MA, Wolfe F, Kleinheksel SM, Miller S, Pitetti KH. Functional ability and work status in patients with fibromyalgia. Arthritis Care Res 1988; 1:85–98.

76. Cathey MA, Wolfe F, Roberts FK, Bennett RM, Caro X, Goldenberg DL, Russell IJ, Yunus MB. Demographic, work disability, service utilization and treatment characteristics of 620 fibromyalgia patients in rheumatologic practice. Arthritis Rheum 1990; 33:S10.

77. Hudson JI, Goldenberg DL, Pope HG Jr, Keck PE Jr, Schlesinger L. Comorbidity of fibromyalgia with medical and psychiatric disorders. Am J Med 1992; 92:363–7.

78. Goldenberg DL. Diagnostic and therapeutic challenges of fibromyalgia. Hosp Pract 1989; Sept 30:45.

13

The Relevance of Psychiatric Research on Somatization to the Concept of Chronic Fatigue Syndrome

Michael R. Clark
Johns Hopkins University,
Baltimore, Maryland

Wayne Katon
University of Washington Medical School,
Seattle, Washington

This chapter will review recent research describing the association between anxiety and depressive disorders, the personality trait of neuroticism, medical utilization, functional disability, and medically unexplained physical symptoms. The relevance of this research to the presentation by primary care patients of common physical symptoms, such as fatigue, abdominal pain, or sleep problems, will be discussed. Finally, we will present the results of four studies of patients with chronic fatigue in which our group has been involved. These studies include (1) research on the symptom prevalence of chronic fatigue in the general population and its association with anxiety, depression, and somatization; (2) the association between psychiatric disorders, functional disability, the number of medically unexplained physical symptoms and personality factors in patients with chronic fatigue; (3) the results of structured psychiatric interviews in patients with chronic fatigue compared with patients with rheumatoid arthritis; and (4) a 2-year follow-up study of patients with chronic fatigue, which examined the factors at initial presentation that were associated with persistent symptoms.

This chapter will present data on patients with chronic fatigue and not limit findings to patients who meet the case criteria for chronic fatigue syndrome (CFS). Thus far, studies have not confirmed that patients meeting case criteria for CFS differ immunologically or virologically from patients with chronic fatigue who do not meet these criteria. In fact, as we will present, the requirement for multiple somatic symptoms in the case criteria tend to identify a chronic fatigue sample of patients with recurrent anxiety and depressive disorders.

DEFINITIONS

Both somatization and chronic fatigue syndrome (CFS) have roots in Beard's syndrome of neurasthenia [1]. Similar to chronic fatigue syndrome, neurasthenia was described as consisting of a myriad of somatic symptoms (fatigue, headache, aches, and pains), cognitive symptoms (decreased concentration and memory), and emotional symptoms (depression and anxiety). Also, analogous to CFS, neurasthenia was posited to be due to an organic cause and the "rest cure" was often applied. The term gradually fell into disfavor in the late 19th century as Freud and other psychiatric researchers described and removed depressive and anxiety disorders from this undifferentiated disorder. Psychiatrists became exclusively interested in the psychodynamic and, later, biologic underpinning of the anxiety and depressive disorders, and only in recent years did they rediscover that these disorders are associated with a myriad of somatic symptoms.

The term *somatization* was first used by Stekel [2]. Although he considered it a type of bodily disorder arising from a deep-seated neurotic cause and essentially identical with Freud's concept of conversion, he also referred to it as the "organ speech" of the mind or the organic expression of mental processes. The term *illness behavior* has also been used in recent years to depict both the adaptive and maladaptive ways patients deal with somatic symptoms and disease. Mechanic described illness behavior as the more general "ways in which given symptoms may be differentially perceived, evaluated and acted upon by different kinds of persons" [3].

Currently, *somatization* is conceptualized as at least three overlapping, distinct patterns of illness behavior. These three definitions of somatization have been operationalized by Kirmayer and Robbins [4] and include (1) high levels of medically unexplained symptoms in multiple physiologic systems [5–7]; (2) levels of somatic preoccupation or illness worry beyond what is expected from demonstrable disease [8–10]; and (3) the predominantly or exclusively somatic clinical presentation of psychiatric disorders, such as depression or anxiety (Fig. 1) [11–13]. These definitions of somatization can be understood as distinct forms of abnormal illness behavior. Pilowski describes abnormal illness behavior as resulting when "the patient is uninfluenced by the doctor's explanation of what he believes to be the problem and the way in which it should be managed." In other words, "the doctor does not believe that the patient's objective pathology entitles him to be placed in the type of sick role he expects for the reasons which he claims it" [14].

The first form of somatization described in the foregoing is typified by the *Diagnostic and Statistical Manual of Mental Disorders*, 3rd ed., revised

Multiple functional symptoms 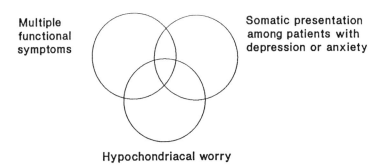 Somatic presentation among patients with depression or anxiety

Hypochondriacal worry

Figure 1 Venn diagram of relationship between three forms of somatization. (From Ref. 3).

(*DSM-III-R*) diagnosis of *somatization disorder*. Patients with somatization disorder have experienced 13 or more medically unexplained physical symptoms in multiple organ systems, with at least some occurring before aged 30. The prevalence of this strictly defined condition is less than 1% of the general population and occurs in about 1–2% of women [4,6,15]. There is also an inverse relation with education, income, and occupational status. Although it is a chronic condition, with a fluctuating course and increased morbidity, patients with somatization disorder do not have significantly higher rates of mortality [16]. A subsyndromal form of somatization has been defined by Escobar and colleagues and requires only 4–12 unexplained physical symptoms for men and 6–12 for women [17]. The prevalence of this condition ranges from 9 to 20% of community samples [18]. Many studies have demonstrated that individuals with both somatization disorder and subsyndromal somatization have significantly increased utilization of health care services and more functional impairment or disability compared with community controls [19,20]. Both the subsyndromal definition of somatization as well as somatization disorder have been shown to be highly correlated with anxiety and depressive disorders.

The *DSM-III-R* diagnosis of *hypochondriasis* characterizes the second form of somatization. Although individuals with hypochondriasis do report increased levels of current unexplained physical symptoms, the essential features of this syndrome are excessive concern about disease and preoccupation with the belief of having a serious illness. In primary care or general medical practice, the prevalence of hypochondriasis ranges from 3 to 14% [20–24]. It occurs in roughly equal numbers of men and women, but the age of onset is usually in the fourth or fifth decade, as compared with the teens for somatization disorder. In studies of hypochondriasis in primary care, most patients had comorbid anxiety and depressive disorders on structured psychiatric interview. Some authorities have labeled patients with hypochondriasis and associated psychiatric comorbid diagnosis as secondary hypochondriasis. Many authorities have suggested that primary hypochondriasis or hypochondriasis occurring without comorbid psychiatric disorder is relatively rare.

A current model of hypochondriasis is built on the process of *somatosensory amplification*. This term refers to the tendency of individuals to experience somatic sensation as intense, noxious, and disturbing. Barsky and colleagues described amplification as involving the following elements: (1) hypervigilance or heightened attentional focus on bodily sensation; (2) the tendency to select out and concentrate on certain relatively weak, infrequent sensations; and (3) the disposition to react to somatic sensations with affect and cognitions that intensify them and make them more alarming, ominous, and disturbing [7,25–28]. Subsequently, the hypochondriac misinterprets bodily sensations and incorrectly attributes them to a serious disease, rather than a more benign and common cause. In this model, somatic symptoms continue to increase as the individual, who already has heightened bodily preoccupation, screens for somatic perceptions that confirm the hypothesis of disease, and ignores the sensory inputs that disconfirm illness. Additional physical symptoms are also produced directly by increased levels of psychological distress, which are then again attributed to the presumed illness.

Finally, the third form of somatization is the presentation of *DSM-III-R* diagnoses, other than the somatoform disorders, as primarily somatic symptoms. The most common psychiatric disorders associated with the presentations of medically unexplained complaints to primary care physicians are anxiety and depressive disorders. The prevalence of these common psychiatric conditions are significantly increased in primary care populations compared with the community [10,29–34]. Approximately 50–70% of patients meeting criteria for anxiety and depressive diagnoses present with unexplained somatic symptoms. From another perspective, 11 common symptoms, such as fatigue, chest pain, dizziness, abdominal pain, and edema, are associated with one-third to 40% of primary care visits. Only approximately 10% of people with these common symptoms are found to have an organic disorder over a 1-year period in primary care [35–37]. As will be more fully described later, studies of homogeneous populations of patients with the medically unexplained symptoms of tinnitus, dizziness, syncope, pelvic pain, chest pain, and irritable bowel syndrome, find significantly increased prevalences of anxiety and depressive diagnoses when these patients are compared with patients with a well-verifiable organic disease [38–44].

The foregoing definitions of somatization and hypochondriasis suggest that these are disorders that one categorically has, or meets criteria for, or does not. In actuality, somatization or hypochondriasis should be thought of as continuous measures of symptom perception that form a bell-shaped curve in the general population (Fig. 2). The terms *amplifiers* and *minimizers* may be used to describe

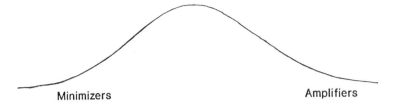

Minimizers   Amplifiers

Figure 2   Symptom perception in the general population.

patients at either end of this continuum of symptom perception. Amplifiers may pick up and worry about minor sensations and utilize more medical care for symptoms that would not bring the average person to a doctor. Thus, minor stomach discomfort may lead the amplifier to perceive more pain, visit the doctor, and take more medicine. On the other hand, the minimizer may disregard bodily symptoms or signals of severe illness, which also may endanger his or her health.

In a recent study, patients with chest pain were given a brief test to measure amplification or somatization before an angiogram [45]. Patients who scored the highest on these scales had the least coronary artery disease and, in fact, were usually found to have negative workups. On the other hand, patients with the lowest scores (the minimizers or dampeners of symptoms had the most severe coronary artery disease, often three- and four-vessel disease. These minimizers probably did not sense bodily signals of ischemic pain that most people would have perceived, worried about, and sought medical care for and, therefore, did not present to physicians until they were in a later stage of illness. The degree of minimization or amplification is probably a long-term trait, but aversive life events and psychological distress, in general, as well as specific psychiatric disorders, can also produce *state* amplification [12,13]. The state of distress pushes the patient's normal level of perception of symptoms toward the amplifier end of the bell-shaped curve. Also, acute medical illnesses, such as myocardial infarction, may transiently push a patient's perception of symptoms toward the amplifier end of the bell-shaped curve. The amplification associated with acute medical illness is often time-limited and associated with a sense of personal vulnerability and some degree of psychological distress.

The overlap or cooccurrence of these three types of somatization is important to appreciate. As will be discussed later, there is a linear relation between the number of medically unexplained physical symptoms and the prevalence of depression and anxiety disorders. Almost all patients with depressive or anxiety disorders have somatic complaints that include pain or other vegetative symptoms [29,46,47]. Hypochondriacal fears and disease conviction are significantly increased in 50–70% of patients with major depression or anxiety disorders [6,46–49]. Patients with hypochondriasis have significant psychiatric comorbidity, ranging from 42 to 88% [48–51]. Finally, hypochondriacal symptoms were found in 38% of family practice patients with somatization disorder [49], and 39% of hypochondriacal patients referred to psychiatry from general practitioners satisfied the criteria for somatization disorder [52].

More specifically, in a study of patients meeting *DSM-III-R* criteria for hypochondriasis, the number of lifetime axis I psychiatric diagnoses was twice that of controls [50]. Both the current and lifetime prevalence of major depression (current 33.3 vs 6.6%; lifetime 42.9 vs 18.4%) and dysthymic disorder (45.2 vs 9.2%) were significantly increased compared with controls. The anxiety disorders were also more common in hypochondriasis. These results included the diagnoses of generalized anxiety disorder (current 24.4 vs 13.2%; lifetime 71.4 vs 27.6%), panic disorder (lifetime 16.7 vs. 26%), phobias (current 33.3 vs 13.2%; lifetime 42.9 vs 21.0%), and obsessive–compulsive disorder (lifetime 9.5 vs 2.6%). Thus, many patients in primary care with hypochondriasis may suffer from a coexisting affective or anxiety disorder, and the hypochondriacal tendency may be cured by treatment of their coexisting anxiety or depressive disorder.

Patients with full or subsyndromal somatization also have high prevalences of depression and anxiety disorders. Escobar et al. found more than 60% of patients with subsyndromal somatization had a lifetime history of major depression or an anxiety disorder [5]. The overlap of depressive and anxiety diagnoses is also found with patients meeting criteria for somatization disorder. Seventy-six percent of patients diagnosed with somatization disorder by *DSM-III* criteria reported lifetime depressive symptoms, compared with only 30% of the general population. In this same sample, 88% of somatization disorder patients had lifetime anxiety symptoms compared with only 25% of the total community [53]. Thus, the epidemiological data suggest that there is substantial overlap in the three types of syndromes associated with medically unexplained symptoms. All three are associated with anxiety and depressive disorders that, in most patients, are either relapsing, recurrent, or chronic disorders. We will now describe the epidemiology of anxiety and depressive disorders and their relation to medical utilization, somatization, and disability.

PREVALANCE OF DEPRESSIVE AND ANXIETY DISORDERS IN PRIMARY CARE

Within the primary care sector, the prevalence of psychiatric disorders is difficult to estimate based on physician notation or billing codes. Frequently, physicians do not accurately make the diagnosis of depression [54,55]. Another problem occurs when the diagnosis is accurate, but is intentionally miscoded to avoid social stigmatization or poor insurance coverage. Depression has been estimated to be coded as a diagnosis in 1.5–4.5% of patient visits to primary care physicians

[5], but other studies indicate one-third to one-half of patients with major depression are purposefully miscoded (to avoid stigma and to increase potential third-party payments) [56]. When specific depression rating scales are used to assess prevalence, 9–30% of primary care patients score in the moderate to severe depressed range [54]. Structured psychiatric interviews provide more reliable estimates and find a point prevalence of major depression between 4.8 and 8.6%. These findings are consistent across four different countries, using three different structured psychiatric interviews [31–33,57].

Anxiety is also a common problem in primary care patients. A study, using a self-rating anxiety scale developed by Zung, found that 32% of primary care patients versus 9% of the general population scored in the pathological range [58]. The most common severe anxiety disorder, panic disorder, is present in 1.6–2.9% of women and 0.4–1.7% of men in the community [59]. However, 3.6–10% of people report having suffered panic attacks that were just not frequent enough to meet formal diagnostic criteria [59]. These individuals are more likely to report significant levels of anxiety and depression at their baseline when compared with patients who have never experienced a panic attack. Studies with structured psychiatric interviews have found the prevalence of panic disorder within the primary care population to be 6.5–8% [60–62].

RELATION OF PSYCHIATRIC DISORDERS TO MEDICAL UTILIZATION

When patients suffer from a mental disorder, their use of nonpsychiatric medical care is double that of patients without a mental disorder [63]. Other studies of high-utilizers of primary care further characterize these patients as having more psychological distress and a greater number of chronic medical illnesses than low-utilizers [64,65]. One study of an HMO primary care population found high-utilizers represented 10% of all patients, but used 29% of all outpatient primary care visits, 52% of outpatient specialty visits, 48% of all inpatient hospital days, and 26% of all prescriptions over a 1-year period. Half of these high-utilizers demonstrated significant psychological distress [65]. Structured psychiatric interviews detected quite high prevalence rates of recurrent major depression (68%) as well as anxiety disorders, somatization disorder, and alcohol abuse. Similar results were reported by The National Institute of Mental Health (NIMH) Epidemiologic Catchment Area Study, which studied the prevalence of mental illness and the utilization of medical services in five major United States cities [66]. In this study, high medical utilization was defined as six or more visits for general medical services in a 6-month period [66]. Odds ratios for the high use of any general medical services ranged from 1.2 to 8.2 depending on sex and the specific mental disorder (Table 1).

Table 1 Odds Ratio for High Use of Medical
Services (Six or More Visits in a 6-Month Period)

Psychiatric diagnosis	Odds ratio	
	Male	Female
Somatization disorder	3.3	2.5
Panic disorder	8.2	5.2
Major depression	1.5	3.4
Phobias	2.7	1.6
Alcohol abuse	1.6	1.6
Drug abuse	1.8	1.2

Source: Ref. 66.

THE RELATION OF PSYCHIATRIC DISORDERS TO MEDICALLY UNEXPLAINED SOMATIC SYMPTOMS

In the Epidemiologic Catchment Area Study, somatic symptoms such as fatigue, headache, or bodily pain occur in one-quarter to one-third of the community throughout the lifetime. In over 80% of these individuals, symptoms have resulted in seeking medical care, taking medication, or substantially changing normal activities [67] In this study, respondents with five or more current functional somatic symptoms had significantly increased prevalence of current psychiatric diagnoses (50 vs 6%) when compared with those with no current somatization symptoms [68]. Over a 1-year period, only 10% of patients with these common physical symptoms are found to have a medical disorder explaining their symptoms [67]. Our group has had a long-term interest in patients with one or more medically unexplained symptoms. We have used similar methodology to study these subgroups of patients. In each study, we have used the Diagnostic Interview Schedule (DIS), a structured psychiatric interview, to compare patients with a medically unexplained symptom with a control group with a homogeneous medical illness, such as rheumatoid arthritis. Patients with one aversive complaint (e.g., back pain, chest pain, pelvic pain, tinnitus, fatigue, irritable bowel) in each study were compared with a medical control group with a well-defined medical disease or problem. These studies have demonstrated a significantly higher prevalence of current and lifetime major depression in the patients with subjective aversive symptoms compared with medical controls (Table 2) [38–44,69]. In addition, patients with noncardiac chest pain or irritable bowel syndrome (IBS) were more likely to meet criteria for panic disorder. The IBS and chronic fatigue patients also were more likely to have somatization disorder than the medical controls with whom they were compared.

Research has also demonstrated that when psychiatric disorders and minor

Table 2 Prevalence Rates of Major Depression as Related to Chronic Pain, Tinnitus, and Fatigue

	Current major depression (%)	Lifetime major depression (%)	Number of depressive episodes	Associated psychiatric or medical illness
Back pain	33	57	3	Alcoholism
Chest pain vs controls	35 vs 3	64 vs 16	5	Panic disorder
Pelvic pain vs controls	34 vs 10	66 vs 16	5	Substance abuse, sexual abuse
Tinnitus vs controls	60 vs 7	75 vs 15	3.5	Mild sensorineural hearing loss
Fatigue vs controls	15 vs 3	76.5 vs 42	2	Somatization disorder
Irritable bowel syndrome vs controls	21 vs 5.5	61 vs 17	2.5	Panic disorder, somatization disorder
Dizziness vs peripheral ear	12 vs 5	42 vs 18	2	Panic disorder

somatic symptoms, such as chronic tinnitus, dizziness, syncope, or migraine headache, cooccur, the patient has significantly more functional disability, with decrements in both social and vocational function and poorer view of their physical health [70–73]. Patients with depressive symptoms or major depression have as much or more functional disability as patients with chronic medical illnesses, such as diabetes, hypertension, arthritis, or coronary artery disease [74]. When patients have both depressive symptoms and a comorbid medical illness, they experience equal and additive disability from these medical and psychiatric disorders. In addition, functional disability and depressive symptoms change in a synchronous fashion over a prospective period of follow-up [75,76]. As depressive symptoms decrease, social and vocational functioning tend to improve, and the patient also rates his or her health status as improved. These findings are further supported by a double-blind, placebo-controlled trial showing successful treatment of depression associated with medical illness with antidepressant medications resulted in significant decreases in functional disability [77,78]. Primary care physicians have the opportunity to impinge on both patient functional disability as well as health care utilization through the recognition and appropriate treatment of psychiatric illness in their patients presenting for the evaluation and treatment of chronic, unexplained physical symptoms.

In the following sections, we will describe four studies that we have carried out on patients with chronic fatigue and how data from these studies are associated with the large body of research described in the foregoing on somatization.

Community and Primary Care Data

Only one report has examined the comorbidity of fatigue and psychiatric illness in the community using structured psychiatric interviews. Using the public-use data tape from the 1984 NIMH Epidemiologic Catchment Area Study [79], we have examined the relation between the current report of experiencing the symptom of fatigue, and psychiatric diagnoses, in a community sample of 18,571 people [80]. The current or 1-month prevalence of medically unexplained fatigue was 6.6%. Women were significantly more likely than men to report the symptom of fatigue (71 vs 57%).

Significantly higher rates of lifetime and current psychiatric diagnoses were found in subjects with *current* (1 month) fatigue, compared with respondents who did not report current fatigue. As seen in Table 3, men with current fatigue had significantly higher odds ratios of having experienced affective, anxiety, and somatoform disorders, including significantly higher prevalence rates of lifetime and current major depression, dysthymic disorder, and both lifetime and current panic disorder. They were also more likely to have somatization disorder and an abridged diagnosis of somatization. When fatigue was removed as a criterion for

Table 3 Prevalences of Current and Lifetime Psychiatric
Diagnoses in Men and Women with Current (1 mo) Complaints
of Fatigue Compared with Those Without Fatigue

	Fatigue subjects n (%)	Comparison subjects n (%)	Odds ratio
Men			
Major Depression			
Lifetime[a]	30 (18.0)	106 (2.6)	8.2
Current 1 mo[a]	4 (2.4)	7 (0.2)	14.7
Lifetime[b]	21 (12.6)	90 (2.2)	6.5
Current 1 mo[b]	2 (1.2)	7 (0.2)	7.2
Dysthymia	23 (13.8)	63 (1.5)	10.2
Panic			
Lifetime	9 (5.5)	29 (0.7)	8.1
Current 1 mo	1 (0.6)	4 (0.1)	6.3
Somatization D/O	1 (0.6)	1 (0.0)	24.9
Abridged somatization	25 (15.0)	82 (2.0)	8.8
Women			
Major Depression			
Lifetime[a]	92 (19.9)	244 (4.4)	5.4
Current 1 mo[a]	10 (2.2)	20 (0.3)	6.3
Lifetime[b]	68 (14.7)	201 (3.5)	4.7
Current 1 mo[b]	8 (1.7)	15 (0.3)	6.7
Dysthymia	72 (15.6)	169 (3.0)	5.9
Panic			
Lifetime	34 (7.4)	74 (1.3)	5.9
Current 1 mo	10 (2.2)	10 (0.2)	12.6
Somatization D/O	13 (2.8)	12 (0.2)	13.4
Abridged somatization	220 (47.5)	945 (16.5)	4.6

[a]Diagnoses allow fatigue in the count of depression symptoms.
[b]Diagnoses exclude fatigue in the count of depression symptoms.
Source: Ref. 80.

the diagnosis of major depression, the significantly higher prevalence of current
and lifetime major depression remained.

As seen in Table 3, women with current fatigue also had significantly higher
odds ratios of having experienced affective, anxiety, and somatoform disorders,
including a higher prevalence of lifetime and current major depression, dysthymic
disorder, as well as lifetime and current panic disorder. They were also more
likely to have somatization disorder and an abridged diagnosis of somatization.
When fatigue was excluded as a criterion for the diagnosis of major depression,
the increased prevalence of current and lifetime major depression remained
significantly different.

Respondents with current fatigue reported a significantly greater mean number of medically unexplained symptoms than respondents not reporting current fatigue (men: 2.5 vs 0.7; women: 4.5 vs 1.6). Moreover, patients with fatigue not only reported a higher mean number of medical symptoms believed to be common in the chronic fatigue syndrome (myalgias, arthralgias, headaches, difficulty walking, weakness, inability to continue with daily activities because of illness), but were significantly more likely to have almost every one of the other 37 medically unexplained symptoms about which the Diagnostic Interview Schedule (DIS) inquires. These data suggest that, rather than suffering from the more delimited somatic symptoms associated with chronic fatigue syndrome, patients with fatigue have a tendency to somatize or amplify all physical symptoms.

We also examined the effect of comorbid psychiatric disorders in respondents with fatigue. Compared with subjects who reported fatigue, but no lifetime history of depression or anxiety diagnoses, subjects with both fatigue and one or more of these psychiatric diagnoses had made a significantly higher number of medical visits in the last 6 months (4.3 vs 2.2 for men; 4.2 vs 2.6 for women) and had had significantly more medically unexplained physical symptoms (2.4 vs 1.3 for men; 4.2 vs 2.6 for women).

These data suggest that anxiety and depressive disorders, as well as the tendency to somatize, are significantly associated with the symptom of fatigue in community respondents. Patients with fatigue and psychiatric illness had higher rates of medical utilization which, at least partially, explains the findings of even higher psychiatric comorbidity in primary and tertiary care patients with chronic fatigue [81].

The Relation of Lifetime Psychiatric Disorders, Personality Traits, and Unexplained Physical Symptoms

To investigate this interaction between somatization, psychiatric disorder/psychological distress, and disability in chronic fatigue patients, Katon and Russo also analyzed data on 285 patients presenting to a chronic fatigue clinic [92]. These patients were separated into four groups according to the number of unexplained somatic symptoms they reported on the DIS. Overlapping symptoms with CFS were deleted from the analysis. The four groups differed significantly with greater numbers of unexplained somatic symptoms associated with a higher number of total *current* psychiatric diagnoses, total *lifetime* psychiatric diagnoses and *lifetime* depressive symptoms. All of these differences were *linear* relative to the number of unexplained physical symptoms. In addition, the extent of impairment in activities of daily living and the tendency to amplify somatic symptoms also increased *linearly* with the number of medically unexplained physical symptoms. These findings are consistent with the results of our studies of patients who are high utilizers of primary care clinics [93]. High-utilizers of primary medical care with the gretest number of unexplained physical symptoms, despite similar burden of medical illness, have the highest prevalence of current and lifetime psychiatric illness, the greatest medical care utilization, and the most functional impairment. Moreover, psychiatric illness and disability increase linearly with unexplained physical symptoms [93].

Somatization is also affected by personality traits. The personality trait of neuroticism or negative affectivity is characterized by increased sensitivity to signals of punishment and greater likelihood of developing a negative affect when confronted with aversive stimuli [97]. Patients with high neuroticism tend to describe more worry, anxiety, low self-esteem, feelings of guilt, shyness, moodiness, and sense of vulnerability. Both cross-sectional and prospective studies have demonstrated an association between somatization and neuroticism [94,99]. Presumably, the enduring trait of neuroticism predisposing an individual to negative affective states would then result in increased reporting of physical complaints. Several research reports have reported an increasing linear association between neuroticism and the number of anxiety and depressive diagnoses experienced by patients [100,101].

Although the number of medically unexplained physical symptoms has been significantly increased in patients with anxiety and depressive disorders, and these patients are more likely to have higher neuroticism, the question of *independent* contributions of personality and psychiatric illness to the severity of somatization needed to be answered. Russo and colleagues studied three different populations of medical patients [95]. One group was composed of patients undergoing evaluation for the complaint of dizziness, the second was made up of patients with disabling tinnitus, and the third suffered from chronic fatigue. The subjects underwent structured psychiatric interviews to determine the presence of *DSM-III-R* psychiatric diagnoses and personality assessment with the Tridimensional Personality Questionnaire (TPQ) [102,103]. The dimension of harm-avoidance on the TPQ is similar to the trait of neuroticism. Cloninger conceptualizes *harm-avoidance* as an individual's "tendency to respond intensely to aversive stimuli and to avoid punishment, novelty, and non-reward passively" [103]. The dimension of harm-avoidance comprises four subscales: worry–pessimism, fear of uncertainty, shyness with strangers, and fatigability–asthenia. The other dimensions of the TPQ are reward–dependence, which is similar to extroversion as described by Eysenck [99], and novelty-seeking, which is an individual's tendency toward excitement in response to novel stimuli [103,105].

The results of this study showed that the number of current and past anxiety and depressive diagnoses and the personality factor of harm-avoidance both contributed independently to the reporting of multiple medically unexplained physical symptoms across all patient groups. Further analyses demonstrated that the two subscales of worry–pessimism and impulsiveness (a subscale of the novelty-seeking dimension) were significantly associated with greater numbers of medically unexplained symptoms. These subscales focus attention on the chronic dysphoria and inability to tolerate negative emotions characteristic of neuroticism [106,107]. These personality traits appear to independently contribute to the development of and the seeking of medical care for unexplained physical symptoms.

Tertiary Care Studies of Psychiatric Illness, Somatization, and Chronic Fatigue Syndrome

The relation between psychiatric disorders, somatization, and chronic fatigue syndrome has been quite controversial. Several hypotheses have been considered. Psychiatric disorders and somatization could be a cause of CFS, the consequence of CFS, or an artifact of overlapping symptom criteria. In an attempt to address these issues, the prevalence of psychiatric disorders have been studied in patients with chronic fatigue. Unfortunately, many studies have not included a medical comparison group. If psychiatric disorders are secondary to the burden of medical illness, than these patients would be expected to have similar prevalences of psychiatric conditions when compared with patients with chronic fatigue. Wessely and Powell found a significantly higher prevalence of psychiatric disorders in patients with chronic fatigue (CF) when compared with those with neuromuscular disorders (72 vs 36%) [82]. Katon et al. compared chronic fatigue patients with rheumatoid arthritis (RA) patients and also found a significantly higher prevalence of psychiatric disorders in patients suffering from chronic fatigue (86 vs 48%) [81]. Wood et al. demonstrated a significantly higher prevalence of definite and probable psychiatric cases among patients with chronic fatigue compared with patients with chronic muscular illness (41 vs 12.5% and 26.5 vs 4%, respectively) [83]. Patients with chronic fatigue in the Katon et al. study also had a significantly higher mean number of unexplained medical symptoms (many of which were not symptoms in the case criteria for CFS) and a higher prevalence of somatization disorder. Both patients with chronic fatigue and those with rheumatoid arthritis who had associated affective illness had a significantly higher mean number of unexplained symptoms than patients with CF and RA without affective illness. The studies by Wessely el al. and Katon et al. also controlled for overlapping symptoms of somatization disorder, depression, and CFS. Their results support the conclusions that psychiatric disorders found in CFS are not a psychologic reaction to having a debilitating medical disorder. If the psychiatric symptoms were simply a secondary psychologic reaction to illness, then we would have expected similar rates of psychiatric disorders in patients with CFS and medical controls.

Other studies have also found a high prevalence of psychiatric disorders in chronic fatigue patients, and most patients had the onset of psychiatric disorders before the onset of chronic fatigue [84–87]. Further research will clarify the relation between psychiatric disorder and chronic fatigue. One hypothesis is that psychiatric disorders could lead to complex physiological changes in the immunological or neuroendocrine systems. These physiological changes may lead to the reactivation of latent viruses or, alternatively, decreases in "stress" hormones such as cortisol, and result in the distinct affective, cognitive, and somatic symptoms of chronic fatigue syndrome. Another possibility is that psychiatric disorders are the main cause of the symptoms of chronic fatigue syndrome, with the psychophysiological abnormalities that are secondary to major depression, such as disturbed sleep, autonomic dysregulation, and muscle tension problems expressed as the multiple physical symptoms associated with CFS.

A PROSPECTIVE LONGITUDINAL STUDY OF PROGNOSIS

Identifying etiological or precipitating causes of chronic fatigue, such as major depression, allows the institution of effective therapy and prevention, but it is also important to clarify the factors that have a role in sustaining CFS and result in prolonged disability and suffering. Frequently, the duration of chronic fatigue symptoms in individual patients is so long that the initiating factors may be difficult to detect or are no longer present. For instance, in our study comparing patients with chronic fatigue with those with rheumatoid arthritis, patients with chronic fatigue had been ill a mean of 5 years. Longitudinal follow-up studies of chronic fatigue patients have been limited, but are necessary to determine which aspects of their initial presentation to health care providers are associated with the persistence of significant disabling symptoms.

Clark et al. performed a 2-year follow-up study of a cohort of patients with chronic fatigue [88]. The patients were separated into two groups, based on their self-report of change in chronic fatigue symptoms at the time of follow-up, compared with the time of initial presentation to a chronic fatigue clinic. Overall, 41% of patients with chronic fatigue described themselves as moderately to completely recovered at a mean of 2.5 years of follow-up. This was labeled the "recovery" group and the patients with persistent symptoms the "no-recovery" group. The no-recovery group was found to have been significantly more likely to have met criteria for at least one current, as well as one lifetime, psychiatric diagnosis at initial presentation, when compared with the recovery group. Patients classified as having recovered from chronic fatigue showed significantly fewer numbers of all medically unexplained physical symptoms at initial presentation, even when overlapping symptoms with CFS were deleted. In addition, initial self-report measures of somatization, somatic distress, and heightened awareness of bodily functioning, all were significantly elevated in the no-recovery group at initial presentation. Initial physical examination findings (except pharyngeal inflammation and a positive Romberg sign) and laboratory test results were not associated with recovery status. After controlling for age, education, and the duration of chronic fatigue symptoms, the factors at time 1 which best predicted persistent chronic fatigue were a history of dysthymic disorder and the number of medically unexplained physical symptoms.

Both psychological distress and a tendency to report multiple physical symptoms have been demonstrated to be risk factors for prolonged disability from other illnesses. In chronic brucellosis and influenza, patients who reported more depressive and somatic symptoms before becoming ill had significantly longer times to recovery [89,90]. In ambulatory patients with upper respiratory tract infections, the two most important predictors of overall physical discomfort and both social and vocational disability were somatization and somatosensory amplification [91]. Predicting the course of symptoms is an important aspect of medical care. Once factors have been identified as significant predictors, interventions can be implemented to alter risk factors for developing chronic symptoms and decrease the duration of symptoms. The chances of recovery would be increased and quality of life in addition to functional impairment would improve. The evidence is growing that psychiatric illness and somatization play a role in prevention, treatment, and rehabilitation of a subset of patients with chronic fatigue.

CONCLUSION

In summary, anxiety and depressive disorders are extremely common in the community and in primary care patients, and are associated with the tendency to report multiple medically unexplained symptoms and high medical utilization. The personality trait of neuroticism or harm-avoidance is also associated with both anxiety and depressive disorders and the tendency to experience and report multiple medically unexplained symptoms.

Results of community and tertiary care studies have found high associations between chronic fatigue and anxiety and depressive disorders and somatization. The robust association of the symptom of chronic fatigue with anxiety, depression, and somatization is similar to the findings of studies of other unexplained aversive symptoms, such as chronic pain, irritable bowel syndrome, and dizziness. Moreover, patients with chronic fatigue in tertiary care who have associated current or lifetime disorders and high numbers of somatic symptoms were most likely to remain disabled from their chronic fatigue 2.5 years later. Thus, psychiatric illness may not only be important in causing the symptom of fatigue in some patients, but appears to be a risk factor in prolonging the disability associated with chronic fatigue.

REFERENCES

1. Beard GM. American nervousness. New York: Putnam's, 1869.
2. Steckel W. The interpretation of dreams. New York: Liveright, 1943.
3. Mechanic D. The concept of illness behavior. J Chronic Dis 1962; 15:189–94.
4. Kirmayer LJ, Robbins JM. Three forms of somatization in primary care: prevalence, co-occurrence, and sociodemographic characteristics. J Nerv Ment Dis 1991; 179:647–55.
5. Escobar JL, Burnam A, Karno M, et al. Somatization in the community. Arch Gen Psychiatry 1987; 42:821–33.
6. Kellner R. Functional aomatic symptoms and hypochondriasis. Arch Gen Psychiatry 1985; 42:821–33.
7. Swartz M, Blazer D, George L, et al. Somatization disorder in a community population. Am J Psychiatry 1986; 143:1403–08.
8. Barsky AJ, Klerman GL. Overview: hypochondriasis, bodily complaints, and somatic styles. Am J Psychiatry 1983; 140:273–83.
9. Barsky A, Wyshak G, Klerman G. Hypochondriasis—an evaluation of the *DSM-III* criteria in medical outpatients. Arch Gen Psychiatry 1986; 43:493–500.
10. Pilowsky I. Dimensions of hypochondriasis. Br J Psychiatry 1967; 113:89–93.
11. Bridges KW, Goldberg DP. Somatic presentation of *DSM-III* psychiatric disorders in primary care. J Psychosom Res 1985; 29:563–9.
12. Goldberg DP, Bridges K. Somatic presentations of psychiatric illness in primary care setting. J Psychosom Res 1988; 32:137–44.
13. Katon W, Ries RK, Kleinman A. The prevalence of somatization in primary care. Compr Psychiatry 1984; 25:208–15.
14. Pilowsky I. Abnormal illness behavior. Br J Med Psychol 1969; 42:347–51.
15. Swartz M, Blazer D, George L, et al. Somatization disorder in a southern community. Psychiatr Ann 1988; 18:335–9.
16. Kaplan HI, Sadock BJ, eds. Comprehensive textbook of psychiatry. 5th ed. Baltimore: Williams & Wilkens, 1989.
17. Escobar JL, Rubio-Stipec M, Canino G, et al. Somatic symptom index (SSI). A new and abridged somatization construct. J Nerv Ment Dis 1989; 177:140–6.
18. Escobar JI, Canino G. Unexplained physical complaints: psychopathology and epidemiologic correlates. Br J Psychiatry 1989; 154:24–7.
19. Escobar JI, Golding JM, Hough RI, et al. Somatization in the community: relationship to disability and use of services. Am J Public Health 1987; 77:837–40.
20. Smith GR, Monson RA. Patients with multiple unexplained symptoms: their characteristics, functional health, and health care utilization. Arch Intern Med 1986; 146:69.
21. Barsky AJ, Wyshak G, Klerman GL, et al. The prevalence of hypochondriasis in medical outpatients. Soc Psychiatry Psychiatr Epidemiol 1990; 25:89–94.
22. Kellner R, Wiggins RG, Pathak D. Hypochondriacal fears and beliefs in medical and law students. Arch Gen Psychiatry 1986; 43:487.
23. Barsky A, Wyshak G, Klerman G. Hypochondria—an evolution of the *DSM-III* criteria in medical outpatients. Arch Gen Psychiatry 1986; 43:493–500.
24. Kellner R. Hypochondriasis and somatization. JAMA 1987; 258:2718–22.
25. Barsky AJ, Goodson JD, Lane RS, Cleary PD. The amplification of somatic symptoms. Psychosom Med 1988; 50:510–9.

26. Barsky AJ. Patients who amplify bodily sensations. Ann Intern Med 1979; 91:63–70.

27. Barsky AJ, Wyshak G. Hypochondriasis and somatosensory amplification. Br J Psychiatry 1990; 157:404–9.

28. Barsky AJ, Wyshak G. Hypochondriasis and related health attitudes. Psychosomatics 1989; 30:412–20.

29. Katon W, Vitaliano PP, Russo J, et al. Panic disorder: a spectrum of severity and somatization. J Nerv Ment Dis 1987; 175:12–9.

30. Katon W. The epidemiology of depression in medical care. Int J Psychiatry Med 1987; 17:93–112.

31. Barrett JE, Barrett JA, Oxman TE, et al. The prevalence of psychiatric disorders in a primary care practice. Arch Gen Psychiatry 1988; 45:1100–6.

32. Blacker CVR, Clare AW. Depressive disorder in primary care. Br J Psychiatry 1987; 150:737–51.

33. Schulberg HC, Burn BJ. Mental disorders in primary care: epidemiologic, diagnostic, and treatment research directions. Gen Hosp Psychiatry 1988; 10:79–87.

34. Von Korff M, Shapiro S, Burke JD, et al. Anxiety and depression in a primary care clinic: comparison of diagnostic interview schedule, general health questionnaire, and practitioner assessments. Arch Gen Psychiatry 1987; 44:152–6.

35. Koch KH. The national ambulatory medical care survey: 1975 summary. Hyattsville, MD: (DHHS Publication No. PHS 78-1784), 1978.

36. Braun JW, Robertson LS, Kosa J, Albert JJ. A study of general practice in Massachusetts. JAMA 1971; 2216:301–6.

37. Kroenke K, Mangelsdorff AD. Common symptoms in ambulatory care: incidence, evaluation, therapy and out-care. Am J Med 1989; 86:262–6.

38. Sullivan M, Clark M, Katon W, et al. Psychiatric and otologic diagnoses in patients complaining of dizziness. Arch Intern Med 1993; 153:1479–84.

39. Katon W, Egan K, Miller D. Chronic pain: lifetime psychiatric diagnoses and family history. Am J Psychiatry 1985; 142:1156–60.

40. Walker E, Katon W, Harrop-Griffiths J, et al. Relationship of chronic pelvic pain to psychiatric diagnosis and childhood sexual abuse. Am J Psychiatry 1988; 145:75–80.

41. Walker E, Roy-Byrne P, Katon W, et al. Psychiatric illness and irritable bowel syndrome: a comparison with inflammatory bowel disease. Am J Psychiatry 1990; 147:565–72.

42. Katon W, Hall M, Russo J, et al. Chest pain: relationship of psychiatric illness to coronary arteriographic results. Am J Med 1988; 84:1–9.

43. Sullivan M, Katon W, Dobie R, et al. Disabling tinnitus: association with affective disorder. Gen Hosp Psychiatry 1988; 10:285–91.

44. Linzer M, Varia I, Pontinen M, et al. Medically unexplained syncope: relationship to psychiatric illness. Am J Med 1992; 92(suppl A):18–26S.

45. Frasure-Smith N. Levels of somatic awareness in relation to angiographic findings. J Psychosom Res 1987; 31:545–54.

46. Matthew RJ, Largen J, Claghorn JL. Biological symptoms of depression. Psychosom Med 1979; 41:439–43.

47. Lipowski ZJ. Somatization and depression. Psychosomatics 1990; 31:13–21.

48. Hamilton M. Frequency of symptoms in melancholia (depressive illness). Br J Psychiatry 1989; 154:201–6.
49. Oxman TE, Barrett J. Depression and hypochondriasis in family practice patients with somatization disorder. Gen Hosp. Psychiatry 1985; 7:321–9.
50. Barsky AJ, Wyshak G, Klerman GL. Psychiatric comorbidity in *DSM-III-R* hypochondriasis. Arch Gen Psychiatry 1922; 49:101–8.
51. Kenyon FE. Hypochondriasis: a clinical study. Br J Psychiatry. 1964; 110:478–88.
52. Cloninger CR, Sigvardsson S, Von Knorning AL, Bohman M. An adoption study of somatoform disorders, II: identification of two discrete disorders. Arch Gen Psychiatry 1984; 41:863–71.
53. Swartz M, Hughes D, Blazer D, George L. Somatization disorder in the community: a study of diagnostic concordance among three diagnostic systems. J Nerv Ment Dis 1987; 175:26–33.
54. Katon W, Schulberg H. Epidemiology of depression in primary care. Gen Hosp Psychiatry 1992; 14:237–47.
55. Katon W. The epidemiology of depression in medical care. Int J Psychiatry Med 1987; 17:93–112.
56. Rost K, Smith GR. Deliberate miscoding of depression in primary care: an obstacle for outcomes management. Presented at the fifth annual NIMH international research conference on the classification, recognition and treatment of mental disorders in general medical settings. Bethesda, Maryland, 1991.
57. Kirmayer LJ, Robbins JM, Dworkind M, Yaffe M. Somatization and the recognition of depression and anxiety in primary care. Paper presented at the annual meeting of the American Psychiatric Association. New Orleans, May 15, 1991.
58. Zung WWK. Assessment of anxiety disorder. Qualitative and quantitative approaches. In: Fann WE, Karacan I, Pokorney AD, Williams RL, eds. Phenomenology and treatment of anxiety. New York: Spectrum, 1979:1–17.
59. Katon W. Panic disorder in the medical setting. Washington, DC: APA Press, 1991.
60. Katon W, Vitaliano PP, Russo J, Jones M, Anderson K. Panic disorder: epidemiology in primary care. J Fam Pract 1986; 23:233–9.
61. Finley-Jones R, Brown GW. Types of stressful life events and the onset of anxiety and depressive disorders. Psychol Med 1981; 11:803–15.
62. Taylor CB, Russiter EM, Agras WS. Utilization of health care services by patients with anxiety and anxiety disorders. (in press).
63. Hankin J. Oktay JS. Mental disorder and primary medical care. An analytic review of the literature. In: National Institute of Mental Health, series D, No. 7 (DHEW Publication No. ADM 78-661). Washington, DC: Supt. of Docs., US Government Printing Office, 1979.
64. McFarland GH, Freeborn DH, Mullooley JP, Pupee CR. Utilization patterns among long-term enrollees in a prepaid group practice health maintenance organization. Med Care 1985; 23:1221–33.
65. Katon W, Von Korff M, Lin E. Distressed high utilizers of medical care: *DSM-III-R* diagnoses and treatment needs. Gen Hosp Psychiatry 1990; 12:355–62.
66. Simon G. Psychiatric disorder and functional somatic symptoms as predictors of health care use. Psychiatr Med 1992; 10:49–59.

67. Kroenke K. Symptoms in medical patients: an untended field. Am J Med 1992; 92(suppl 1A):315–45.
68. Simon GE, Von Korff M. Somatization and psychiatric disorder in the NIMH Epidemiologic Catchment Area study. Am J Psychiatry 1991; 148:1494–500.
69. Katon W. The development of a randomized trial of consultation–liaison psychiatry trial in distressed high utilizers of primary care. Psychiatric Med 1991; 9:577–91.
70. Sullivan M, Katon W, Dobie R, et al. Disabling tinnitus. Association with affective disorder. Gen Hosp Psychiatry 1988; 10:285–91.
71. Linzer M, Varia I, Pontinen M, et al. Medically unexplained syncope: relationship to psychiatric illness. Am J Med 1992; 92(suppl 1A):18–26.
72. Stewart WF, Scheter A, Liberman J. Physician consultation for headache pain and history of panic. Results from a population-based study. Am J Med 1992; 92(suppl 1A):355–405.
73. Clark MR, Sullivan MD, Katon WJ, et al. Psychiatric and medical factors association with disability in patients with dizziness. Psychosomatics 1993; 34:409–15.
74. Wells KB, Stewart A, Hays RD, et al. The functioning and well-being of depressed patients. JAMA 1989; 262:914–9.
75. Von Korff M, Ormel J, Katon W, Lin EHB. Disability and depression among high utilizers of health care: a longitudinal analysis. Arch Gen Psychiatry 1992; 49:91–100.
76. Katon W, Sullivan M, Russo J, et al. Depressive symptoms and measures of disability. A prospective longitudinal study. J Affect Disorders 1993; 27:245—54.
77. Borson S, McDonald GH, Gayle T, et al. Improvement in mood, physical symptoms and function with nortriptyline for depression in patients with chronic obstructive pulmonary disease. Psychosomatics (in press).
78. Sullivan M, Katon W, Russo J, et al. A randomized trial of nortriptyline in severe, chronic tinnitus: effects on depression, disability and symptoms. Arch Int Med 1993; 153:1–9
79. Myers JK, Weissman MM, Tischler GE, et al. Six-month prevalence of psychiatric disorder in three communities. Arch Gen Psychiatry 1984; 41:959–70.
80. Walker E, Katon W, Jemelka RP. Psychiatric disorders and medical care utilization among people who report fatigue in the general population. J Gen Intern Med 1993; 8:436–40.
81. Katon WJ, Buchwald DS, Simon GE, Russo JE, Mease PJ. Psychiatric illness in patients with chronic fatigue and those with rheumatoid arthritis. J Gen Intern Med 1991; 6:277–85.
82. Wessely S, Powell R. Fatigue syndromes: a comparison of chronic "post-viral" fatigue with neuromuscular and affective disorder. J Neurol Nurosurg Psychiatry 1989; 52:940–8.
83. Wood GE, Bentall RP, Gofert R, et al. A comparative psychiatric assessment of patients with chronic fatigue syndrome and muscle disease. Psychol Med 1991; 21:619–28.
84. Gold D, Bowden R, Sixby J, et al. Chronic fatigue: a prospective clinical and virologic study. JAMA 1990; 264:58–3.
85. Manu P, Matthews DA, Lane TJ. The mental health of patients with a chief complaint of chronic fatigue: a prospective evaluation and follow-up. Arch Intern Med 1988; 148:2213–7.

86. Taerk GS, Thone BB, Sulit JE, et al. Depression in patients with neuromyasthenia (benign myalgic encephalomyelitis). Int J Psychiatry Med 1987; 13:49–52.

87. Kruesi MJP, Dale J, Straus S. Psychiatric diagnoses in patients who have chronic fatigue. J Clin Psychiatry 1989; 50:53–6.

88. Clark MR, Katon WJ, Russo JE, Buchwald DS. Chronic fatigue: predictors of persistent symptoms in a three-year follow-up study. (submitted).

89. Imboden JB, Center A, Cluff LE, Trever RW. Brucellosis. III. Psychologic aspects of delayed convalescence. Arch Intern Med 1959; 103:406–14.

90. Imboden JB, Center A, Cliff LE. Convalescence from influenza: at study of the psychological and clinical determinants. Arch Intern Med 1961; 108:393–9.

91. Lane RS, Barsky AJ, Goodson JD. Discomfort and disability in upper respiratory tract infection. J Gen Intern Med 1988; 3:540–6.

92. Katon WJ, Russo JE. Chronic fatigue syndrome criteria: a critique of the requirement for multiple physical complaints. Arch Intern Med 1992; 152:1604–9.

93. Katon WJ, Lin E, Von Korff M, et al. Somatization: a spectrum of severity. Am J Psychiatry 1991; 148:34–40.

94. Pennebaker JW. The psychology of physical symptoms. New York: Springer-Verlag, 1982.

95. Russo JE, Katon WJ, Sullivan M, Clark MR, Buchwald D. Severity of somatization and its relationship to psychiatric disorders and neuroticism. Psychosomatics (in press).

96. Larsen R, Kasimatis M. Day-to-day physical symptoms: individual differences in the occurrences, duration, and emotional concomitants of minor daily illnesses. J Pers 1991; 59:387–423.

97. Watson D, Pennebaker J. Health complaints, stress, and distress: exploring the central role of negative affectivity. Psychol Rev 1989; 96:234–54.

98. Larsen R, Kefelarr T. Personality and susceptibility to positive and negative emotional states. J Pers Soc Psychol 1991; 61:132–40.

99. Eysenck H, Eysenck S. Manual of the Eysenck personality questionnaire. London: Hodder & Stoughton. 1979.

100. Andrews G. Neurosis, personality and cognitive behavior therapy. In: McNaughton N, Andrews G, eds. Anxiety. Dunedin: Otago University press, 1990.

101. Andrews G, Stewart G, Morris-Yates A, Holt P, Henderson S. Evidence for a general neurotic syndrome. Br J Psychiatry 1990; 157:6–12.

102. Cloninger C. A unified biosocial theory of personality and its role in the development of anxiety states. Psychiatr Dev. 1986; 3:167–226.

103. Cloninger C. A systematic method for clinical description and classification of personality variants. Arch Gen Psychiatry 1987; 44:573–88.

104. Surakic D, Przybeck T, Cloninger C. Further contribution to the conceptual validity and the unified biosocial model of personality: US and Yugoslav data. Compr Psychiatry 1991; 32:195–209.

105. Earleywine M, Finn P, Peterson J, Pihl R. Factor structure and correlates of the tridimensional personality questionnaire. J Stud Alcohol 1992; 53:233–8.

106. Watson D, Clark L. Negative affectivity: the disposition to experience aversive emotional states. Psychol Bull 1984; 96:465–90.

107. Gray J. Perspectives on anxiety and impulsivity: a commentary. J Res Pers 1987; 21:493–509.

V

AN INTERNATIONAL PERSPECTIVE

14

Studies of the Pathophysiology of Chronic Fatigue Syndrome in Australia

Andrew Lloyd, Ian Hickie, and Denis Wakefield
The Prince Henry Hospital, Little Bay,
New South Wales, Australia

The principal focus of our research program in Australia has been to elucidate the pathophysiological basis of chronic fatigue syndrome (CFS). As a preliminary to our studies, we developed a hypothesis of the pathophysiology of the disorder (Fig. 1). We proposed that CFS results from a disordered immune response to antigenic challenge (usually in the form of viral infection), occurring in genetically predisposed individuals [1]. The disturbance of cell-mediated immunity may allow persistence of viral antigen(s) resulting in chronic and excessive production of cytokines, such as interferon-alpha (IFN-α) in localized sites, particularly in the brain. The fatigue and neuropsychiatric symptoms of CFS may be directly mediated by the effects of these cytokines on the function of cells in the immediate microenvironment (i.e., within the muscle or brain).

To examine this hypothesis, we undertook studies initially to define and characterize the patients presenting with a chronic fatigue state. We sought to develop diagnostic criteria for CFS to define a relatively homogeneous patient group who were suitable for further study [2]. An epidemiological study was performed to examine the nature and prevalence of the illness in a primary care setting, potentially contrasting with tertiary referral centers where ours and other research is based [3,4]. Studies of the possible pathophysiology of CFS, were initiated by examining the relation of preexisting and intercurrent psychiatric morbidity to CFS [5], and subsequently the potential relevance of psychiatric morbidity to immunological disturbances [6,7]. The nature of the subjective

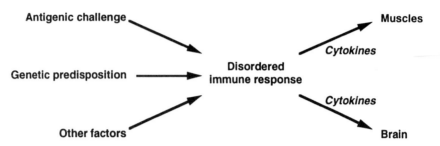

Figure 1   The proposed pathophysiology of CFS.

complaint of fatigue was evaluated as an important step in the process of defining the site of the hypothesized immunological disturbance (i.e., the muscle of the brain) [8,9]. The studies central to our hypothesis were those examining humoral and cellular immunity in patients with CFS and control subjects [6,7,10–14].

DIAGNOSTIC CRITERIA FOR CHRONIC FATIGUE SYNDROME

Patients who were referred to one of four physicians in the Infectious Diseases or Immunology Departments of The Prince Henry and Prince of Wales Hospitals in Sydney, Australia, with a primary symptom complaint of chronic fatigue were assessed clinically and investigated using a standard protocol to exclude alternative explanations for their symptoms. These investigations included a blood count, differential count and film; renal, liver, and thyroid function tests, including estimation of thyroid-stimulating hormone; measurement of creatine kinase, serum immunoglobulins, antinuclear antibody, and rheumatoid factor assays, as well as serological tests for syphilis, hepatitis B, and human immunodeficiency virus (HIV). In addition, selected patients underwent further investigations, such as muscle biopsy and standard electromyography, to exclude primary muscle disorder, or psychiatric referral to evaluate the possibility of an alternative primary psychiatric diagnosis.

The clinical features of 100 consecutive patients in whom this assessment revealed no alternative diagnosis and in whom the fatigue and other symptoms had been present for at least 6 months were discussed by the four physicians. For the criteria, consensus was reached among these physicians on the major features of history and examination consistent with the diagnosis of CFS. A minimum time of 6 months was arbitrarily imposed for the duration of symptoms, so that patients with transient fatigue and constitutional symptoms associated with infection would be excluded, and also so that specific signs indicative of alternative diagnoses could manifest in this period (e.g., fevers and weight loss in a patient with chronic suppurative infection or malignancy). As there is no objective measure available for the severity of the symptoms of CFS, emphasis was placed on the association of disability with the cardinal symptom of fatigue.

In addition, these 100 patients and 100 healthy control subjects underwent assessment of cell-mediated immunity, including peripheral blood T-cell subset analysis, delayed-type hypersensitivity (DTH) skin testing, and lymphocyte proliferation in response to phytohemagglutinin (PHA) in vitro [10]. Evidence of abnormal cell-mediated immunity was found in most patients with CFS, including reduced DTH skin responses in 88% (discussed later). T-lymphocyte counts were significantly reduced in the patients with CFS, in comparison with healthy control subjects, in both the CD4 and CD8 subsets.

On the basis of these clinical and laboratory data a preliminary set of diagnostic criteria were formulated (Table 1). These criteria were designed to highlight the positive clinical features of the syndrome, and to be used in conjunction with appropriate investigations to exclude alternative diagnoses [2].

A further 100 patients defined by these diagnostic criteria were followed up for a period of at least 12 months, as a measure of the temporal stability of the diagnosis of CFS. In only two patients was a 'possible alternative diagnosis reached—one of melancholic depression and one of chronic active hepatitis (probable hepatitis C).

The requirement for all three of the major features of CFS (i.e., chronic and

Table 1 Australian Criteria for the Diagnosis of CFS

To fulfil the criteria for chronic fatigue syndrome (CFS), a patient must have no alternative diagnosis reached by appropriate investigations and

1. *Chronic persisting of relapsing fatigue* of a generalized nature, exacerbated by minor exercise, causing significant disruption of usual daily activities, present for longer than 6 months.
2. *Neuropsychiatric dysfunction*, including impairment of concentration evidenced by difficulty in completing mental tasks that were easily accomplished before the onset of the syndrome, or new onset of short-term memory impairment.
3. *Abnormal cell-mediated immunity*, evidenced by reduced delayed-type hypersensitivity skin responses or by a reduction in the absolute count of CD4 or CD8 lymphocyte subsets or both.

In addition the following findings are supportive of a diagnosis of CFS:

1. *Symptoms* (persistent for longer than 6 months, with no other cause found on investigation): myalgia, arthralgia, headaches, depression, tinnitus, paresthesia, sleep disturbance.
2. *Signs* (present on two or more occasions subsequent to an initial illness): lymphadenopathy, localized muscle tenderness, pharyngitis.

disabling fatigue, neuropsychiatric dysfunction, and abnormal cell-mediated immunity) was intended to provide a set of restrictive criteria to define a uniform patient group for research studies examining evidence for an immunopathological basis for CFS. The criteria for use in clinical practice, in the diagnosis and management of patients with CFS, could reasonably be modified to require only chronic, disabling fatigue, neuropsychiatric dysfunction, and the exclusion of alternative medical and psychiatric diagnoses.

Subsequent to the formulation of the criteria, a questionnaire was developed to provide a standardized data record of the clinical features of patients with CFS. The questionnaire included a 50-item section (see Appendix at end of this chapter) asking the subjects to rate the severity of their symptoms in the last month on a scale of 0 ("never suffer from it") to 3 ("severe or very frequent, making you unable to perform your usual daily activities") and 4 ("suffered from it previously . . . but not now"). Thirty of the questions were prepared by consensus from our review of the pattern of symptomatology of the first 100 consecutive, exhaustively investigated patients with CFS. Ten questions were designed as "distractors," to detect symptoms suggestive of alternative diagnoses, including arthritis ("redness and swelling localized around joints"), dyspnea, incontinence, and dysphagia. Ten questions taken from the 20-item Zung self-report scale of depression [15] were incorporated specifically to detect psychiatric morbidity in the cases, the specific items being those that best-discriminated between cases of CFS and subjects with major depression [5]. The remaining questions sought information concerning other features of the syndrome, including onset after infection, duration of symptoms, and so on.

This questionnaire was completed by 625 patients with CFS (defined by the presence of chronic fatigue and neuropsychiatric dysfunction, and the exclusion of alternative diagnoses), who were drawn from the practices of the four physicians (83.3% of the total number of patients with CFS). There were 440 women (70.4%) and 185 men (29.6%), with a mean age of 38 years (SD 13 years) and a median duration of symptoms (from onset to the time of reporting) of 4.0 years (range 6 months to 46 years). The profile of the symptoms reported by these patients is summarized in Table 2.

In contrast with our diagnostic criteria, a Centers for Disease Control (CDC) working party of epidemiologists and physicians formulated a set of consensus criteria that were not based directly on the assessment of a characterized patient group, nor were they subsequently evaluated [16]. These criteria recommend the specific exclusion of over 30 diseases, by at least 20 laboratory investigations, before the complex clinical requirements may be considered. The criteria do emphasize the same clinical features as our own, including debilitating fatigue and associated disability as a major criterion, as well as neuropsychological complaints ("forgetfulness, inability to concentrate, irritability, and depression . . .") as a minor criterion.

Table 2 Symptoms Most Commonly Reported by Patients with CFS[a]

Symptom	Responses to questionnaire % of subjects ($N = 625$)	
	Symptom present (score 1, 2 or 3)[b]	Symptom severe (score 3)
Prolonged fatigue after activity	92.6	44.3
Concentration impairment	90.0	30.2
Excessive fatigue with minor activity	86.6	32.6
Headache	85.6	25.0
Myalgia—after activity	84.9	26.7
Disturbed sleep or disrupted sleep pattern	81.0	30.9
Memory impairment	80.2	19.8
Speech disturbance (anomia)[c]	80.0	16.9
Prolonged sleep requirements	79.7	33.1
Myalgia—at rest	76.1	15.6
Disturbance of balance	71.7	16.3
Nausea	70.6	12.5
Sore throat	69.2	11.9
Arthralgia	68.8	11.6
Blurring of vision	68.6	16.3

[a]The 15 most commonly reported items are included.
[b]Rated as 1, mild; to 3, severe or very frequent, on questionnaire
[c]Difficulty with speech—lost for the word.

Importantly, one of the *exclusion* sets in the CDC criteria is the presence of "psychiatric disease, either newly diagnosed or by history," or "chronic use of . . . antidepressant medications," despite the *inclusion* of "depression" as an accepted minor symptom criterion. Apart from its ambiguity, this approach effectively prevents study of the potential relevance of both psychological and biological determinants of CFS. The assumption was made that the presence of psychological dysfunction excludes the presence of a medical disorder. These limitations were later recognized, and modifications were suggested in a National Institutes of Health conference [17].

PREVALENCE OF CHRONIC FATIGUE SYNDROME

The aims of this study were to ascertain the point prevalence of CFS in the population of a potentially representative Australian community, and to characterize the clinical and demographic features of the cases [3]. We sought to identify individuals suffering from chronic, unexplained fatigue of at least 6-months duration in the 114,000 population of the Richmond Valley in northern New

South Wales, on the eastern seaboard of Australia. The CFS cases were identified in three stages: (1) notification of cases by local medical practitioners; (2) notified cases were screened further using a detailed questionnaire forwarded by mail; (3) most cases then attended for a medical interview, examination and investigation, as well as a psychiatric interview. At the conclusion of the study, the adequacy of notification was assessed by a look-back survey of a random selection of approximately 50% of the local medical practitioners.

Forty-two subjects fulfilled the case criteria and included 24 females (57%) and 18 males, a female/male ratio of 1.3:1.0, in comparison to a 1.0:1.0 ratio in the population of the Richmond Valley. The ages ranged from 9 to 58 years, with a mean of 33.7 years (median 34; standard deviation [SD] 13.5 years). The crude point prevalence rate for all persons was 37.1 cases per 100,000 (95% confidence interval [CI] 26.8–50.2), with a rate of 42.2 (CI 27.0–62.8) cases in females and 32.0 (CI 19.0–50.6) cases per 100,000 in males. Age-standardizing these crude rates to the Australian population marginally increased the prevalence rate for all persons to 39.6 cases per 100,000.

The mean age at onset of symptoms was 28.6 years (SD 12.3 years), with an essentially normal distribution in the 42 cases (Fig. 2). The median duration of symptoms from onset to sampling date was 30 months, with a range of 6 months to 25 years.

At the medical interview, 21 of 28 (75%) cases gave a history of an acute "viral" illness immediately preceding the onset of the chronic fatigue and other symptoms. In seven cases (25%), serological studies performed at the time of this original illness had confirmed the nature of the infection. Seroconversion to

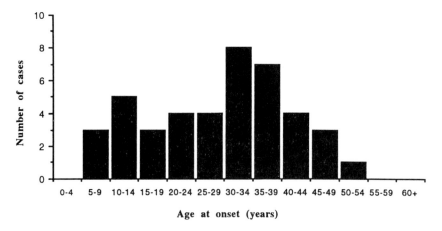

Figure 2   Age at onset of symptoms of CFS in the 42 cases from the prevalence survey in the Richmond Valley, New South Wales, Australia. (From Ref. 3.)

Ross River virus (an Australian arbovirus) had been demonstrated in three cases, to Coxsackie B and to mumps virus in one case each; the Monospot test had been positive in two cases, suggesting Epstein–Barr virus infection. Delayed-type hypersensitivity skin testing was performed on 26 of the 28 interviewed cases. Twenty-three of the 26 patients (88%) had an abnormal DTH response, being reduced in 50%, and absent in 38% (anergic).

The distribution of the social status of the 42 cases, measured using the Congalton socioeconomic scale, was preponderantly that of lower and middle classes (Fig. 3). Twenty-two cases (53%) had a rating of 5–7 on the scale, corresponding with occupations such as unskilled laborer, truck driver, and dress-maker. Only six cases (14%) came from families in which the principal wage-earner was a professional (e.g., research scientist or psychologist; Congalton rating 1–2). This distribution was similar to that of the Richmond Valley population as a whole, in which 51% of individuals had occupations ranking 5–7 on the Congalton scale, and 16% of the principal wage-earners were professionals (see Fig. 3).

The economic impact of CFS on the individual, the government, and the community was studied by calculating the direct and indirect costs arising from the disorder [4]. Data concerning utilization of health resources, income, and employment were obtained by questionnaire from the Richmond Valley cases. In addition, aggregate data from Medicare (the Australian universal health care organization) on the incidence and fees charged for each schedule item for the

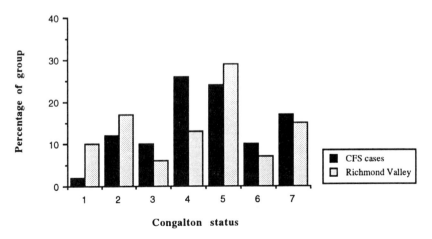

Figure 3   Social status of the cases of CFS and the Richmond Valley population as a whole. The social status of the 42 cases of CFS, determined by the occupation of the principal wage-earner in the family of the cases, rated on the Congalton scale, closely resembles that of the Richmond Valley population as a whole. (From Ref. 3.)

cases was obtained. The conservative estimate of the per assum costs of CFS in the Richmond Valley was 396,000 dollars Australian. Approximately 2000 dollars Australian of direct medical costs attributable to CFS were recorded per patient per annum (approximately 1400 US dollars). If extrapolated to the Australian population, we estimated CFS would generate an annual cost of at least 59 million dollars Australian (1988–1989 dollars).

These remain the only published data examining the prevalence of CFS in the community and its economic impact. Our findings suggest that the disorder is relatively common (comparable in prevalence with multiple sclerosis in the same region). In contrast with the female preponderance noted in tertiary referral settings, CFS appears to affect young adults in the community in an approximately equal sex distribution. We did not document a predisposition of CFS among so-called yuppies, as individuals from all social strata were affected. The disorder typically affected individuals in the peak of their productive years, with resulting disability for prolonged periods. Thus, CFS contributes a substantial area of health resource use and economic burden.

Preliminary reports from the three United States centers of the CDC epidemiological survey have provided minimum prevalence estimates of approximately 2–6 cases per 100,000 [18]. However, if cases excluded from the CFS diagnosis on the basis of previous or intercurrent depression were included, the prevalence estimates in the United States would be remarkably similar to those we have determined in Australia.

PSYCHIATRIC FACTORS IN THE PATHOGENESIS OF CHRONIC FATIGUE SYNDROME

This study was designed to determine the prevalence of psychiatric morbidity in patients with carefully defined CFS, both *during* and *before* the illness episode. Cases were enrolled after exhaustive investigation to exclude alternative medical explanations for the chronic fatigue state. We sought to clarify whether the syndrome is associated with an increase in psychological disturbance, and whether subjects had a high premorbid rate of psychiatric disorder. Psychiatric diagnoses were applied according to established *(DSM-III-R)* diagnostic criteria. A relative of each patient with CFS was interviewed independently to corroborate the patient's report. The study included a control group of subjects with nonmelancholic depression to assess whether patients with CFS resembled those with typical depression, either during the illness episode, or in the features of their premorbid psychiatric health.

All subjects completed several psychometric measures, including (1) the 30-item General Health Questionnaire [19] (GHQ)—a screening instrument for psychiatric morbidity; (2) the Zung Self-Rating Depression Scale [15]; (3) the Eysenck Personality Inventory [20], which is particularly relevant for the assessment of neurotic personality traits; and (4) the Illness Behaviour Questionnaire [21] (IBQ), which generates scores on seven dimensions to indicate the subject's attitudes toward illness, and has been used in the standardized assessment of patients with somatization disorder. The 17-item Hamilton Rating Scale for Depression [22]; which is designed to assess current severity of depression, was administered by the psychiatrist.

Of the 48 patients with CFS, 19 (40%) spontaneously reported psychological and 29 (60%) reported neuropsychological complaints among their key symptoms (Table 3). Twenty-four patients (50%) warranted a psychiatric diagnosis during the course of their illness. The most common disorder was major (nonmelancholic) depression (8 men, 14 women). Six of these 22 patients with CFS and concurrent depression also experienced panic attacks, although these were frequent enough in only one patient to justify an additional diagnosis of panic disorder. Only one patient, who also met criteria for major depression, fulfilled criteria for somatization disorder.

Patients with CFS were markedly dissimilar to the control subjects with depression on each of the standardized measures. Eight of the 33 patients with CFS and 37 of the 48 depressive control subjects scored in moderately affected range (greater than 48) on the Zung scale ($\chi^2 = 22.06$, $p < 0.001$). This established that depressive disorders of clinical severity were rare in the CFS sample. This distinction was supported by the findings of lower mean scores in the patients with CFS on the Hamilton (10.6 vs 19.0; $p < 0.001$) as well as the

Table 3 Neuropsychological and Psychological Symptoms Spontaneously Reported as "Key" Features by Patients with CFS

Symptoms		Number of patients	%
Neuropsychological impairments			
Concentration/attention		25	52
Short-term memory		13	27
Speech disturbance		4	8
Planning tasks		2	4
	Total	29	60
Psychological symptoms			
Depression		18	38
Irritability		8	17
Anxiety/worry/tension		4	8
	Total	19	40
Neuropsychological or psychological	TOTAL	38	80

Source: Ref. 5.

Zung scales (40.7 vs 55.2; p < 0.001). Importantly, patients with CFS also reported lower levels of neuroticism, measured on the Eysenck Personality Inventory (7.3 vs 15.8; p < 0.001), suggesting that any psychiatric morbidity in the CFS sample was less severe, in addition to being less prevalent than in depressed subjects.

There was substantial agreement between the patients' and relatives' estimates of psychological morbidity before the onset of CFS (kappa = 0.81; Table 4). Thirty of the 48 depressive control subjects (63%) had a history of a previous episode that met *Diagnostic and Statistical Manual of Mental Disorders,* 3rd ed, revised *DSM-III-R* [25] criteria for major depression, compared with 6 of the 48 (13%) patients with CFS (χ^2 = 25.6; p < 0.001).

We concluded from this study of well-defined patients that although depression and anxiety are common symptoms, CFS is unlikely to simply be a somatic presentation of an underlying psychological disorder. In particular, the evidence did not support the concept that CFS was equivalent to primary or typical depression. Instead, this study lends support to the hypothesis that current psychological symptoms in patients with CFS may be a consequence of the disorder, rather than evidence of antecedent vulnerability.

Several other groups have completed similar studies examining the prevalence of premorbid and intercurrent psychiatric diagnoses in patients with CFS [23–27]. Comparison between these studies is difficult because of different sampling techniques (notably primary versus tertiary care), methodological differences, and potential heterogeneity of patient groups. All studies have demonstrated that depression and anxiety are common in patients with CFS, and they are severe enough in at least half of the cases to justify treatment. Direct comparisons with patients with depression or with neuromuscular disorders confirm, however, that patients with CFS do not present psychological profiles similar to either of those

Table 4 Premorbid Psychiatric Diagnoses in the Patients with CFS and Control Subjects with Depression

DSM-III-R diagnoses	Number (%) of subjects (N = 48 each group)		Depressive control subjects
	Patients		
	Self-report	Relatives' report	
Major depression	6 (12.5)	6 (12.5)	30 (62)
Panic disorder	1 (2)	1 (2)	3 (6)
Alcohol dependence	4 (8)	4 (8)	18 (38)
Benzodiazepine dependence	0 (0)	0 (0)	5 (10)
Psychotic episode	1 (2)	1 (2)	0 (0)
Total previous morbidity	12 (45)	12 (45)	43 (90)

Source: Ref. 5.

groups [5,24]. Therefore, from a psychological perspective, suggestions that patients with CFS simply have typical depression or, alternatively, the understandable psychological sequelae of chronic neuromuscular disorder, are not supported. Furthermore, in all studies, there are a substantial number of patients with CFS who have neither premorbid nor intercurrent psychiatric diagnoses.

It is more likely that the range of mood, cognitive, and motor symptoms presented by patients with CFS arise directly from a pathophysiological process involving the central nervous system (CNS). Therefore, further studies were undertaken to seek evidence implicating the CNS as the principal site of the pathophysiological disturbance.

MUSCLE PERFORMANCE IN PATIENTS WITH CHRONIC FATIGUE SYNDROME

In conjunction with the indications from the psychiatric studies that the CNS should be examined further in patients with CFS, we evaluated "the muscle" as the site from which the fatigue was originating in patients with CFS. Therefore, we studied muscle strength, endurance, and recovery in various protocols of isometric exercise in patients with CFS and in healthy, matched control subjects. Patients were enrolled after exhaustive assessment and investigation to exclude alternative medical or psychiatric explanations for the chronic fatigue state. The hypothesis was tested that the "fatigue" in patients with CFS can be equated with the neurophysiological definition (i.e., a failure of the muscle to maintain maximal force during sustained or repeated contractions [28]).

The protocols chosen were designed to test the integrity of each aspect of the physiological mechanisms underlying skeletal muscle fatigue, including the descending voluntary drive to the motoneuronal pool, the neuromuscular and excitation–contraction-coupling mechanisms, metabolic factors within the muscle, as well as inhibitory stimuli from peripheral afferent pathways. These mechanisms are illustrated in Figure 4. In normal subjects each of these factors may potentially contribute to the inability to maintain a maximal voluntary effort during the different forms of physical activity that produce fatigue in usual daily life [29]. Isometric, rather than isotonic, exercise was chosen for the studies, as the physiological basis of fatigue in this form of exercise has been extensively characterized. In addition, in contrast with isotonic exercise testing (e.g., on a treadmill), isometric studies allow careful assessment of the potential role of inadequate motivation in findings of impaired performance by the technique of twitch interpolation [9].

In protocols of repetitive, maximal, and submaximal isometric exercise undertaken by normal subjects, the force-generating capacity declines rapidly, yet the muscles can be kept fully activated by the CNS, and force production is not limited by failure of neuromuscular transmission. The mechanism responsible

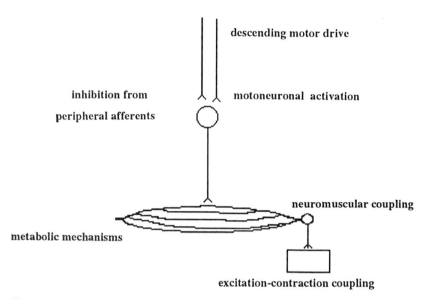

Figure 4   A diagrammatic representation of the motor chain. Failure at the major points shown will be associated with a decline in the force of a maximal voluntary contraction, and the development of "neurophysiological fatigue."

lies within the muscle itself. During all sustained contractions at force levels greater than 25% of the determined maximal voluntary contraction (MVC), large biochemical changes are observed in the muscle [for review, see 29]. Almost total depletion of creatine phosphate and glycogen stores, as well as a profound increase in muscle lactate concentration, have been demonstrated. Thus, decreased muscle strength has been attributed to low-energy substrate availability and to decreased pH from lactic acidosis. Similarly, during dynamic exercise, exhaustion has been attributed to either depletion of energy supplies or to intracellular accumulation of metabolites.

In protocols of repetitive submaximal exercise in normal subjects, at force levels of 30% of MVC, the decline in force-generating capacity after 30 min of exercise was unassociated with accumulation of lactic acid or depletion of energy substrate. Hence, in this setting, failure of excitation–contraction mechanisms is thought to be the basis for the initial development of fatigue.

Protocols of maximal and submaximal isometric exercise were employed to compare the performance of normal subjects and patients with CFS to test the integrity of the physiological mechanisms described in the foregoing. Strength and endurance of the elbow flexors were examined, because established techniques exist for this assessment. The specific muscle group selected was thought not to be critical in view of the generalized nature of the muscle fatigue in patients with CFS.

The studies documented normal maximal voluntary strength in patients with CFS when tested at rest. Thus, there is no objective muscle weakness in patients with this syndrome. This finding is consistent with the characteristically normal neurological examination [8]. We showed further that repeated, maximal isometric contractions in patients with CFS, do not produce premature or excessive loss of force, in comparison with healthy control subjects. In addition, the muscle performance of the patients with CFS tested 4 hr after an initial exercise sequence was not significantly impaired (Fig. 5), at a time when subjective fatigue has typically become a prominent symptom.

The findings of our second study using submaximal isometric exercise, did not support the possibility that failure of the link between motor drive and the metabolic mechanisms of the muscle (including excitation–contraction coupling) is the site of the pathophysiological disturbance producing fatigue in patients with CFS [9]. Muscle performance in response to both voluntary and electrically induced contractions was similar in patients with CFS and control subjects (Fig. 6).

Subjects recorded the level of exertion they felt was required to achieve the target force on a modified Borg scale [30] during the prolonged exercise. The patients' mean score did not differ significantly from that of the control subjects

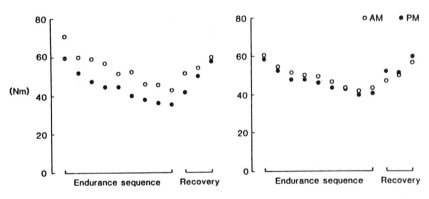

Figure 5 Endurance and recovery sequences in a maximal isometric exercise regimen repeated after a 3-hr interval. Data from a single experiment (of five performed) including a male control subject (left) and a male patient (right) are represented. The absolute force values are shown from the first testing session (open circles, labeled AM, for the morning session) and from the second testing session (closed circles, labeled PM, for the afternoon session). The mean of consecutive pairs of contractions in the endurance sequence of 18 contractions are shown, as are each of the contractions in the recovery phase (1 min, 5 min, and 10 min). There was no significant difference in the performance between the two testing periods for either patients or control subjects. (From Ref. 8.)

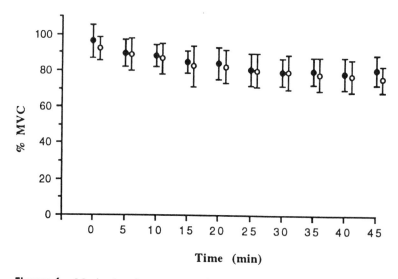

Figure 6 Maximal voluntary strength (MVC) of the elbow flexors in ten static contractions recorded at 5-min intervals during a sequence of 45 min of repetitive submaximal isometric exercise at 30% of the initial MVC. Each data point represents the mean ± SD for the peak force attained in each contraction, expressed as a percentage of the control MVC. Data for patients with CFS (closed circles) and 13 healthy control subjects (open circles). (From Ref. 9.)

at any stage during the exercise. Thus, both groups recorded the perceived effort as being approximately "mild" to "moderate" after 4.5 min of exercise, and at the completion of the submaximal contractions, both groups had increased to a "large" to "very large" level of perceived exertion required to complete each submaximal contraction.

Our findings of normal muscle performance in patients with CFS were supported by subsequent studies involving other muscle groups [31,32]. We concluded that the essential symptom of "fatigue," which provides the basis for current nomenclature for CFS, should not be equated with failure of contractile force. We found no evidence that the centrally generated commands associated with the "sense of effort" increase abnormally in the patients, even during a prolonged period of exercise. The pathophysiological abnormality responsible for the prominent subjective fatigability, appears likely to lie within the CNS. The prevalence of neuropsychiatric and cognitive symptoms in patients with CFS suggests that the abnormality involves high-level integrative functions, rather than the executive pathways for motor performance. These data stimulated the focus of our further research into the pathogenesis of CFS towards the CNS, rather than the muscle.

IMMUNOLOGICAL FUNCTION IN PATIENTS WITH CHRONIC FATIGUE SYNDROME

As both cell-mediated and humoral immune responses are essential for effective resolution of the viral and other infections thought to precipitate CFS, these immune parameters were assessed using standard laboratory measures. Three separate studies were completed evaluating immune function in patients with CFS in comparison with healthy subjects, as well as control subjects with nonmelancholic depression [6,10,11]. We also studied cytokine activity in patients with CFS, healthy control subjects, and patients with acute viral illnesses, to critically examine previous circumstantial evidence implicating cytokines such as IFN-α in the pathogenesis of CFS [12–14].

Cellular Immunity in Patients with Chronic Fatigue Syndrome and Healthy Control Subjects

In our initial study, 100 patients in whom CFS was producing significant morbidity, frequent medical consultation, and considerable time lost from work were studied [10]. They were compared as a group to 100 healthy control subjects, who were recruited from the hospital and laboratory staff. None of the patients or control subjects were receiving medications known to produce immune deficiency. The degree of disability produced by CFS was evaluated by questionnaire assessing the ability to participate in work, recreation, and social activities during the illness, in comparison with the premorbid situation.

Cellular immunity was assessed by measurement of peripheral blood T-lymphocyte counts, lymphocyte proliferation in vitro in response to phytohemagglutinin (PHA), and DTH skin testing. The DTH assessment was performed using a commercially available kit that employs seven antigens (tetanus, diphtheria, streptococcus, purified protein derivative [PPD], candida, trichophyton, and proteus) and a glycerine control (Multitest; CMI, Merieux, France). Both the application and measurement of DTH were conducted by trained personnel. Results of the DTH skin testing were categorized according to previously determined reference ranges generated by the examination of healthy adult populations [33]. Abnormal results (hypoergy or anergy) using these ranges are generally limited to fewer than 10% of healthy adults.

The total lymphocyte count was significantly lower in the patients, as were the CD2 (total T-cell), CD4 (helper T-cell), and CD8 (suppressor–cytotoxic T-cell) subset counts. As a group, the patients with CFS had significantly elevated numbers of peripheral blood mononuclear cells displaying class II major histocompatibility complex (MHC) antigens, suggesting activation of these immune cells. Lymphocytes from all of the patients with CFS responded to stimulation by PHA, with counts that fell within the normal range (mean ± 2 SD) of the response obtained in the control subjects. However, the response to

PHA in the patients with CFS, when analyzed as a group, was significantly lower than in the control subjects. Impaired T-cell function in vivo was demonstrated with reduced DTH responses in 50 of 57 patients tested (88%). Thirty-one patients (54%) were anergic and 19 (33%) were hypoergic. Seventeen of the 18 patients who had repeated DTH testing over several months had persistently reduced DTH responses. Patients with suppressed DTH had significantly lower absolute CD2 and CD4 cell counts ($p < 0.05$).

Regression analysis did not demonstrate that any clinical variables (age, sex, disease duration, or disease severity) predicted the abnormal measures of cellular immunity.

Cellular Immunity in Patients with Chronic Fatigue Syndrome and Subjects with Major Depression

Research over the last decade has suggested an association between depressive disorders and impaired cell-mediated immunity, although the results have not been consistent [for review, see 34]. Therefore, it was important to clarify whether the immunological disturbances demonstrated in our initial study may be attributable to the concurrent psychiatric morbidity, notably depression, in patients with CFS.

Although our evaluation of the psychiatric morbidity in patients with CFS [5], did not support the contention that the disorder is a depressive equivalent, patients with the nonmelancholic or neurotic subtype of major depression remain the most relevant and comparable psychiatric control group. These patients have demographic features similar to patients with CFS, and their depression is usually less severe than in patients with the melancholic subtype of depression.

Accordingly, cell-mediated immunity was examined in patients with CFS, and compared with that of matched patients with typical major depression as well as matched, healthy control subjects. Potential patients and control subjects (including the patients with depression) were excluded if they had taken any psychotropic medication other than benzodiazepines, or any other medication known to impair cell-mediated immunity (e.g., corticosteroids) in the 2 weeks before testing, or if they had a history of any other physical illness associated with abnormal cell-mediated immunity (e.g., autoimmune disease, malignancy, or recent viral infection).

Significant differences in the lymphocyte subset counts were demonstrated only in the CD8 counts, which were lower in the patients with CFS and the subjects with nonmelancholic depression, in comparison with their matched healthy control subjects (Table 5). There was a similar nonsignificant trend toward lower CD3 and CD4 lymphocyte counts in patients with CFS.

Significantly more patients with CFS than subjects with nonmelancholic depression or healthy control subjects had abnormal DTH skin responses. Ten

Table 5 Peripheral Blood Lymphocyte Counts in Patients with CFS, Matches Subjects with Major Depression, and Healthy Control Subjects

Subjects	Absolute number of cells $\times$ 10^3/mm^{3a}				
	Lymph.	CD3	CD4	CD8	HLA DR[b]
Controls ($n = 20$)	2.2 (0.5)	1.5 (0.5)	1.1 (0.4)	0.6 (0.1)	0.36 (0.18)
Depression ($n = 20$)	2.2 (0.5)	1.4 (0.4)	1.0 (0.4)	0.5 (0.2)[c]	0.30 (0.13)
CFS ($n = 20$)	2.0 (0.5)	1.3 (0.4)	0.9 (0.3)	0.4 (0.2)[c]	0.31 (0.18)

[a]Mean (1 SD).
[b]Mononuclear cells displaying class II MHC antigens.
[c]$p < 0.05$ paired t-test versus healthy control subjects.
Source: Ref. 6.

of the 20 patients with CFS had abnormal results, 4 patients (20%) had cutaneous anergy, and 6 (30%) demonstrated hypoergic responses, in comparison to 2 subjects with nonmelancholic depression and 2 healthy control subjects (10%) who had hypoergic DTH responses ($\chi^2 = 5.83$, $p = 0.02$). Cutaneous anergy was not seen in either of the control groups.

The proliferation of lymphocytes in response to PHA from patients with CFS (Fig. 7) was significantly lower than that seen in healthy control subjects (F = 4.47, $p = 0.005$; repeated measures ANOVA) and less than that in patients with nonmelancholic depression (F = 2.49, $p = 0.06$). The plateau response in the assay was significantly lower in the patients with CFS than that obtained in the subjects with nonmelancholic depression ($p < 0.05$, unpaired t-test), who demonstrated the highest mean plateau response.

In these two studies, we evaluated the immunity of a large number of carefully defined patients with CFS. The patients preponderantly had a long-standing disorder that was causing major disruption of their usual daily lives. The abnormal cellular and humoral immunity documented, supports the hypothesis that an immunological disturbance may be important to the pathogenesis of CFS. The abnormalities demonstrated may represent a "marker" of an underlying disruption of the regulation of the immune response to a precipitating infection in patients with CFS.

The finding of significantly increased numbers of peripheral blood mononuclear cells expressing class II MHC antigens (HLA-DR–positive cells), in the initial study implies activation of these cells in the patients. These cell surface antigens may have been induced by interferon or other cytokines. Subsequent studies measuring peripheral blood lymphocyte subpopulations in patients with CFS have suggested that T-cell lymphopenia may be restricted to the CD8 subset

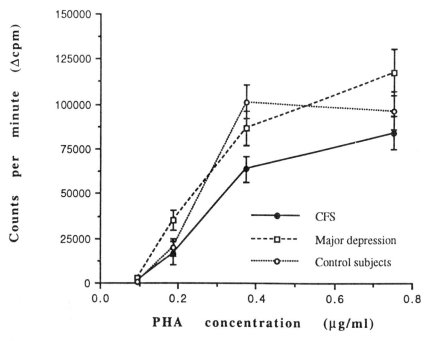

Figure 7　Phytohemagglutimin (PHA)-induced lymphocyte stimulation in patients with CFS (closed circles), subjects with major depression (open squares), and healthy control subjects (open circles). Each point represents group mean ± SEM (*n* = 20) of Δcpm (value minus background cpm) at various concentrations of PHA. (From Ref. 6.)

and that activation markers such as HLA-DR, CD38, and CDw26 may be persistently elevated on CD8 T lymphocytes [35,36].

The demonstration of impaired lymphocyte proliferation in response to PHA in patients with CFS in our studies and those of others [35–38] also suggests disordered immune regulation in patients with this syndrome. The reduction in the response in our studies was mild (characteristically 1 SD or less from the mean of the response in normal subjects) and, hence, the results indicate immune dysfunction, rather than clinically significant immunodeficiency.

The finding of reduced DTH responses in 88% of patients in the initial study and 50% of the smaller group of patients in our second study, provides in vivo evidence of disordered cell-mediated immunity in patients with CFS. Two of the 20 healthy control subjects (10%) and 2 patients with nonmelancholic depression (10%) in the second study had hypoergic responses. Although the numbers of healthy subjects tested were small, these data are consistent with the reference data from the US population study [33] and with preliminary data from a population survey conducted in Sydney [Hickie C, personal communication].

The demonstration of essentially normal cell-mediated immunity in subjects with major depression, when compared with healthy control subjects, indicates that the evidence of disordered immunity found in closely matched patients with CFS, is unlikely to be attributable to intercurrent depression during the illness.

Factors affecting standard measures of cell-mediated immunity, such as diurnal variation in lymphocyte counts, the effect of medication, and intercurrent viral illness, were controlled for in our studies. Other potentially significant variables known to alter measures of cell-mediated immunity, which were not controlled for in the studies, include sleep deprivation and alcohol abuse. Prolonged sleep deprivation has been shown to induce impaired lymphocyte stimulation in response to mitogen [39], and heavy alcohol abuse is associated with cutaneous anergy, decreased lymphocyte responses to PHA, and altered T-lymphocyte subset numbers [40]. However, the patients with CFS in our studies were unlikely to have had either adequately severe sleep disruption or significant alcohol misuse, enough to account for the abnormalities demonstrated.

The alterations in immunological function demonstrated in patients with CFS are also characteristically seen in association with many acute viral infections. In this context, the activity of soluble factors of viral or host origin, such as interferon gamma (IFN-γ) are likely to be at least partially responsible for the disturbances in immune profiles [41]. T-cell lymphopenia and impaired lympho-cyte proliferative responses to mitogen are common during acute viral infection [42–45] and are also reduced in association with administered IFN-α [46]. Viral infections with cytomegalovirus (CMV) or Epstein–Barr virus (EBV) are commonly associated with the development of reduced or absent DTH responses, including responses to unrelated antigens [43,44]. Both IFN-α and IFN-γ modulate DTH and variably affect the response in humans [42].

Humoral Immunity in Patients with Chronic Fatigue Syndrome and Healthy Control Subjects

Humoral immune mechanisms are also important in the host response to the viral and other intracellular infections thought to precipitate CFS. Neutralizing antibodies may be generated in this response to bind antigens of the infecting organism and prevent attachment to susceptible cells. The IgG1 and IgG3 subclass antibodies (and less so IgG2) produced in the response, may fix complement and, thereby, mediate lysis. Antibody-dependent cellular cytotox-icity (ADCC) is facilitated by binding of T lymphocytes by the Fc portion of IgG antibodies of all four subclasses. Therefore, we examined the serum levels of the immunoglobulin subclasses in patients with CFS and healthy control subjects.

Seventy-eight patients with CFS who had not participated in previous studies were included in this analysis [11]. They were compared with a group of 71 healthy control subjects who were recruited from the hospital and laboratory staff, as well as volunteers from the local community who had agreed to participate in studies of immunity. The control subjects were selected with an age and sex distribution similar to that of the patients.

Total IgG levels were within the laboratory reference range (7–16 g/L; mean ± 2 SD) in all subjects. The level of total IgG was significantly lower in the patients than in the control subjects (Table 6). The patients had significantly lower levels of IgG1, IgG2, and IgG3 when compared with the control subjects (see Table 6). Essentially all reductions in immunoglobulin levels were partial. Levels of total immunoglobulin and immunoglobulin subclasses were not significantly correlated with age or sex in the patients and control subjects, nor with duration or severity of symptoms in the patients.

This degree of reduction in serum immunoglobulin levels is not typical of that seen in patients with clinically significant humoral immunodeficiency, but rather, suggests a mild abnormality in the synthesis of immunoglobulin. Mild reductions in immunoglobulin levels may occur transiently in association with acute viral infections, including with EBV [47], and are likely to be due to alteration in the T-cell control of immunoglobulin production and isotype switching by B cells [48]. Both IFN-α and IFN-γ, as well as other cytokines, notably interleukin-4, modulate immunoglobulin synthesis [49].

Cytokines in Serum and Cerebrospinal Fluid in Patients with Chronic Fatigue Syndrome and Control Subjects

The most significant, although circumstantial, evidence for the possible role of cytokines in the pathogenesis of CFS has come from the observation that a syndrome resembling CFS results from the administration of recombinant IFN-α

Table 6 Serum Immunoglobulin (IgG) Subclass Levels in Patients with CFS and Healthy Control Subjects

Subjects	Immunoglobulin level (g/L), mean (SD)				
	Total IgG	IgG1	IgG2	IgG3	IgG4
Controls (n = 71)	13.2 (3.1)	7.4 (2.6)	4.2 (1.7)	0.63 (0.31)	0.34 (0.21)
CFS (n = 78)	11.3 (3.2)	6.3 (2.1)	3.5 (2.1)	0.49 (0.27)	0.38 (0.26)
Significance level[a]	$p < 0.05$	$p < 0.01$	$p < 0.01$	$p < 0.01$	$p > 0.1$

[a]Unpaired t-test.

for therapeutic purposes [50]. The studies already outlined in this chapter have provided data concerning the prevalence of neuropsychiatric symptoms in patients with CFS, and evidence has been presented for the CNS as the most likely pathophysiological site of the "fatigue," which is foremost in the symptom complex. Evidence for a disturbance of cellular immunity in patients with CFS has also been outlined. Thus, an abnormal immunological process (i.e., persistent cytokine activity) occurring particularly within the CNS, which may give rise to the fatigue and neuropsychiatric symptoms, was sought. Levels of cytokines that may potentially be relevant to the pathogenesis of the disorder were measured in the serum and cerebrospinal fluid of patients with CFS and in control subjects.

The cytokines selected for study included IFN-γ and IFN-α, as both are secreted in response to viral infection and have been associated with fatigue when administered therapeutically. Tumor necrosis factor-alpha (TNF-α) and interleukin-1β (IL-1β) were also measured, as both are secreted in response to viral stimuli, but also because both of these cytokines are released by monocyte–macrophages early in the development of a cellular immune response to antigen; hence, their detection would provide evidence of an ongoing immune response. In addition, neopterin, an intermediate in the synthetic pathway of biopterin and a reliable marker of recent IFN-γ activity was measured [51]. Commercially available radioimmunoassay (RIA) and enzyme-linked immunosorbent assay (ELISA) kits were used for detection of cytokines.

Twenty-five patients with CFS were enrolled. Control subjects included a negative control group, consisting of 25 individuals undergoing elective myelography for investigation of noninflammatory neurological disorders (predominantly disk prolapse). A second control group (positive controls) included 10 subjects with aseptic meningitis or encephalitis. In addition, serum and cerebrospinal fluid was available from three subjects with major depression participating in a separate study of possible immunological factors in the pathogenesis of depression.

For each cytokine measurement, samples were thawed on only one occasion, immediately before assay. Internal control samples of high, intermediate, and low concentration for each cytokine were assayed repetitively with each run of the individual cytokine kits to ensure interassay reliability. The coefficient of variation in the levels obtained was less than 15%. Samples obtained from patients with CFS and from both negative and positive control subjects were included in each run of the cytokine assays. The minimum detectable level of each cytokine was defined as the concentration corresponding to the sum of the mean value of the counts per minute in the RIA assays (or optical density in the ELISA assays) of the zero standard plus 2 SD from the mean.

The cerebrospinal fluid was clear and colorless in all subjects. In the 25 patients with CFS, cells were found in only four cases (one red blood cell per cubic millimeter in three cases, and three mononuclear cells per cubic millimeter in one case). The glucose estimation was normal in all cases, and the protein level was mildly elevated in three cases (values: 0.47, 0.50, 0.57 g/L; NR 0.15–0.45 g/L). A single band of oligoclonal IgG was detected in the cerebrospinal fluid of one patient (who had no cells and a normal protein level estimation).

The serum and cerebrospinal fluid concentrations of the cytokines are presented in Table 7. The cerebrospinal fluid concentration of IFN-α (Fig. 8) was significantly greater in the patients with CFS who had a mean of 3.3 IU/ml (SD 0.5 IU/ml), than in the negative control subjects who had a mean of 2.9 IU/ml (SD 0.7 IU/ml; $p < 0.05$, Mann Whitney U test), and was significantly less than that found in the positive control group (mean 5.5, SD 3.3 IU/ml; $p < 0.01$).

Several recent studies have measured cytokines in the serum of patients with CFS and control subjects. Elevated serum levels of IFN-α (2.4–3.2 IU/ml) were reported in 3 of 15 patients with CFS and none of 10 healthy control subjects [52]. Other controlled studies have not found elevations of the serum levels of IFN-γ, IFN-α, IL-1β, IL-2, IL-6, or TNF-α [53,54], although the serum level of transforming growth factor-beta (TGF-β) was found to be elevated [54].

Previous studies of the cerebrospinal fluid levels of cytokines, such as IFN-γ and IFN-α, in patients with viral illness and with meningitis, have shown that even at the peak of the clinical illness, levels of IFN vary from 1 to 100 IU/ml in patients with viral meningitis and are often undetectable in patients with simple

Table 7 Cytokine Levels Serum and Cerebrospinal Fluid in Patients with CFS and Control Subjects[a]

		Subject groups, mean (SD)		
Cytokine	Sample	CFS	Myelogram	CNS infections
IFN-γ (IU/ml)	Serum	0	0	0
	CSF	0	0	1.4 (1.9)
Neopterin (nmol/l)	Serum	6.7 (4.0)	11 (6.3)	
	CSF	2.9 (3.0)	3.1 (1.7)	
IFN-α (IU/ml)	Serum	0.5 (0.9)	0.6 (0.9)	7.5 (4.7)
	CSF	3.3 (0.5)[b]	2.9 (0.7)[b]	5.5 (3.3)
IL-1β (pg/ml)	Serum	17.1 (4.4)	17.7 (5.5)	
	CSF	20.5 (4.1)	20.5 (4.1)	
TNF-α (pg/ml)	Serum	10.0 (2.6)	9.7 (1.6)	
	CSF	5.0 (7.6)	4.1 (0.9)	

[a]Values below the calculated minimum detection limit for the assays are included in these figures, except for the IFN-γ assay in which all values were zero apart from those obtained in four positive control subjects.
[b]$p < 0.05$.

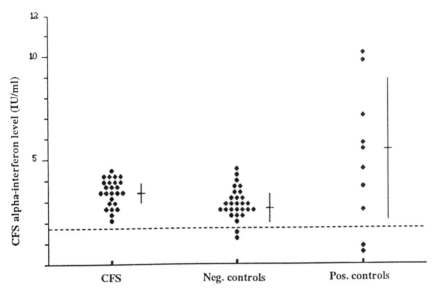

Figure 8 Cerebrospinal fluid levels of IFN-α in 25 patients with CFS, 28 negative control subjects (elective myelography patients), and 10 positive control subjects with CNS infections. The mean and standard deviation are indicated for each group. The minimum detection limit of the assay (1.8 IU/ml) is indicated with the dotted line. Patients with CFS had significantly elevated levels in comparison with negative control subjects ($p < 0.05$).

viral infections [55–57]. Serum levels of IFN-γ and IFN-α in the same conditions are frequently minimally elevated or undetectable [56].

Chronic fatigue syndrome is not associated with the classic hallmarks of an inflammatory process, such as fever, leukocytosis in the peripheral blood, and elevated protein levels and pleocytosis in the cerebrospinal fluid. Hence, it is likely that if recognized cytokines are important in mediating the symptoms of the disorder, they will be present in small amounts in cerebrospinal fluid (or serum), or present only within a local microenvironment, such as in specific areas within the CNS.

Cytokine Production in Response to Exercise in Patients with Chronic Fatigue Syndrome and Healthy Control Subjects

The fatigue experienced by patients with CFS is often reported to be exacerbated by disproportionately minor physical activity and followed by a prolonged period (of hours or days) before which resolution of the fatigue (to the baseline level) occurs. Our studies of exercise performance suggest that the muscle strength, endurance, and recovery in patients with CFS is no different from those of healthy control subjects, and that the CNS is, therefore, the most likely site of the pathophysiological process producing the fatigue. Exercise may induce a fatigue state in patients with CFS by an effect on the CNS, and this effect may persist for a prolonged period after the cessation of muscular activity (and the normal recovery of muscle strength). This phenomenon may be mediated by a circulating factor (such as a cytokine) produced in response to exercise, which acts on CNS target(s).

Previous studies have demonstrated that IL-1 and IFN-α are released in response to vigorous exercise in healthy subjects and can be detected in the serum [58,59]. Therefore, a study was undertaken to examine the cytokine and symptomatic fatigue response to prolonged isometric exercise in patients with CFS and healthy control subjects [14]. Male subjects were chosen for this study to avoid the potential confounding effects of the variation in menstrual cycle on the psychological and immunological measures.

Twelve male patients and 13 male control subjects participated in this study. The control subjects were drawn from healthy members of the hospital and laboratory staff and were matched as a group by age, height, weight, and training status to the patients with CFS. A protocol of submaximal isometric exercise was undertaken, as our previous studies have shown that this form of exercise is associated with the development of neurophysiological fatigue (i.e., the failure to maintain maximal force) in an identical fashion in patients with CFS and healthy control subjects, and is unassociated with deficits in motivation or other factors producing a failure of central motor drive to the muscle in both patients with CFS and healthy control subjects. Subjects undertook the exercise protocol simultaneously in patient and control pairs to encourage similar levels of performance in the exercise.

Hand-grip exercise utilizing dynamometers (Lafayette, USA) was chosen for this study, as it enabled blood sampling (for cytokine estimation) from the venous drainage of the exercising limb. The signals from the dynamometers were displayed for each subject on an oscilloscope, to provide visual feedback throughout the exercise. The subjects performed repeated contractions of 5 sec duration separated by 5 sec of rest for 30 min of exercise. At the completion of the protocol a brief MVC was performed to measure the decline in maximal force during the exercise.

Blood samples were collected immediately before the exercise, after 15 min of exercise, and immediately before cessation of exercise. In addition, samples were collected 4 and 24 hr after the initial specimen. The systolic and diastolic blood pressure were recorded at regular intervals to calculate the mean arterial pressure (MAP) and its change in response to the exercise. Before, and immediately after completing the 30 min of exercise, and at 4 and 24 hr subjects completed a standardized 65-item questionnaire—the Profile of Mood States

(POMS; Educational and Industrial Testing Service, California). This assessment includes six subscales that provide quantitative measures of the symptoms of "depression," "confusion," "anger," and "anxiety." The questionnaire was particularly intended to evaluate the subjective feeling of fatigue before, during, and after the exercise.

There was no significant difference in the percentage decline in the MVC measured at the completion of 30 min of exercise between the patients with CFS and the control subjects (mean 61.8, SD 11.0% versus mean 63.8, SD 11.3%). The MAP rose progressively in all subjects during the period of exercise. The increase MAP for the final recording (at 30 min) was 25 mmHg (SD 6 mmHg) in the patients with CFS, which was not significantly different from the control subjects who had a mean increase of 22 mmHg (SD 8 mmHg).

Serum levels of IL-1β, -γ and IFN-α and -γ, and TNFα remained at or below the minimum detection limit of the assays in all subjects, in each of the samples taken before, during, and after the exercise protocol.

The patients with CFS were significantly different from healthy control subjects in the responses on the POMS scale recorded before the exercise. In particular, the patients scored highly on the "fatigue" subscale with a mean of 18.1 (SD 7.8) in comparison with the control subjects who had a mean score of 2.2 (SD 3.3). The patients also rated highly on the "confusion" subscale with a mean of 14.8 (SD 7.3) versus a mean of 2.4 (SD 1.3) in the control subjects, and on the "depression" subscale with a mean of 21.5 (SD 16.9) versus a mean of 0.6 (SD 0.9) in the control subjects. Surprisingly, the level of fatigue, depression, and confusion measured on the POMS, decreased marginally in the patients in response to the exercise. In contrast, (as would be expected) the mean value recorded on each of these subscales in the control subjects increased transiently following the exercise.

The normal control subjects in this study did not have a detectable increase in the level of circulating cytokines. Hence, the results did not confirm the previous reports of IFN-α and IL-1β production after vigorous exercise [58,59]. This discrepancy may be related to the nature and severity of the exercise performed by the subjects in the previous reports—being dynamic exercise and involving multiple large muscle groups, unlike in our study.

The self-report of fatigue before the isometric exercise in patients with CFS showed that the subjective complaint of fatigue was markedly greater in the patients than in the control subjects. Following exercise, the patients had relatively unchanged (or mildly reduced) levels of reported fatigue, in contrast with the control subjects, who had the expected increase in their reported fatigue immediately after the exercise, which had returned to baseline by the time of the 4-hr recording. These data are not consistent with the common report of fatigue being exacerbated by exercise in patients with CFS, but rather suggest that the major disturbance is a continuing abnormally high level of symptomatic fatigue that alters relatively little in response to physical activity. Limitations of the POMS scale as a monitor of fatigue in patients with CFS may also account for the findings.

Production of IFN-γ, IFN-α, and IL-1 from peripheral blood mononuclear cells (PBMC) in vitro has also been studied recently in patients with CFS. Apparently conflicting data have been published on the in vitro production of IL-1β, with one study suggesting increased [54] and one normal levels [60]. An increased level of IFN-α production in vitro from PBMC stimulated by Sendai virus was demonstrated in eight children who had protracted symptoms after an outbreak of Coxsackie B4 infection, in comparison with four healthy classmates (two seropositive for Coxsackie B4) [61].

Multiple factors may have contributed to the difficulties and discrepancies in the detection of cytokine activity in patients with CFS. Different assay systems were used in each of the reported studies. Samples were taken on a single occasion, whereas an evolving cascade of production of various cytokines is a feature of the immune response. Many of the cytokines of potential interest have naturally occurring inhibitors (such as soluble forms of the receptor) that may interfere with the detection of the factor in body fluids. Localized production within a CNS microenvironment may make detection virtually impossible with current techniques in living patients.

CONCLUSION

In the light of the findings of our studies and those of other groups, our hypothesis of the pathophysiology of CFS can be reexamined. A growing body of evidence now indicates that patients with CFS have alterations in standard measures of cellular and humoral immune function. These changes cannot be easily attributed to the psychological disturbances recognized as commonly associated with the clinical course of CFS. The immunological changes are characteristically mild and do not clarify the nature of a potential underlying immunological disease process. No clear evidence of chronic and excessive cytokine activity has yet been obtained, although technical and methodological limitations have not allowed definitive studies to be completed. It clearly remains possible that the immunological changes in patients with CFS are secondary to an unrecognized cofactor in the pathophysiological process and, therefore, that CFS is not primarily an immunopathological disorder. On the other hand, strong evidence now implicates the CNS as the site of the abnormalities and, in this setting, the hypothesis of persistent antigen and a disordered cellular immune control of cytokine production, allowing continued cytokine activity, remains consistent with the available data. At this site, many of the known effects of cytokines on specialized cellular functions, including either the induction or inhibition of various cellular enzymes, may produce the characteristic symptoms of CFS, that is "fatigue" and neuropsychiatric dysfunction.

ACKNOWLEDGMENTS

This work was supported by research grants from the National Health and Medical Research Council of Australia (for AL) and the New South Wales Institute of Psychiatry (for IH). In addition, several projects were made possible only by generous funding from the CFS/ME Societies of NSW and the other Australian states.

REFERENCES

1. Wakefield D, Lloyd A. Pathophysiology of myalgic encephalomyelitis. Lancet 1987; 2:918–9.
2. Lloyd A, Wakefield D, Boughton C, Dwyer J. What is myalgic encephalomyelitis? Lancet 1988; 1:1286–7.
3. Lloyd AR, Hickie I, Boughton CR, Spencer O, Wakefield D. The prevalence of chronic fatigue syndrome in an Australian population. Med J Aust 1990; 153:522–8.
4. Lloyd AR, Pender H. The economic impact of chronic fatigue syndrome. Med J Aust 1992; 157:599–601.
5. Hickie I, Lloyd A, Wakefield D, Parker G. The psychiatric status of patients with chronic fatigue syndrome. Br J Psychiatry 1990; 156:534–40.
6. Lloyd A, Hickie I, Hickie C, Wakefield D. Cell-mediated immunity in patients with chronic fatigue syndrome, healthy control subjects and patients with major depression. Clin Exp Immunol 1992; 87:76–9.
7. Hickie I, Lloyd A, Wakefield D. Immunological and psychological dysfunction in patients receiving immunotherapy for chronic fatigue syndrome. Aust NZ J Psychiatry 1992; 26:249–56.
8. Lloyd A, Hales J, Gandevia S. Muscle strength, endurance and recovery in the post-infection fatigue syndrome. J Neurol Neurosurg Psychiatry 1988; 51:1316–22.
9. Lloyd AR, Gandevia SC, Hales JP. Muscle endurance, twitch properties, voluntary activation and perceived exertion in normal subjects and patients with chronic fatigue syndrome. Brain 1991; 114:85–98.
10. Lloyd A, Wakefiled D, Boughton C, Dwyer J. Immunological abnormalities in the chronic fatigue syndrome. Med J Aust 1989; 151:122–4.
11. Wakefield D, Lloyd A, Brockman A. Immunoglobulin subclass abnormalities in patients with chronic fatigue syndrome. Pediatr Infect Dis J 1990; 9:S50–3.
12. Lloyd A, Hickie I, Brockman A, Dwyer J, Wakefield D. Serum and cerebrospinal fluid cytokine levels in patients with chronic fatigue syndrome and control subjects. J Infect Dis 1991; 164:1023–4.
13. Lloyd A, Abi-Hanna D, Wakefield D. Interferon and myalgic encephalomyelitis. Lancet 1988; 1:471.
14. Lloyd A, Gandevia S, Brockman A, Hales J, Wakefield D. Cytokine production

and "fatigue" in response to exercise in patients with chronic fatigue syndrome. Clin Infect Dis. 1993; (in press).

15. Zung WWK. A self-rating depression scale. Arch Gen Psychiatry 1965; 12:63–70.

16. Holmes GP, Kaplan JE, Gantz NM, et al. Chronic fatigue syndrome: a working case definition. Ann Intern Med 1988; 108:387–9.

17. Schluederberg A, Straus SE, Petersen P, et al. Chronic fatigue syndrome research— definition and medical outcome assessment. Ann Intern Med 1992; 117:325–31.

18. Gary H, Reyes M, Fukuda K. Estimated prevalence of chronic fatigue syndrome in four surveillance cities. Clin Infect Dis 1993; (in press).

19. Goldberg DP. Manual of the general health questionnaire. Windsor: NFER Publishing, 1979.

20. Eysenck HJ, Eysenck SB. Manual of the Eysenck personality inventory. London: Hodder & Stoughton, 1964.

21. Pilowsky I, Spence ND. Manual for the illness behaviour questionnaire (IBO). 2nd ed. Adelaide: University of Adelaide, 1983.

22. Hamilton M. A rating scale for depression. J Neurol Neurosurg Psychiatry 1960; 23:56–62.

23. Taerk GS, Toner BB, Salit IE, et al. Depression in patients with neuromyasthenia (benign myalgic encephalomyelitis). Int J Psychiatry Med 1987; 17:49–56.

24. Wessely S, Powell R. Fatigue syndromes: a comparison of chronic "postviral" fatigue with neuromuscular and affective disorders. J Neurol Neurosurg Psychiatry 1989; 52:940–8.

25. Kruesi MJP, Dale J, Straus SE. Psychiatric diagnoses in patients who have chronic fatigue syndrome. J Clin Psychiatry 1989; 50:53–60.

26. Manu P, Lane TJ, Matthews DA. The frequency of the chronic fatigue syndrome in patients with symptoms of persistent fatigue. Ann Intern Med 1988; 109:554–6.

27. Katon WJ, Buchwald DS, Simon GE, Russo JE, Mease PJ. Psychiatric illness in patients with chronic fatigue and rheumatoid arthritis. 1992.

28. Merton PA. Voluntary strength and fatigue. J Physiol London 1954; 123:553–64.

29. Edwards RHT. Human muscle function and fatigue. In: Porter R, Whelan J, eds. Human muscle fatigue: physiological mechanisms. London: Pitman Medical, 1981 (Ciba Foundation Symposium 82).

30. Borg G, Ljunggren G, Ceci R. The increase of perceived exertion, aches and pain in the legs, heart rate and blood lactate during exercise on a bicycle ergometer. Eur J Appl Physiol 1985; 54:343–9.

31. Stokes MJ, Cooper RG, Edwards RHT. Normal muscle strength and fatiguability in patients with effort syndromes. Br Med J 1988; 297:1014–7.

32. Rutherford OM, White PD. Human quadriceps strength and fatiguability in patients with postviral fatigue. J Neurol Neurosurg Psychiatry 1991; 54:961–4.

33. Kniker W, Anderson C, McBryde J, Roumiantzeff M, Lesourd B. Multitest CMI for standardised measurement of delayed cutaneous hypersensitivity and cell-mediated immunity. Normal values and proposed scoring system for healthy adults in the USA. Ann Allergy 1984; 52:75–82.

34. Hickie I, Hickie C, Silove D, Wakefield D, Lloyd A. Is there significant immune dysfunction in depressive disorders? Psychol Med 1990; 20:755–61.

35. Klimas NG, Salvato FR, Morgan R, Fletcher MA. Immunologic abnormalities in chronic fatigue syndrome. J Clin Microbiol 1990; 28:1403–10.

36. Landay AL, Jessop C, Lennette ET, Levy JA. Chronic fatigue syndrome: clinical condition associated with immune activation. Lancet 1991; 338:707–12.

37. Jones JF, Ray CG, Minnich LL, Hicks MJ, Kibler R, Lucas DO. Evidence for active Epstein–Barr virus infection in patients with persistent, unexplained illnesses: elevated early antigen antibodies. Ann Intern Med 1985; 102:1–7.

38. Behan PO, Behan WMH, Bell EJ. The postviral fatigue syndrome—an analysis of the findings in 50 cases. J Infect 1985; 10:211–22.

39. Palmblad J, Petrini B, Wasserman J, et al. Lymphocyte and granulocyte reactions during sleep deprivation. Psychosom Med 1979; 41:273–8.

40. Watson RR, Eskelson C, Hartman BR. Severe alcohol abuse and cellular immune functions. Ariz Med 1984; 41:665–8.

41. Schattner A, Meshorer A, Wallach D. Involvement of interferon in virus-induced lymphopenia. Cell Immunol 1983; 79:11–25.

42. Toy JL. The interferons. Clin Exp Immunol 1983; 54:1–13.

43. Rinaldo CR, Carney WP, Richter BS, Black PH, Hirsch MS. Mechanisms of immunosuppression in cytomegaloviral mononucleosis. J Infect Dis 1980; 141:488–95.

44. Haider S, Coutinho M de L, Edmond RTD, et al. Tuberculin anergy and infectious mononucleosis. Lancet 1973; 2:74.

45. Rouse B, Horohov D. Immunosuppression in viral infections. Rev Infect Dis 1986; 8:850–73.

46. Einhorn S, Blomgren H, Einhorn N, Strander H. In vitro and in vivo effects of interferon on the response of human lymphocytes to mitogens. Clin Exp Immunol 1983; 51:369–77.

47. Reinherz E, O'Brien C, Rosenthal P, Schlossman S. The cellular basis for viral-induced immunodeficiency: analysis by monoclonal antibodies. J Immunol 1980; 125:1269–74.

48. Sissons JGP, Borysiewicz LK. Viral immunopathology. Br Med Bull 1985; 41:34–40.

49. Peters M, Ambrus JL, Zhelenznyak A, et al. Effect of alpha interferon on immunoglobulin synthesis by human B cells. J Immunol 1986; 137:3153–7.

50. McDonald EM, Mann AH, Thomas HC. Interferons as mediators of psychiatric morbidity. An investigation in a trial of recombinant alpha interferon in hepatitis B carriers, Lancet 1987; 2:1175–9.

51. Huber C, Batchelor JR, Fuchs D, et al. Immune response-associated production of neopterin. J Exp Med 1984; 160:310–16.

52. Ho-Yen DO, Carrington D, Armstrong AA. Myalgic encephalomyelitis and alpha-interferon. Lancet 1988; 1:125.

53. Straus SE, Dale JK, Peter JB, Dinarello CA. Circulating lymphokine levels in the chronic fatigue syndrome. J Infect Dis 1989; 160:1085.

54. Chao CC, Janoff EN, Hu S, et al. Altered cytokine release in peripheral blood mononuclear cell cultures from patients with the chronic fatigue syndrome. Cytokine 1991; 3:292–8.

55. Ho-Yen DO, Carrington D. alpha-Interferon in cerebrospinal fluid of patients with suspected meningitis. J Clin Pathol 1987; 40:83–6.

56. Abbott RJ, Bolderson I, Gruer PJK. IFN-γ and IFN-α in CSF in viral meningitis. Lancet 1985; 2:456–7.

57. Lebon P, Boutin B, Dulac O, Ponsot G, Arthuis M. Interferon γ in acute and subacute encephalitis. Br Med J 1988; 296:9–11.

58. Cannon JG, Evans WJ, Hughes VA, Meredith CN, Dinarello CA. Physiological mechanisms contributing to interleukin-1 secretion. J Appl Physiol 1986; 61:1869–74.

59. Viti A, Muscettola M, Paulescu L, Bocci V, Almi A. Effect of exercise on plasma interferon levels. J Appl Physiol 1985; 59:426–8.

60. Morte S, Castilla A, Civiera MP, Serrano M, Prieto J. Production of interleukin-1 by peripheral blood mononuclear cells in patients with chronic fatigue syndrome. J Infect Dis 1989; 159:362.

61. Lever AM, Lewis DM, Bannister BA, Fry M, Berry N. Interferon production in postviral fatigue syndrome. Lancet 1988; 2:101.

APPENDIX

This document is designed to record the details of the symptoms of your illness, particularly the *current* symptoms, but also those in the past.

Please answer *every question*, do not leave any question blank. *Read carefully* the scale below, then *score* each of the symptoms listed (Questions 1–40) by entering in the righthand column a single number from the scale:

O *Never* suffer from it.

1 *Mild or rare* symptoms during the last month, causing minor disruption to your usual daily activities

2 *Moderate or frequent* symptoms during the last month, causing major disruption to your usual daily activities

3 *Severe or very frequent* symptoms during the last month, making you unable to perform your usual daily activities

4 Suffered from it *previously* (for a period of at least 1 month), but *not now*.

Symptoms

1. Excessive muscle fatigue with minor activity   [   ]
2. Prolonged feeling of fatigue after physical activity (lasting hours or days)   [   ]
3. Muscle pain (not joint pain) after activity   [   ]
4. Muscle pain (not joint pain), even when doing nothing   [   ]
5. Joint pain   [   ]
6. Redness and swelling localized around joints   [   ]

7.   Repetitive muscle twitching—on the face   [   ]
8.   Repetitive muscle twitching—elsewhere (arms, legs)   [   ]
9.   Sudden involuntary jerking of one arm or leg—in sleep   [   ]
10. Sudden involuntary jerking of one arm or leg—when awake   [   ]
11. Headache   [   ]
12. Nausea   [   ]
13. Stomach pain   [   ]
14. Difficulty swallowing foods   [   ]
15. Recurrent diarrhea (more than four loose stools per day)   [   ]
16. Repeated fevers and sweats   [   ]
17. Painful, red eye(s)   [   ]
18. Tender glands—in the neck   [   ]
19. Tender glands—elsewhere   [   ]
20. Sore throat (without "common cold" symptoms)   [   ]
21. Feeling of disturbed balance   [   ]
22. Difficulty in focusing vision   [   ]
23. Repeated tingling sensations (fingers, toes, or elsewhere)   [   ]
24. Persistent ringing in the ears   [   ]
25. Memory loss   [   ]
26. Loss of concentrating ability   [   ]
27. Difficulty with speech: "lost for the word"   [   ]
28. Palpitations (feeling the heart racing)   [   ]
29. Recurrent chest pain   [   ]
30. Persistent cough   [   ]
31. Shortness of breath with minor activity   [   ]
32. Persistent dryness in the eyes and mouth   [   ]
33. Needing to sleep for long periods   [   ]
34. Disturbed sleep or disrupted sleep pattern   [   ]
35. Vivid dreams or nightmares   [   ]
36. Episode(s) of complete loss of vision in one or both eyes   [   ]
37. Loss of interest in sex   [   ]
38. Loss of sexual performance   [   ]
39. Episode(s) of loss of control of the bladder or bowel   [   ]
40. Episodes of abrupt anxiety or panic   [   ]

Circle the single most appropriate response to the following statements (41–50) concerning how you have been *in the last month*:

| 41. | Morning is when I feel the best | None or a little | Some of the time | Good part of the time | Most of the time |
| 42. | I have crying spells or feel like it | None or a little | Some of the time | Good part of the time | Most of the time |

43.	I eat as much as I used to	None or a little	Some of the time	Good part of the time	Most of the time
44.	I notice that I am losing weight	None or a little	Some of the time	Good part of the time	Most of the time
45.	My heart beats faster than usual	None or a little	Some of the time	Good part of the time	Most of the time
46.	I get tired for no reason	None or a little	Some of the time	Good part of the time	Most of the time
47.	My mind is as clear as it used to be	None or a little	Some of the time	Good part of the time	Most of the time
48.	I find it easy to do the things I used to do	None or a little	Some of the time	Good part of the time	Most of the time
49.	I am restless and I can't keep still	None or a little	Some of the time	Good part of the time	Most of the time
50.	I feel that others would be better off if I were dead	None or a little	Some of the time	Good part of the time	Most of the time

VI

APPROACHES TO TREATMENT

15

Medical Therapy of Chronic Fatigue Syndrome

Cheryl A. I. Hirata-Dulas and Charles E. Halstenson
Hennepin County Medical Center and the University of Minnesota College of Pharmacy, Minneapolis, Minnesota

Phillip K. Peterson
Hennepin County Medical Center and the University of Minnesota Medical School, Minneapolis, Minnesota

> The practice of physic is jostled by quacks on the one side, and by science on the other.
>
> Peter Mere Latham [1]

The medical entity that is currently termed the chronic fatigue syndrome (CFS) has been referred to by various other names throughout the centuries. The different terminologies in part reflect the different approaches to treatment of this disorder, which were largely driven by the prevailing concepts of its pathogenesis [2]. Even today, there is continued debate about whether CFS is an organic or psychological disease.

Neurasthenia, a disorder that is probably identical with CFS, was described by Beard in the 1800s. Beard introduced the notion that the illness was due to an organic disease and recommended electrical treatments for replacement of deficient nerve energy [3]. Rest cure was also recommended [4], as overwork was thought to contribute to the illness. Subsequently, rest cure fell out of favor, and physical activity or exercise was recommended [5]. Moral treatment, or rational psychotherapy, was advocated for neurasthenia as well [6]. Other remedies were mineral and herbal tonics described by Da Costa for treatment of "irritable heart" [7]. A variety of therapies for "effort syndrome" and "hyperventilation syndrome," including sedatives, acidifying drugs, and special diets,

387

were suggested as temporary measures of treatment, until psychiatric evaluation could be performed [8]. Others promoted the use of vitamins, alcohol, and sympathomimetic drugs in depressed or significantly fatigued patients [9]. Additional unproved alternative therapies for CFS include herbal remedies, homeopathy, acupuncture, aromatherapy, Bach flower remedies, royal jelly, reflexology, colonic irrigation, yoga, hypnosis, and hydrotherapy [10,11].

Antimicrobial agents were used unsuccessfully in the past to treat "chronic brucellosis" [12] and, more recently, to eradicate *Candida albicans*, in accord with the "yeast connection" hypothesis that candidal overgrowth is the explanation for the inability to recover from CFS [13]. In a recent study of women diagnosed with "candidiasis hypersensitivity syndrome," characterized by recurrent or persistent candidal vaginitis, premenstrual tension, menstrual irregularities, fatigue, gastrointestinal symptoms, and depression, the investigators reported no improvement in systemic or psychological symptoms with long-term vaginal or oral nystatin treatment compared with placebo [14]. Other unproved treatments for the eradication of presumed candidal infection are avoidance of yeast-containing products in the diet, use of the antifungal agents ketoconazole and amphotericin B, and reconstitution of the gut with "beneficial bacteria" such as *Lactobacillus acidophilus* with yogurt ingestion or enemas [15].

At the present time, there continues to be no specific cure established for CFS. Therefore, the mainstay of therapy is supportive. Many pharmacological remedies for symptomatic treatment of CFS have been proposed; however, most reports of treatment of CFS are anecdotal, and few controlled clinical trials have been performed. Information from published reports about treatment is difficult to generalize to all patients owing to variable case definitions of CFS, different outcome measures used, difficulty interpreting therapeutic responses owing to the cyclic nature of the symptoms, and possibly because of the heterogeneous nature of the disease itself [16]. In addition, because the etiology and pathogenesis of CFS are unknown, rational therapeutic strategies are difficult to design.

Despite our lack of understanding of the pathogenesis of CFS, researchers agree that this illness is often disabling. Although some patients appear to recover normal health, many suffer from ongoing fatigue and the associated symptoms of CFS. At the Minnesota Regional CFS Research Program, for example, a recent survey revealed that most of the respondents had been ill for longer than 5 years (Fig. 1). A large number of medications had been prescribed for treatment of these patients and, although symptomatic benefit was reported with many of these drugs (Table 1), the mean ($\pm$ SEM) severity of fatigue using a visual analog scale was 5.49 ± 0.21, with a range of 0 (only one patient) to 10 (four patients) (see Fig. 1). Patients also reported taking another 153 medications or remedies not listed in Table 1, including everything from "A (acidophilus) to Z (zinc)."

The data from our research program underscores the urgent need for more

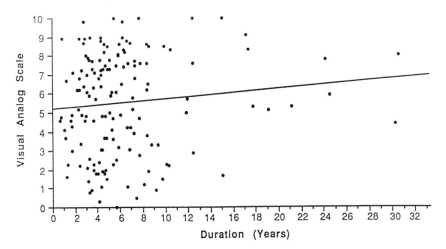

Figure 1 Severity of fatigue by length of illness. Responses are plotted for 153 of 190 patients in the Minnesota Regional CFS Research Program who responded to a mailed questionnaire in June 1992. The level of fatigue over the previous month was rated on a visual analog scale with 0 cm representing "none" and 10 cm representing "couldn't be worse." The regression line of severity of fatigue by duration of illness is shown (r = 0.099).

effective therapy of this disorder. Although many drugs have been touted to be beneficial, only a small fraction of the medications taken by patients with CFS have been subjected to rigorous clinical trials. The primary purpose of this chapter is to review the information that has been learned from these trials. A summary of the randomized clinical trials in patients with CFS is presented in Table 2.

CLINICAL TRIALS

Antiviral Agents

In the mid-1980s, the pathogenesis of CFS was thought to be related to infection by Epstein–Barr virus (EBV) and, thus, it was hypothesized that acyclovir therapy might be effective in ameliorating CFS. Twenty-seven adults, who met the Centers for Disease Control (CDC) criteria for CFS [17] and who had titers of antibodies to diffuse or restricted early antigens of EBV of 1:40 or higher, or lacked antibodies to Epstein–Barr virus nuclear antigens (<1:2), were enrolled [18], as this selected group of patients was believed to have the greatest chance of benefiting from acyclovir therapy. Placebo or acyclovir (500 mg/m^2) was administered intravenously every 8 hr for 7 days, then orally (acyclovir 800 mg four times daily) for 30 days. After a 6-week washout period, each patient was

Table 1 Medications Used by 153 CFS Patients[a]

Medication (trade name)	No. (%) of patients	No. (%) reporting benefit[b]
Antimicrobial agents		
Ceftriaxone (Rocephin)	13 (8)	6 (46)
Nystatin	26 (17)	10 (38)
Immunomodulatory agents		
Immunoglobulin	20 (13)	6 (30)
Vitamins		
Vitamin C	79 (51)	16 (20)
Vitamin B_{12} injections	13 (8)	4 (31)
Psychiatric agents		
Antidepressants		
Fluoxetine (Prozac)	64 (42)	25 (39)
Amitriptyline (Elavil)	50 (32)	16 (32)
Doxepin (Sinequan)	44 (29)	19 (43)
Nortriptyline (Pamelor)	17 (11)	5 (29)
Desipramine (Norpramin)	16 (10)	2 (13)
Bupropion (Wellbutrin)	5 (3)	1 (20)
Anxiolytics		
Alprazolam (Xanax)	20 (13)	11 (55)
Diazepam (Valium)	14 (9)	5 (36)
Neuroendocrine agents		
Prednisone	33 (21)	9 (27)
Other		
Ibuprofen (Motrin)	103 (67)	64 (62)
Terfenadine (Seldane)	73 (47)	29 (40)

[a]Partial listing of medications reported to be used currently or in the past by 153 (83%) of 190 patients in the Minnesota Regional CFS Research Program who responded to a questionnaire mailed in June 1992.
[b]Patients who reported having taken the drug who "found it helpful."

crossed over to the alternative treatment. The power of the study was 0.80 to detect a difference at $p < 0.05$ between acyclovir and placebo, assuming improvement with acyclovir of 65% and with placebo of 20%.

The primary outcome measurements were weekly self-assessment forms and psychological tests. Every evening patients recorded oral temperatures and scored their levels of activity, energy, and sense of wellness, on arbitrarily defined numerical scales. A standardized Profile of Mood States questionnaire was administered once during each of the 28 study weeks.

The investigators reported that 21 of the 24 patients who completed the trial scored themselves as improving during one treatment phase. Improvement occurred with similar frequency during acyclovir (11 of 24 patients) and placebo

Table 2 Summary of Recent Prospective, Double-Blind, Placebo-Controlled Trials in Chronic Fatigue Syndrome and Related Disorders[a]

Drug, year, country [Ref.]	Treatment groups and dosage regimen	No. pts completed/ enrolled	Inclusion criteria	Patient characteristics			Results		Adverse events
				Age (yr) [range]	Sex (M/F)	Disease duration (yr) [range]	Clinical	Laboratory	
Acyclovir, 1988, USA [18]	AC, 1500 mg/m²/d IV × 7d + 3200 mg/d PO × 30 d; PL, saline IV + oral (not described)	24/27 (crossover study, 6-wk washout phase)	CDC criteria for CFS [17], and EBV titer ≥1:40 or antibodies to EBNAs < 1:2	34.1 ± 1.5 (SEM)	8/19	6.8 ± 1.4 (SEM)	Improvement: 11/24 AC vs 10/24 PL (p = NS).	No changes in body temperature, EBV titers, circulating immune complexes, or leukocyte 2',5'-oligoadenylate synthetase.	3 dropouts due to reversible AC-induced renal failure. Greater GI and CNS adverse events in AC vs PL.
Gamma-globulin, 1986, USA [19]	IgG 0.13 ml/kg IM self-determined at ≥1-wk intervals (max 10 doses); PL, bacteriostatic water	19/19 (crossover study?)	Chronic mononucleosis syndrome [49]	Not stated	Not stated	Not stated	Improvement: 39/73 IgG courses vs 19/60 PL courses (p < 0.001).	6/19 pts with mild deficiency of ≥1 immunoglobulin isotopes.	Not stated.
Gamma-globulin, 1990, USA [20]	IgG 1 g/kg monthly × 6 doses; PL, equivalent volume of albumin 1% solution	14/15 14/15	CDC criteria for CFS [17]	45.3 ± 12.7 (SD), (p = 0.02 vs PL) 36.2 ± 7.3 (SD)	8/22	3.8 ± 2.2 (SD)	Improvement at 30, 60, 90, 120, and 150 d: IgG vs PL, p = NS.	Baseline: low total IgG and IgG1 in 43% pts; low IgG3 in 64% pts; normal B-cell counts in all pts; low T-cells and CD4+ T-cell subset in 18% pts. Post-study: IgG1 within normal range in all IgG pts, IgG3 increased, but remained low in 6 IgG pts.	20% major adverse events in both groups. Significant increase in headaches in IgG (14/15) vs PL (9/15), p = 0.03. 2 dropouts due to adverse events (1 IgG, 1 PL).

Table 2 Continued

Drug, year, country [Ref.]	Treatment groups and dosage regimen	No. pts completed/ enrolled	Patient characteristics				Results			Adverse events
			Inclusion criteria	Age (yr) [range]	Sex (M/F)	Disease duration (yr) [range]	Clinical	Laboratory		
Gamma-globulin, 1990, Australia [22]	IgG 2 g/kg monthly × 3 doses;	21/23	≥6 mo fatigue, decreased ability to perform usual daily activities, chronic and persisting symptoms	39 ± 10 (SD)	9/14	6.1 ± 4.4 (SD)	Response at 3 mo after final infusion by physician assessment: 10/ 23 IgG vs 3/26 PL ($p < 0.05$); psychiatrist assessment: 6/ 16 IgG vs 2/17 PL (p = NS).	Prestudy: Reduced T-cell subset counts in 43% and reduced DTH in 67%. In responders vs nonresponders: greater change in CD4 count and increase in DTH response ($p < 0.01$).		2 IgG dropouts due to elevated LFTs and phlebitis. Greater phlebitis, headache, worsened fatigue, and concentration impairment in IgG vs PL (p = 0.001).
	PL, equivalent volume of maltose 10% solution	26/26		33 ± 12 (SD)	15/11	5.1 ± 3.6 (SD)				
Liver extract–folic acid–cyanocobalamin, 1989, USA [25]	Bovine liver extract 20 μg, folic acid 0.8 mg, cyanocobalamin 200 μg IM daily × 7 d (self-administered); PL, identical appearing fluid, not described	14/15 (crossover study, no washout phase)	CDC criteria for CFS [17]	40.4 ± 7.1 (SD)	3/11	[0.5– >10]	Improvement in daily activity, mental health, energy level, symptoms: LEFAC vs PL, p = NS.	None reported		None reported
Essential fatty acids, 1990, United Kingdom [29]	EFA: γ-linoleic acid 288 mg, eicosapentanoic acid 136 mg, docosahexanoic acid 88 mg, linoleic acid 2040 mg, vitamin E 80 IU/d × 3 mo;	39/39	Postviral fatigue syndrome	Males: 40.6 [21–63] Females: 39.6 [22–56]	27/36	1–3 yr by study criteria	Symptomatic improvement at 1 mo: EFA 74% vs PL 23% ($2p < 0.0002$); at 3 mo: EFA 85% vs PL 17% ($2p < 0.0001$).	Baseline: decreased n-6 EFA, arachidic acid and adrenic acid vs normal controls. End of trial (EFA gp): increased n-3 EFA in red cell membranes; shift to normal for other EFAs.		None reported
	PL, linoleic acid 400 mg, vitamin E 80 IU/d	24/24								

| Magnesium sulfate, 1991, United Kingdom [32] | MG 1 g IM weekly × 6 wk; PL, injectable water | 15/17 17/17 | Australian criteria for CFS | 35.7 [18–56] 37.1 [22–51] | 5/10 5/12 | 0.5–1.5 yr by study criteria | Improvement in energy, pain, emotional reactions at 6 wk: MG > PL ($p = 0.0015$). Overall response at 6 wk: 12/15 MG vs 3/17 PL ($p < 0.05$). | Baseline red blood cell MG: lower in CFS pts vs normal subjects; poststudy, all MG pts had RBC MG within normal range vs 1 PL pt. | 1 dropout due to rash in MG gp. |
| Amitriptyline, 1986, Canada [36] | AM 10 mg at bedtime for 1 wk, 25 mg at bedtime for 3 wk, then 50 mg at bedtime for 5 wk; PL, identical capsules | 27/34 32/36 | Primary fibrositis (Smythe's criteria, [38]) | 41.8 ± 10.4 (SD) 40.1 ± 10.5 (SD) | 2/25 3/29 | 5.9 ± 4.8 (SD), ($p < 0.05$ vs PL) 8.1 ± 7.2 (SD) | Overall improvement: 77% AM vs 43% PL at 5 wk ($p = 0.008$); 70% AM vs 50% PL at 9 wk ($p = 0.11$). Sleep improvement at 5 and 9 wk, AM > PL, $p < 0.05$. | None | 19/27 AM vs 4/32 PL (including dry mouth, drowsiness). Dosage reduction in 3 AM pts. 2 AM dropouts for adverse events. |

Table 2 Continued

Drug, year, country [Ref.]	Treatment groups and dosage regimen	No. pts completed/ enrolled	Patient characteristics				Results		
			Inclusion criteria	Age (yr) [range]	Sex (M/F)	Disease duration (yr) [range]	Clinical	Laboratory	Adverse events
Amitriptyline and naproxen, 1986, USA [37]	AM 25 mg at bedtime + NAP 500 mg twice daily (Gp 1); PL (not described) + NAP 500 mg twice daily (Gp 2); AM 25 mg at bedtime + PL (not described) (Gp 3); PL (double doses, not described) (Gp 4)	62 total enrolled/ no. pts in each group not stated	Fibromyalgia (Yunus' criteria, [50])	43.8 (21–69)	3/59	3.5 (0.25–20)	Improvement at 6 wk: AM-treated pts had significant improvement in tender point score, pain, fatigue, sleep difficulties, patient and physician global assessments. No synergy between AM and NAP was observed.	None	Dry mouth, 4 pts (Gps 1 and 3); dyspepsia, 2 pts (Gps 2 and 4); diarrhea, 2 pts (Gps 2 and 4). 1 dropout in each group.

aAC, acyclovir; AM, amitriptyline; CDC, Centers for Disease Control; CNS, central nervous system; DTH, delayed-type hypersensitivity; EBNAs, Epstein–Barr virus nuclear antigens; EBV, Epstein–Barr virus; EFA, essential fatty acids; GI, gastrointestinal; IgG, immunoglobulin G; IM, intramuscular; IV, intravenous; LEFAC, liver extract–folic acid–cyanocobalamin; LFTs, liver function tests; MG, magnesium sulfate; NAP, naproxen; NS, not significant; PL, placebo; PO, oral; RBC, red blood cells; SD, standard deviation; SEM, standard error of the mean.

(10 of 24 patients) phases. In most patients the improvement was transient and lasted only a short period after the end of the treatment phase. Four patients reported that their improvement was sustained for a year or more and, of these patients, three reported that improvement began during the placebo phase. All four patients reported that they were not back to baseline and continued to be easily fatigued.

In this study, substantial adverse events were associated with high-dose acyclovir; three patients were withdrawn from the study because of reversible acyclovir-induced nephrotoxicity. In addition, gastrointestinal and central nervous system (headache, dizziness) symptoms were more frequent with acyclovir treatment than with placebo. There were no changes with acyclovir treatment in antibody titers to EBV, circulating immune complexes, or leukocyte $2',5'$-oligoadenylate synthetase, a measure of immune system activation.

The results of this study suggested that the natural history of CFS includes periods of improvement and exacerbation, and that a placebo effect should be anticipated in drug studies of CFS. Also, a history of an affective disorder was found in some patients. Recent guidelines for inclusion of such patients in therapeutic trials recommend that they be stratified for separate analysis [16].

Immunomodulatory Agents

In three prospective, double-blind, placebo-controlled studies gamma-globulin has been tested. Dubois reported benefit with intramuscular gamma-globulin versus placebo (52 and 32%, respectively, $p < 0.001$) in patients with chronic mononucleosis syndrome, but the duration of benefit was short [19]. The results of the study are difficult to interpret because there were only 19 patients, the frequency of injections was determined by the patient, and the outcome evaluation method was based on a yes or no patient questionnaire.

Peterson et al. hypothesized that pooled immunoglobulin might contain neutralizing antibodies against an etiological virus other than EBV, or that it might correct immunoregulatory defects in patients with CFS [20], as it had been noted that CFS patients may have immunological abnormalities, including immunoglobulin deficiency [21]. Thirty patients from the Minnesota Regional CFS Research Program who satisfied the CDC definition of CFS were randomized to receive either high-dose immunoglobulin (IgG; Gammagard), 1 g/kg, or an equivalent volume of a 1% solution of albumin, intravenously every month for six doses. Two patient self-assessments were completed within 48 hr before each drug administration. Patients were asked to rate on a 4-point scale the severity of symptoms during the previous month, and the Medical Outcome Study Short Form was used to assess physical and social functioning, health perceptions, and mental health.

In the 28 patients who completed the study, there were no significant changes in symptoms at each monthly interval within each group, and there were no clinically significant differences in responses of patients who received IgG and placebo. However, there was a small, but statistically significant, improvement in health perceptions at the end of the study in the IgG group, compared with baseline. An improvement in social functioning at the end of the study was observed in the placebo group, but physical functioning declined compared with baseline. The improvement in social functioning in the placebo group was statistically significantly greater than in the IgG group, but the magnitude was small.

A substantial number of patients were hypogammaglobulinemic at baseline; 12 of 28 patients had low IgG1 serum concentrations and 18 of 28 patients had low IgG3 serum concentrations at baseline. The IgG treatment restored IgG1 levels to normal in all patients by the end of the study, but in six patients IgG3 remained low. Adverse events necessitated withdrawal of two patients from the study (one IgG and one placebo patient). The frequency of postinfusion headaches was significantly higher with IgG than with placebo. A sample size of 15 patients in each group was needed to detect a difference between the two groups, assuming improvement of 67% in the IgG group and 25% in the placebo group, a one-tailed p of 0.05, and a power of 0.76.

In contrast to the negative results reported by Peterson et al., Lloyd et al. reported that higher-dose IgG therapy was effective in the treatment of patients with CFS [22]. Forty-nine patients were randomized to receive either IgG (Intragram), 2 g/kg intravenously every month for three doses, or a 10% solution of maltose. Patient enrollment criteria were not as stringent as the CDC criteria. Over half of the patients who underwent psychiatric evaluation were classified with mild depression. An assessment of the severity of symptoms and degree of disability was performed at baseline and at 3 months after the final infusion by a blinded physician investigator. Patients were designated as "responders" if there was a major reduction in severity of symptoms and improvement in functional capacity. Thirty-three patients had a standardized psychiatric interview at baseline and at 3 months posttherapy to evaluate improvement in psychological morbidity. Self-report measures of physical and psychological symptomatology were also performed at entry and at monthly intervals throughout the trial. Cell-mediated immunity was assessed before the first dose, before the third dose, and 3 months after the final infusion. The IgG subclass concentrations in serum were measured at study entry.

Most patients (82%) had reduced cell-mediated immunity at baseline, evidenced by reduced delayed-type hypersensitivity skin-test responses or reduced T-cell subsets.

Two patients in the IgG group were withdrawn from the study after the first dose. These patients were included in an intent-to-treat analysis. At the conclusion of the study, the blinded physician classified 10 of 23 patients who received IgG and 3 of 26 patients in the placebo group as "responders" ($p < 0.05$). Most IgG patients who responded had improvement in symptoms within 3 weeks after the first dose. All responders had an increase in functional and social capacity. The psychiatrist's assessment of responders versus nonresponders was not significantly different between the IgG (6/16) and the placebo (2/17) groups.

There was a significantly greater number of adverse events in the IgG group, including phlebitis (35 of 65 IgG infusions versus 1 of 78 placebo infusions, $p < 0.001$)); constitutional symptoms, such as headache, worsened fatigue, and impaired concentration (53 IgG infusions versus 19 placebo infusions, $p < 0.001$); and transient elevation in serum alanine aminotransferase level. One IgG patient was withdrawn because of phlebitis during the first infusion, and another IgG patient was withdrawn because of increased liver function test values.

Low CD4 lymphocyte counts predicted response to IgG. In addition, all patients who responded had an improvement in markers of cell-mediated immunity.

By 12 months after the last dose, all three placebo responders and eight of the ten IgG responders had a relapse of symptoms and disability. Eight of the initial IgG responders were successfully retreated with IgG. This finding suggests that, in most cases, the beneficial effects of IgG are transient. However, despite the positive results in this study, because of the expense, high incidence of adverse reactions, and limited benefit, immunoglobulin therapy is not currently recommended for treatment of CFS [23].

Another agent that was used widely in Southern California for treatment of CFS was an injectable solution of bovine liver extract containing folic acid and cyanocobalamin (LEFAC). In an open-labeled pilot study of nine patients, all had an improvement in symptoms within 1 week of daily intramuscular administration of LEFAC (20 μg liver extract with 0.8 mg folic acid and 200 μg cyanocobalamin) [24]. In addition, lymphocyte transformation studies on mononuclear cells isolated from healthy adults confirmed that LEFAC had immunomodulatory effects [24]. However, in a placebo-controlled, double-blind, crossover-designed trial of 15 patients who met the CDC criteria for CFS, these investigators reported that responses to LEFAC treatment administered in the same dosage regimen as the pilot study were not significantly different compared with placebo [24]. Indeed, in this study, the placebo effect appeared to be strong.

Double-stranded (ds)RNAs, immunomodulatory compounds with antiviral and antitumor activities, have recently been developed. These dsRNAs are stimulators of cellular defense mechanisms and can induce endogenous interferon production and activate interferon-associated intracellular mediators. The usefulness of the early compounds was limited because of significant toxicity. However, a dsRNA with a high therapeutic ratio, Ampligen, has been developed and is currently undergoing clinical trials in patients with human immunodeficiency virus (HIV) infection [25] and with various types of malignancies [26].

Preliminary results of a randomized, multicenter, double-blind, placebo-controlled trial of Ampligen in CFS have been published in abstract form [27]. In 92 patients who met the CDC criteria for CFS, the preliminary report suggests a benefit of 400 mg of mismatched dsRNA administered intravenously twice weekly for 24 weeks, compared with placebo [28]. Patients randomized to receive Ampligen had increased Karnofsky scores, demonstrating an improved ability to perform daily activities, as well as improved oxygen uptake during exercise tolerance testing. Compared with placebo-treated patients, patients who received mismatched dsRNA had fewer hospitalizations and took fewer pain, anti-inflammatory and central nervous system active drugs. Therapy with mismatched dsRNA was reported to reverse abnormalities of the 2-5A synthase/RNase L antiviral pathway [27]. Notably, the patients who were most likely to respond had an acute onset of symptoms, lesions in the subcortical region on magnetic resonance imaging scans, and elevated circulating interleukin-1 levels. Minor rash and fever were reported by the investigators, but no patient required discontinuation of therapy because of adverse events. On further investigation, it was noted that acute hepatic toxicity occurred in one patient on a single occasion, and severe abdominal pain and arrhythmias were observed in both patients and controls [28]. All serious adverse events observed were self-limited and were reported to resolve without discontinuing treatment. Adequate assessment of these results, however, must await more complete publication of the study and confirmation by other investigators.

Nutritional and Physiological Agents

Agents targeted to treat nutritional and physiological disorders felt to be associated with CFS include essential fatty acids and magnesium. High-dose essential fatty acid therapy was evaluated in patients diagnosed with postviral fatigue syndrome [29]. The investigators hypothesized that disordered metabolism of fatty acids contributed to the disease. In addition, viral infections have been reported to inhibit desaturation of the parent ω-6-linoleic acid and the parent ω-3-α-linolenic acid [30]. Thirty-nine patients were randomized to receive treatment (γ-linolenic acid, 36 mg; eicosapentanoic acid, 17 mg; docosahexanoic acid, 11 mg; linoleic acid, 255 mg; and vitamin E, 10 IU/capsule taken as eight capsules per day), and 24 patients received placebo (linoleic acid, 50 mg; and vitamin E, 10 IU/capsule taken as eight capsules per day). Patients participated for a 3-month period. There were no dropouts in the study, and no adverse events were reported. However, no statements about compliance were made in the report.

Patients were evaluated at baseline, at 1 month, and at 3 months after treatment. Symptoms were scored at each visit on a scale of 0–3. At 1 and 3 months, patients also assessed whether they felt worse, unchanged, or better compared with the beginning of the study. In addition, at baseline and at the end of the study, essential fatty acids were measured by analyzing the fatty acid composition of the red cell membrane phospholipids.

At 1 month, there was a significant self-assessment of patient improvement in the treatment group, compared with placebo [29 (74%) of 39 versus 7 (23%) of 24, respectively, $p < 0.0002$]. At 3 months, 85% of treatment patients were assessed as improved, compared with 17% of placebo patients ($p < 0.0001$). In addition, at 3 months, all symptom scores (fatigue, myalgia, dizziness, poor concentration, and depression) were significantly improved over placebo.

The red cell membrane phospholipid analysis showed that essential fatty acid levels were abnormal in all patients at baseline. Treatment with essential fatty acids corrected all abnormalities with the exception of ω-3 essential fatty acids.

Other possible explanations proposed by the investigators for the improved outcome in patients who received treatment were that essential fatty acids may have reduced cytokine production [31] or inhibited viral replication [30]. Although this study showed a benefit of essential fatty acid therapy, additional confirmatory studies are required before this treatment approach can be recommended. Also, studies of the long-term effects of essential fatty acids in CFS are needed.

Low-dose intramuscular magnesium has been tested in patients who fit the Australian definition for CFS, less stringent than the CDC criteria for CFS [32]. In a pilot study, Cox et al. observed that patients with CFS had low red blood cell magnesium concentrations and that the symptoms of magnesium deficiency can be similar to those of CFS [32]; thus, he hypothesized that supplementation with low-dose magnesium (equivalent to 5% of the recommended daily intake, [33]) may improve symptoms of CFS. Thirty-eight patients were randomized to receive either magnesium sulfate, 1 g, or placebo (injectable water) administered intramuscularly once weekly for 6 weeks. Patients were assessed using the Nottingham health profile prestudy and 1 week after the last injection.

Thirty-two patients completed the trial. Of 15 patients who received magnesium therapy, 12 reported improvement compared with 3 of 17 placebo-treated patients ($p = 0.0015$). In addition, there was a significant improvement in energy, pain, and emotional reactions in the treatment group compared with placebo.

Red blood cell magnesium levels were lower at baseline in patients with CFS than normal subjects. At follow-up, all treated patients evaluated had normalization of red blood cell magnesium levels, compared with only one patient in the placebo group.

The results of the study by Cox have been challenged by several investigators [34,35]. Clague et al. reported that, in 12 patients who met the CDC criteria for CFS, there was no evidence for magnesium deficiency, compared with normal controls [34]. Furthermore, no improvement in symptoms was reported 1 week after a loading test of 24 mmol (2.9 g) of magnesium sulfate in normal saline given over 1 hr. Thus, until more data are available, therapy with magnesium is not recommended, unless a magnesium deficiency can be clearly demonstrated.

Psychiatric Agents

Agents used to treat the psychiatric aspects of CFS include antidepressant agents. Amitriptyline, a tricyclic antidepressant drug with serotonergic and anticholinergic activities, has been evaluated in two randomized, controlled trials in fibrositis [36,37], a syndrome considered by most researchers to be closely related to CFS [16]. In the first study [36], patients who satisfied the criteria proposed by Smythe for primary fibrositis [38] were randomized to receive amitriptyline, 10 mg at bedtime for 1 week, followed by 25 mg at bedtime for 3 weeks, then 50 mg at bedtime for 5 weeks, or placebo. Morning stiffness and pain scores improved significantly in the amitriptyline group, but no improvement in fibrositic point tenderness was observed in either group. Sleep patterns were also improved in the treated group compared with placebo. At 5 weeks, 77% of patients in the amitriptyline group reported improvement, compared with 43% of patients in the placebo group ($p = 0.008$), but at 9 weeks the difference was not significant (70% reported improvement with amitriptyline versus 50% with placebo). In this study, there appeared to be a high placebo response rate.

In the second study, amitriptyline, 25 mg, was administered with and without concomitant naproxen in a 6-week double-blind, placebo-controlled trial of 62 patients with fibrositis [37]. Treatment with amitriptyline was associated with significant improvement in patient and physician global assessments, pain, sleep difficulties, and tender point scores. Naproxen was not felt to be synergistic with amitriptyline.

Another tricyclic antidepressant agent, imipramine, was reported to have a low response rate in an open-label trial in 20 patients with fibrositis [39]. Nortriptyline and buprorion, other antidepressant agents, have been described in case reports to have beneficial effects in patients with CFS [40,41]. Controlled trials are needed for confirmation.

Neuroendocrine Agents

The results of a randomized, crossover trial in 20 patients with fibrositis were reported in abstract form. Prednisone, 15 mg, administered daily for 2 weeks, had no significant benefit over placebo [42]. Despite these preliminary findings, a study at the National Institutes of Health is currently underway to evaluate the efficacy of low-dose prednisone in the treatment of CFS. The rationale for this trial is based on a study performed by Demitrack et al. [43]. In this study of 30 patients with CDC criteria for CFS, basal evening glucocorticoid levels were reduced compared with normal controls, 24-hour urinary free cortisol excretion was also reduced, and basal evening corticotropin (ACTH) concentrations were elevated. The results suggest that a glucocorticoid deficiency occurs throughout the day in patients with CFS. Hyperresponsiveness to low-dose ACTH was also observed, ruling out primary adrenal insufficiency. The investigators propose that the defect is most consistent with a central adrenal insufficiency caused by either corticotropin-releasing hormone or other central stimulus to the pituitary–adrenal axis.

Other Agents

The efficacy of cyclobenzaprine, a tricyclic muscle relaxant, with structural similarity to amitriptyline, was evaluated in patients with fibrositis and reported in abstract form. Patients who received cyclobenzaprine, 10–40 mg daily administered for 12 weeks, had greater improvement in local pain, sleep and muscle tension compared with patients who received placebo [44]. Thus, this agent may have benefit in CFS; however, additional studies are required.

Terfenadine (Seldane) has been reported in abstract form to have no benefit in patients with CFS [45]. Thirty patients who met the CDC criteria for CFS were randomized to receive either terfenadine, 60 mg twice daily or placebo for 2 months, in this double-blind trial. Every 2 weeks, patients rated their physical and social functioning, health perceptions, and mental health. A high percentage (86.7%) of patients had a history of atopy or positive immediate hypersensitivity skin tests. In the 28 patients who completed the study, there were no differences in the patient responses to terfenadine compared with placebo, and there were no differences in responses of the subgroup of patients with atopy.

Another agent that is currently undergoing clinical testing is dialyzable leukocyte extract or transfer factor, a compound that is hypothesized to transfer delayed-type hypersensitivity in humans [33]. In anecdotal reports, nifedipine [46], cimetidine, and ranitidine were reported to have beneficial effects in CFS or EBV infection [47]. Other currently unproved treatments are antimicrobial agents, interferons, interleukin-2, and liver derivative complex (Kutapressin) [33].

CONCLUSIONS

The optimal treatment for CFS has not been found, in no small measure because the pathogenesis of this disorder is unknown. The results of the controlled clinical trials now reported demonstrate the importance of careful monitoring for placebo effects, as well as for adverse events. Also, some commonality in measurements of outcome and agreement among investigators concerning stratification for certain patient characteristics will foster research on treatment of CFS [16]. Clinical trials are continuing to be performed that will, we hope, yield a strategy that promotes recovery from this disabling illness.

While we await the results of well-controlled studies demonstrating clinically significant benefit of a medical therapy, what is a physician caring for a CFS patient to do? Symptomatic therapies can be recommended [33]. For muscle and joint pains and headaches, for example, ibuprofen or other nonsteroidal anti-inflammatory agents can be offered. If these symptoms are particularly troublesome, consultation with a neurologist specializing in pain management should be considered. Although antidepressants are commonly prescribed for CFS patients, our anecdotal experience suggests that these agents do little for the symptom of fatigue. Nonetheless, amitriptyline or doxepin, started at low dosages, may alleviate symptoms of depression, sleep difficulty, or muscle pain. For moderate to severe depression, psychiatric consultation is in order. Finally, and perhaps of greatest importance in the therapeutic armamentarium of the practicing physician, is attentive listening and encouragement of patients that they can recover from CFS. And for the medical profession, the advice of Dr. Walter Alvarez, given nearly three-quarters of a century ago, is relevant: "I beg of you that more of you spend time generously in trying to help these poor people. They deserve better of us than we now often give them" [48].

REFERENCES

1. Bean WB. Aphorisms from Latham. Iowa City: Prairie Press, 1962.
2. Wessely S. History of postviral fatigue syndrome. Br Med Bull 1991; 47:919–41.
3. Beard G. Neurosthenia, or nervous exhaustion. Boston Med Surg J 1869; 3:217–21.
4. Mitchell SW. Fat and blood. 3rd ed. Philadelphia: J B Lippincott, 1883.
5. Hall HJ. The systematic use of work as a remedy in neurasthenia and allied conditions. Boston Med Surg J 1905; 152:29–32.
6. Ferrier D. Neurasthenia and drugs. Practitioner 1911; 86:11–5.
7. Da Costa JM. On irritable heart: a clinical study of a form of functional cardiac disorder and its consequences. Am J Med Sci 1871; 121:17–52.
8. Soley MH, Shock NW. The etiology of effort syndrome. Am J Med Sci 1938; 196:840–51.
9. Wilbur DL. Clinical management of the patient with fatigue and nervousness. JAMA 1949; 141:1199–1204.
10. McCluskey DR, Riley MS. Chronic fatigue syndrome. Compr Ther 1992; 18:13–6.
11. Buchwald D, Blair J, Mease P. Treatment of chronic fatigue syndrome with acupuncture. Int J Clin Acupunct 1991; 2:231–6.
12. Spink WW. What is chronic brucellosis? Ann Intern Med 1951; 35:358–74.
13. Renfro L, Feder HM, Lane TJ, Manu P, Matthews DA. Yeast connection among 100 patients with chronic fatigue. Am J Med 1989; 86:165–8.
14. Dismukes SE, Wade JS, Lee JY, Dockery BK, Hain JD. A randomized, double-blind trial of nystatin for the candidiasis hypersensitivity syndrome. N Engl J Med 1990; 323:1717–23.
15. McBride SJ, McCluskey DR. Treatment of chronic fatigue syndrome. Br Med Bull 1991; 47:895–907.

16. Schluederberg A, Straus SE, Peterson P, Blumenthal S, Komaroff AL, Spring SB, Landay A, Buchwald D. Chronic fatigue syndrome research: definition and medical outcome assessment. Ann Intern Med 1992; 117:325–31.

17. Holmes GP, Kaplan JE, Gantz NM, Komaroff AL, Schonberger LB, Straus SE, Jones JF, Dubois RE, Cunningham-Rundles C, Pahwa S, Tosato G, Zegans LS, Purtilo DT, Brown N, Schooley RT, Brus I. Chronic fatigue syndrome: a working case definition. Ann Intern Med 1988; 108:387–9.

18. Straus SE, Dale JK, Tobi M, Lawley T, Preble O, Blaese M, Hallahan C, Henle W. Acyclovir treatment of the chronic fatigue syndrome: lack of efficacy in a placebo-controlled trial. N Engl J Med 1988; 319:1692–8.

19. DuBois RE. Gamma globulin therapy for chronic mononucleosis syndrome. AIDS Res 1986; 2(suppl 1):S191-5.

20. Peterson PK, Shepard J, Macres M, Schenck C, Crosson J, Rechtman D, Lurie N. A controlled trial of intravenous immunoglobulin G in chronic fatigue syndrome. Am J Med 1990; 89:554–60.

21. Straus SE, Tosato G, Armstrong G, Lawley T, Preble OT, Henle W, Davey R, Pearson G, Epstein J, Brus I, Blaese RM. Persisting illness and fatigue in adults with evidence of Epstein–Barr virus infection. Ann Intern Med 1985; 102:7–16.

22. Lloyd A, Hickie I, Wakefield D, Boughton C, Dwyer J. A double-blind, placebo-controlled trial of intravenous immunoglobulin therapy in patients with chronic fatigue syndrome. Am J Med 1990; 89:561–8.

23. Straus SE. Intravenous immunoglobulin treatment for the chronic fatigue syndrome. Am J Med 1990; 89:551–3.

24. Kaslow JE, Rucker L, Onishi R. Liver extract–folic acid–cyanocobalamin vs placebo for chronic fatigue syndrome. Arch Intern Med 1989; 149:2501–3.

25. Armstrong JA, McMahon D, Huang X-L, Pazin GJ, Gupta P, Rinaldo CR, Schoenfeld DA, Gaccione P, Tripoli CA, Bensasi S, Ho M. A phase I study of ampligen in human immunodeficiency virus-infected subjects. J Infect Dis 1992; 166:717–22.

26. Brodsky I, Strayer DR, Krueger LJ, Carter WA. Clinical studies with ampligen (mismatched double-stranded RNA). J Biol Response Modif 1985; 4:669–75.

27. Suhadolnik RJ, Sobol RW, Reichenbach NL, Strayer DR, Gillespie D, Carter WA. Mismatched dsRNA: clinical applications in HIV disease and chronic fatigue syndrome (CFIDS). Program supplement to the 31st International Conference on Antimicrobial Agents and Chemotherapy. Washington, DC: American Society for Microbiology, 1991:S74.

28. Cotton P. Treatment proposed for chronic fatigue syndrome; research continues to compile data on disorder. JAMA 1991; 266:2667–8.

29. Behan PO, Behan WMH, Horrobin D. Effect of high doses of essential fatty acids on the postviral fatigue syndrome. Acta Neurol Scand 1990; 82:209–16.

30. Horrobin DF. Post-viral fatigue syndrome, viral infections in atopic eczema, and essential fatty acids. Med Hypotheses 1990; 32:211–7.

31. Endres S, Ghorbani R, Kelley VE, Georgilis K, Lonnemann G, van der Meer JWM, Cannon JG, Rogers TS, Klempner MS, Weber PC, Schaefer EJ, Wolff SM, Dinarello CA. The effect of dietary supplementation with n-3 polyunsaturated fatty acids on the synthesis of interleukin-1 and tumor necrosis factor by mononuclear cells. N Engl J Med 1989; 320:265–71.

32. Cox IM, Campbell MJ, Dowson D. Red blood cell magnesium and chronic fatigue syndrome. Lancet 1991; 337:757–60.
33. Klonoff DC. Chronic fatigue syndrome. Clin Infect Dis 1992; 15:812–23.
34. Clague JE, Edwards RHT, Jackson MJ. Intravenous magnesium loading in chronic fatigue syndrome. Lancet 1992; 340:124–5.
35. Gantz NM. Magnesium and chronic fatigue. Lancet 1991; 338:66.
36. Carette S, McCain GA, Bell DA, Fam AG. Evaluation of amitriptyline in primary fibrositis. Arthritis Rheum 1986; 29:655–9.
37. Goldenberg DL, Felson DT, Dinerman H. A randomized, controlled trial of amitriptyline and naproxen in the treatment of patients with fibromyalgia. Arthritis Rheum 1986; 29:1371–7.
38. Smythe HA. Fibrositis and other diffuse musculoskeletal syndromes. In: Kelley WN, Harris ED Jr, Ruddy S, Sledge CB, eds. Textbook of rheumatology. Philadelphia: WB Saunders, 1981:485–93.
39. Wysenbeek AJ, Mor F, Lurie Y, Weinberger A. Imipramine for the treatment of fibrositis: a therapeutic trial. Ann Rheum Dis 1985; 44:752–3.
40. Gracious B, Wisner KL. Nortriptyline in chronic fatigue syndrome: a double blind, placebo-controlled single case study. Biol Psychiatry 1991; 30:405–8.
41. Goodnick PJ. Bupropion in chronic fatigue syndrome. Am J Psychiatry 1990; 147:1091.
42. Clark S, Tindall E, Bennett R. A double blind crossover study of prednisone in the treatment of fibrositis. Arthritis Rheum 1984; 27:S76.
43. Demitrack MA, Dale JK, Straus SE, Laue L, Listwak SJ, Kruesi MJP, Chrousos GP, Gold PW. Evidence for impaired activation of the hypothalamic–pituitary–adrenal axis in patients with chronic fatigue syndrome. J Clin Endocrinol Metab 1991; 73:1224–34.
44. Campbell SM, Gatter RA, Clark S, Bennett RM. A double blind study of cyclobenzaprine versus placebo in patients with fibrositis. Arthritis Rheum 1984; 27:S76.
45. Steinberg P, Peterson PK, McNutt BJ, Marshall P, Schenck C, Lurie N, Pheley A. Double-blind placebo controlled study of the efficacy of oral terfenadine in the treatment of chronic fatigue syndrome [abstract]. J Allergy Clin Immunol 1993; 91:144.
46. Adolphe AB. Chronic fatigue syndrome: possible effective treatment with nifedipine. Am J Med 1988; 85:892.
47. Goldstein JA. Cimetidine, ranitidine, and Epstein–Barr virus infection. Ann Intern Med 1986; 105:139.
48. Alvarez WC. What is wrong with the patient who feels tired, weak and toxic? N Engl J Med 1935; 212:96–104.
49. DuBois RE, Seeley JK, Brus I, Sakamoto K, Ballow M, Harada S, Bechtold TA, Pearson G, Purtilo DT. Chronic mononucleosis syndrome. South Med J 1984; 77:1376–82.
50. Yunus M, Masi AT, Calabro JJ, Miller KA, Feigenbaum SL. Primary fibromyalgia (fibrositis): clinical study of 50 patients with matched normal controls. Semin Arthritis Rheum 1981; 11:151–71.

16

Psychopharmacology and Chronic Fatigue Syndrome

Susan E. Abbey
The Toronto Hospital and the University of Toronto, Toronto, Ontario, Canada

Psychopharmacology can play an important role in the management of patients with chronic fatigue syndrome (CFS). Although there has been little formal research and few clinical reports, a vast experience with psychotherapeutic agents serves to guide the practicing clinician in the appropriate use of psychotropic drugs in this population.

A significant advance in the management of CFS has been the introduction of a rehabilitation approach that emphasizes the importance of differentiating initiating from maintaining or perpetuating factors in the ongoing disability of CFS patients [1,15,87,99,101]. There is a growing understanding that psychopharmacology has a role to play within the context of a comprehensive treatment program of this type, because a wide variety of factors that respond to psychopharmacological treatment (e.g., pain, depression, sleep disturbance, anxiety) would seem to perpetuate the physical and psychosocial disability of CFS and interfere with patient recovery. The potential to ameliorate these factors with medication or specific psychotherapeutic modalities and thereby facilitate or hasten psychosocial rehabilitation is important.

Unfortunately, our culture manifests an enduring ambivalence to the use of psychotropic medication, so that some patients are deprived of effective treatment. This ambivalence seems to be multidetermined and not only affects patients and their families, but also influences physicians and how they practice. Although concerns about pharmacotherapy are understandable, both in terms of

405

less-than-optimal prescription patterns and clear misuse of psychotropic drugs in the past, the ambivalence associated with their use extends beyond these issues and has a much deeper and more pervasive origin.

There continues to be ongoing, substantial stigmatization of psychiatric diagnoses and distress. A review of the CFS patient advocacy literature and newspaper and magazine reports emphasizes the continuing misunderstandings and misinformation that exist in the public mind concerning psychiatric distress and the association between psychiatric diagnoses and personal weakness or inadequacy, faking, lying, and malingering [1,89,100]. Clinicians have noted that even raising the issue of psychopharmacology to their CFS patients may be construed by the patient as evidence that the physician sees them as "not ill," is devaluing or dismissing their symptoms, and is labeling the symptoms as "all in the head" [1,100].

Effective pharmacological treatments may also be underutilized because of widespread patient fears about "addiction," about "mind-numbing" and depersonalizing effects of the drugs, and about the possibility that if the medication did not work at all, it would "doom" them to perpetual distress and dysfunction. The physician may be reluctant to use psychotropic drugs and fear that they do not have sufficient experience to properly prescribe such medications. All of these factors contribute to the undertreatment of depression, anxiety, and sleep disturbance in patients with chronic fatigue and CFS, and this undertreatment is associated with unnecessary impairment and dysfunction.

WHEN SHOULD PHARMACOTHERAPY BE CONSIDERED?

In general, pharmacotherapy is an appropriate consideration when the patient has a clear psychiatric diagnosis (e.g., major depressive episode, panic disorder) and exhibits neurobiological changes that interfere substantially with daily social and occupational functioning. It is important to remember that, for any given diagnosis or symptom, there is a range of potential treatments available. The choice of pharmacotherapy alone or in combination with a nonpharmacological treatment may depend on a number of factors, including patient preference, physician skill, and the availability of other treatment resources. In discussing the use of pharmacotherapy in CFS, the importance of symptoms indicative of a neurobiological disturbance (e.g., alterations in sleep, appetite, libido, concentration, and ability to experience pleasure) have been emphasized [65,67].

There may also be a role for psychopharmacological treatment(s) in the management of patients without comorbid or concurrent mood or sleep disorders. The literature on fibromyalgia suggests that pharmacotherapy with an antidepressant may be effective in controlling myalgias and improving sleep, independent of the mood-altering effects of the drugs, and in patients without a comorbid mood disorder [8,18,19,28,31,33,35,44,50,79,93,105].

PSYCHIATRIC DIAGNOSES AND CHRONIC FATIGUE SYNDROME

Over the past 15 years, there have been significant advances in psychiatric nosology and in attempts to define psychiatric disorders that are both valid and reliably diagnosed. The American Psychiatric Association *Diagnostic and Statistical Manual of Mental Disorders*, 3rd ed., revised (*DSM-III-R* [4]) provides current diagnostic criteria. It is presently under revision, and the next edition is expected in 1994. The proposed draft criteria for the upcoming edition are similar to those shown for the diagnoses that are considered in this chapter [5].

The issue of making psychiatric diagnoses in the presence of medical illness is complex and has occupied the growing attention of psychiatrists who specialize in the psychiatric care of such patients [83]. These clinicians and researchers have emphasized, for example, that the common overlap between the symptoms of some medical illnesses and depression should not be cause to abandon psychiatric assessment and treatment for major depression. In addition to its potential detrimental effect on the management of the medical disorder, depression is a serious condition in its own right with significant morbidity [21] and a long-term mortality rate of as much as 10–15% [82].

Common misunderstandings concerning the occurrence of depressive and anxiety symptoms in medically ill patients include the beliefs that (1) depression and anxiety are an understandable consequence of medical illness and, therefore, do not require treatment (e.g., "You would be depressed or anxious if you had CFS"); (2) the treatment of the underlying medical disorder will ameliorate the mood disturbance; and (3) treatment of depression or anxiety will be ineffective if the medical disorder cannot be effectively treated. Studies of organic mood syndromes and of major depression in patients with major medical illness have demonstrated that the foregoing beliefs are untenable, and the pharmacotherapy of depression in the setting of medical illness in general and in a number of specific organic mood syndromes is effective [83].

Psychiatric Disorders Associated with Chronic Fatigue Syndrome

The psychiatric disorders most likely to occur in association with CFS include, fortunately, several conditions for which effective psychopharmacological treatments exist—major depressive episode (MDE), panic disorder (PD), and generalized anxiety disorder (GAD). Somatization disorder (SD) is also common, but there is no effective drug treatment for this diagnosis. However, the long-term course of SD is often characterized by intervals of time when it is complicated by disorders such as MDE, PD, and GAD that can be treated.

Katon and Walker [56] recently reviewed the literature on the relation between chronic fatigue and psychiatric illness in community, primary care, and tertiary care settings [32,47,54,59,92,98,104]. Seven of the nine studies conducted in tertiary care settings included patients whose clinical presentations are consistent with CFS, although not all studies evaluated their sample using the CDC case definition criteria [48].

The Relation of Psychiatric Diagnoses to Chronic Fatigue Syndrome

The relation between the psychiatric disorders and CFS is problematic and controversial [2,56,80]. Katon and Russo have recently raised concerns that the CDC criteria's requirement for multiple symptoms inadvertently selects for patients with a greater burden of both current and lifetime psychiatric diagnoses [57]. It is unlikely that there is a single unitary explanation for the relation between psychiatric disorders and CFS that is applicable to all patients, just as it is unlikely that there is a single unitary etiology for CFS. Rather, there appear to be at least *four* possible relationships between psychopathology and CFS (Table 1), and it is likely that different relationships are applicable for different patients.

The first possibility is that the primary diagnosis is a psychiatric one, and not CFS. Clinicians working with CFS patients recognize patients in whom a primary psychiatric disorder has been misdiagnosed as CFS. In the case of misdiagnosed primary depressive or anxiety disorders, the patients typically respond promptly to treatments directed toward the primary psychiatric disorder. Evidence supporting the concept of psychiatric disorders arising secondary to CFS, another possible relation between psychopathology and CFS, includes recognition of

Table 1 Potential Relations Between Psychiatric Symptomatology and Chronic Fatigue Syndrome

1. Primary psychiatric symptomatology is misdiagnosed as chronic fatigue syndrome.
2. Psychiatric symptomatology occurs as the result of chronic fatigue syndrome on the basis of either:
   a. An organic mood syndrome (e.g., neurotropic virus, influence of cytokines or lymphokines on the central nervous system)
   b. A reaction to having a poorly understood, controversial diagnosis which is extremely disabling and for which there is no clear treatment
3. Chronic fatigue syndrome and psychiatric symptomatology may be covariate phenomena.
4. Psychiatric diagnosis may be inaccurately made when symptoms that are due to chronic fatigue syndrome are artifactually counted toward a psychiatric diagnosis.

organic mood syndromes following documented viral infections [16,17,42, 46,61] and central nervous system effects of cytokines and lymphokines [3,25,69,88]. Wessely has reviewed the neuropsychiatry of CFS [102]. The third possibility is that psychiatric disorders and CFS are covariates of some other underlying abnormality. The fourth possible explanation, that psychiatric diagnoses may be artifactual findings, does not seem to be borne out by researchers who have statistical techniques to "count" and "not count" symptoms as contributing toward a psychiatric diagnosis when they could be attributable to either CFS or a psychiatric disorder. This approach has been derived from studies of depression in the medically ill [64]. When this technique has been used in CFS studies it has not substantially changed the rates of diagnosed psychiatric disorders [32,59,98].

DEPRESSION AND CHRONIC FATIGUE SYNDROME

Depressive symptoms were recognized in 35–70% of the initial case series of patients with chronic fatigue in whom Epstein–Barr virus was presumed to be responsible [7,12,27,52,84,90]. More recently, attention turned to the prevalence of major depression in CFS per se [32,47,54,59,98,104]. The diagnostic criteria for major depression (MDE) used in these studies are shown in Table 2. The findings concerning the prevalence of MDE in tertiary care samples of CFS patients are shown in Table 3. The significance of these findings for the etiology of CFS remains unclear and controversial [2,80], but recent work by Wessely and his group emphasized the clinical importance of MDE in impeding the successful rehabilitation of CFS patients [15,99,101]. Untreated depression was the leading cause of refusal to participate in their cognitive–behavioral rehabilitation program and the strongest predictor of poor outcome [101].

In addition to advances over the past decade in the understanding of the neurobiology of MDE and its treatment by pharmacotherapy and cognitive and interpersonal psychotherapy, there has also been a new appreciation of the magnitude of dysfunction associated with MDE. Wells et al., in a study of psychosocial morbidity and health care utilization in a variety of chronic disorders, showed that patients with either current MDE or subsyndromal depressive symptoms demonstrated poor social, occupational, and physical functioning comparable with, or worse than, that associated with eight other major chronic medical conditions [96]. For example, the association between depressive symptoms and days in bed was stronger for depression than for hypertension, diabetes, and arthritis. The only chronic condition associated with functional impairment comparable with depressive symptoms was current advanced coronary artery disease.

Table 2 Diagnostic Criteria for Major Depressive Episode

A. At least five of the following symptoms have been present during the same 2-week period and represent a change from previous functioning; at least one of the symptoms is either (1) depressed mood, or (2) loss of interest or pleasure.

1. Depressed mood (or can be irritable mood in children and adolescents) most of the day, nearly every day, as indicated either by subjective account or observation by others

2. Markedly diminished interest or pleasure in all, or almost all, activities most of the day, nearly every day (as indicated either by subjective account or observation by others of apathy most of the time)

3. Significant weight loss or weight gain when not dieting (e.g., more than 5% of body weight in a month), or decrease or increase in appetite nearly every day

4. Insomnia or hypersomnia nearly every day

5. Psychomotor agitation or retardation nearly every day (observable by others, not merely subjective feelings of restlessness or being slowed down)

6. Fatigue or loss of energy nearly every day

7. Feelings of worthlessness or excessive or inappropriate guilt (which may be delusional) nearly every day (not merely self-reproach or guilt about being sick)

8. Diminished ability to think or concentrate, or indecisiveness, nearly every day

9. Recurrent thoughts of death (not just fear of dying), recurrent suicidal ideation without a specific plan, or a suicide attempt or a specific plan for committing suicide

B. 1. It cannot be established that an organic factor initiated and maintained the disturbance

2. The disturbance is not a normal reaction to the death of a loved one

C. At no time during the disturbance have there been delusions or hallucinations for as long as 2 weeks in the absence of prominent mood symptoms

Source: Adapted from Ref. 4. Diagnostic and Statistical Manual of Mental Disorders, Third Edition, Revised. Washington, DC: American Psychiatric Association, 1987 (with permission).

The Neurobiology of Major Depression

Although neuroscience remains in its infancy, there have been major advances in understanding the neurobiology of depression and moving beyond a simple older model of inadequate monoamine neurotransmission as the cause for depression and the presumed effect of antidepressant treatment being increased availability of synaptic neurotransmitter [49]. This early model focused on norepinephrine, but was expanded over time to include serotonin. The model had difficulty reconciling the discrepancy between the finding that the tricyclic antidepressants and monoamine oxidase inhibitors have a very rapid effect on synaptic concentrations of monoamines, but there is a substantial delay (3–6 weeks) in the onset of clinical efficacy. Hyman and Nestler review the newer theoretical models that emphasize the "downstream" neuronal consequences of

Table 3 Studies of Depression in Chronic Fatigue Syndrome

Authors [Ref.]	Year	Structured psychiatric interview and diagnostic criteria	Number of fatigue patients	CDC criteria	% With affective illness before fatigue	% with major depression		
						Current MDE	Lifetime MDE	Over course of illness MDE
Taerk et al. [92]	1987	DIS DSM-III	24	NR	50%	NR	67%	54%
Wessely and Powell [98]	1989	SADS RDC	47	NR	43% "prior psychiatric history"	47%	NR	NR
Kruesi et al. [59]	1989	DIS DSM-III	28	100%	40% depression and anxiety before chronic fatigue	46% 55% of women 25% of men	21%	54%
Gold et al. [32]	1990	DIS DSM-III	26	23% retrospective asst of sample	50% MDE	42%	73%	NR
Hickie et al. [47]	1990	SCID DSM-III-R	48	NR	12.5% MDE	21% (45.8% during course of illness)	NR	46%
Katon et al. [54]	1991	DIS DSM-III-R	98	19% of sample	53%	15.3%	76.5%	45%
Wood et al. [104]	1991	PSE CATEGO	34	NR	20.6%	23.5%	NR	NR

Abbrev: MDE, major depressive episode; DIS, Diagnostic Interview Schedule; DSM-III and III-R, Diagnostic and statistical manual, 3rd ed. and 3rd ed. revised; SADS, Schedule for Affective Disorders and Schizophrenia; RDC, Research Diagnostic Criteria; SCID, Structured Clinical Interview for DSM-III-R; PSE, Present State Examination; CATEGO, Computerized diagnostic system for ICD-9 diagnoses; NR, not reported.
Source: Modified from Ref. 56.

antidepressants (i.e., intracellular effects beyond the synapse and effects on projections of affected neurons) and relate the biology of depression to more complex neuronal events extending beyond the synapse [49].

Continuing research has determined that indolamines (e.g., serotonin) must be added to catecholamines (e.g., norepinephrine) as critical factors in the pathogenesis of depression. Hymen and Nessler noted that both noradrenergic and serotonergic projections are wide and include cortex, limbic system, hypothalamus, and brain stem, and that the symptoms of depression are based in a range of brain structures (e.g., sleep disturbances in brain stem or hypothalamus; depressed mood in the limbic system; altered cognition in cortex; psychomotor changes in the basal ganglion and limbic systems) [49].

Serotonin seems to be particularly worthy of study in CFS, given that it is known to be an important neurotransmitter for sleep, pain, and mood. Serotonin is involved in the genesis and maintenance of slow-wave sleep, which is the most restorative type of sleep and the disturbance of which is associated with musculoskeletal symptoms and fibromyalgia [108]. Low levels of serotonin are associated with heightened pain perception [108]. Serotonin acts peripherally as a vasoactive amine released at sites of inflammation and as a potentiator of nociceptive effects of painful stimuli [106]. Moldofsky and Warsh demonstrated that plasma unbound tryptophan, a precursor of serotonin, was inversely related to the severity of symptoms in fibromyalgia patients [107].

Further background on the neurobiology of CFS has been reviewed by Demitrack (see Chapter 11).

Pharmacotherapy of Depression in Chronic Fatigue Syndrome

Unfortunately, there are few reports of antidepressant use in CFS to guide us, and as yet, there have been no randomized controlled or open trials involving an adequately large group of well-characterized patients meeting the CDC case definition criteria. Thus, clinicians are left to rely on case series, clinical reports of series of patients treated with antidepressants, and reports in the patient support literature to guide them. In addition, there is a literature on the use of antidepressants in the medically ill and in organic affective syndromes that also provides some guidance [83].

Jones and Straus, in the first report of antidepressant drug use, noted that low doses of doxepin resulted in clinical improvement in 70% of treated individuals [53], but they did not characterize the study sample relative to the presence or absence of depression and seemed to be using the doxepin for its anti-inflammatory and antihistaminic effects as much as for its psychopharmacological potential. Lynch et al. reported on the use of fluoxetine and lofepramine (a tricyclic antidepressant not available in North America) and noted that a third of their sample of 52 patients had greater than 50% reduction in the severity of depressive symptoms; an additional third had a 25–50% reduction in the severity of depressive symptoms following 8 weeks of treatment [65]. Twenty-five of the 30 responders were able to discontinue the drug, with no relapse at 6 months. A single case study of the double-blind, placebo-controlled use of nortriptyline in a woman with CFS was reported by Gracious and Wisner [41]. Their patient experienced significant, but incomplete, relief of both affective and physical symptoms during treatment with nortriptyline. The authors noted that the improvement in mood and cognition contributed to diminished perception of physical impairment, but they felt that the decrease in symptoms, such as fever and lymphadenopathy, was more difficult to explain by such a mechanism. However, it could be argued that these symptoms are subjective experiences that would be less troublesome without the added somatic amplification of depression. Goodnick reported on two patients with CFS who had previously failed other antidepressants and in whom the use of bupropion produced "rapid relief of all symptoms at minimal dosages" [38]. He noted that bupropion has been reported to be particularly effective in forms of depression characterized by prominent fatigue and hypersomnia [37]. The case report is also important in reminding us to continue to pursue pharmacotherapy with different classes of medication if initial trials are unsuccessful. Manu et al. summarized their experience with pharmacotherapy with psychotropic medications in patients with CFS and noted that, occasionally, augmentation of antidepressants with lithium or thyroid hormone was required [67]. Klimas conducted open trials of fluoxetine, 20 mg daily in two series of patients with CFS (sample sizes of 25 and 35) [58]. The samples were heterogeneous for the presence and intensity of depressive symptomatology, and there was no assessment for MDE. Changes in group mean natural killer cell cytotoxicity were documented and all patients showed clinical improvement. A similar beneficial effect was reported for sertraline [40].

There is a question about the validity of the uncontrolled studies of antidepressant use in CFS. Prior controlled trials of other medications, such as acyclovir [91], immunoglobulin [62,78], and dialyzable leukocyte extract [63] in this population have demonstrated high rates of placebo response. There is also a question about the type and magnitude of benefit that the patient with CFS may expect to achieve with antidepressant therapy. Lynch et al. emphasized that the expectation of "total cure" is unrealistic and argued that there is no evidence to substantiate this view [65]. In their patient series, it was noted that symptoms of fatigue and myalgia may improve concurrently with symptoms of depression and anxiety in some patients with CFS, whereas in others, there is an improvement in depressive symptoms, but much less benefit for fatigue and myalgia. They speculated that depression may heighten or amplify the perception of fatigue and myalgia by a process called somatic amplification [6]. Thus, an improvement in depressive symptoms may result in a reduction in the perceived intensity of the symptoms and a sense that the other symptoms have also improved.

Goodnick and Sandoval theorized that there is differential symptom response with different antidepressants [40]. They assert that more serotonergic compounds were more helpful with symptoms of pain than depression whereas those compounds that were more catecholaminergic seemed more effective with symptoms of depression. This hypothesis is intriguing, but their work awaits replication.

The question of the degree to which antidepressants modulate immune functioning has been raised by Goodnick and Sandoval [40] and by Klimas et al. [58] as one possible basis for their beneficial effects, if any. Goodnick and Sandoval described the influence of various antidepressants on immune function, as reported in studies of patients with major depression, or in their own studies of patients with CFS [40]. Nonetheless, this issue still remains poorly studied and does not appear to be clearly supportable, given the ongoing controversy over the role and clinical significance of immune dysfunction in CFS. It is premature to make decisions about pharmacotherapy based on such issues as these.

Antidepressant Pharmacotherapy of Fibromyalgia

Fibromyalgia (FM) is a closely aligned condition to CFS, for which there is some research literature on pharmacotherapy with antidepressants (see Chapter 12). The similarity of the two syndromes has been commented on by several observers, and it has been suggested that up to 67–70% of CFS patients have tender points, as in FM [34–36], and that up to 55% of FM patients have an acute onset following a viral illness [12].

Over the past 10 years researchers assessed the efficacy of antidepressant therapy in FM. Goldenberg noted that tricyclic antidepressants have a range of actions and possible mechanisms of action, both central and peripheral, that may be of benefit in FM [35]. The proposed mechanisms include central analgesia by modification of endogenous opiates and serotonin, a direct effect on peripheral nociceptors, and effects on sleep that, in turn, modulate the pain experience in FM patients [35]. An early trial of the tricyclic antidepressant, imipramine, in 20 patients with FM was unsuccessful [105]. Goldenberg et al. reported a placebo-controlled, double-blind trial of amitriptyline and naproxen in FM and found that the use of 25 mg of amitriptyline was associated with a significant reduction in patients' complaints of pain, sleep disturbance, fatigue on awakening, and tenderpoint score [33]. In another placebo-controlled trial of amitriptyline, Carette et al. found that its use was associated with a significant improvement in pain and sleep complaints, morning stiffness, and global clinical assessment, but not in tenderpoint score [18]. Interestingly, the size of the effect diminished from weeks 5 through 9 of the study. Goldenberg, in reporting on his follow-up of patients, found that a clinically meaningful response was achieved in only one-third of patients [35].

Positive results also have been reported for other tricyclic compounds including dothiepin [19] and cyclobenzaprine [8,44,79], as well as for S-adenosylmethionine, a methyl donor known to have antidepressant properties [93]. Jaeschke et al. conducted an innovative N-of-1 randomized, controlled trial of amitriptyline in which patients responding to an initial open trial were then enrolled in the N-of-1 randomized controlled trial [50]. They found that one-third of patients responded to the open trial of amitriptyline. In the N-of-1 trial, differences in questionnaire measures of functioning and symptomatology favored amitriptyline in 18 of 23 trials and placebo in 5, although statistically significant differences in favor of amitriptyline were found in only 7 of 18 trials. A change in tenderpoint count favoring amitriptyline occurred in 15 patients, although this was statistically significant in only 4 of the 15. These authors argued that this methodology might be useful to identify those patients with FM who will benefit from medication and avoid unnecessary treatment of those who do not [50]. A similar methodology could be useful in assessing the use of antidepressants in CFS.

Anecdotal reports of the benefits of the selective serotonin reuptake inhibitors in patients with FM suggested that fluoxetine and sertraline have a role to play. The literature contains several case reports of beneficial effect of fluoxetine in FM at doses between 20 and 40 mg daily [28,31]. Interestingly, fluoxetine has been reported to be beneficial in relieving the prolonged fatigue that is associated with recovery from ciguatera fish poisoning [9].

ANXIETY DISORDERS AND CHRONIC FATIGUE SYNDROME

A wide variety of cognitive and somatic anxiety symptoms have been described in patients with CFS. The most common anxiety diagnoses in CFS are panic disorder and generalized anxiety disorder (Table 4). The prevalence of anxiety disorders in groups of patients with CFS (Table 5) is substantially lower than that of major depression, but is generally reported to be elevated in contrast with community samples. The prevalence relative to that found in other medical disorders is more equivocal. For example, panic disorder is diagnosed in 0.4–2.9% of individuals in the community and in 1.4–6.5% in medical clinics [55]. Manu et al. reported an even higher rate of 13.5% in patients with chronic fatigue [66].

Anxiety disorders are an important differential diagnosis in CFS and are treatable. Clinical experience suggests that some patients with primary anxiety disorders may attribute the episodic and fluctuating somatic symptoms of anxiety

Table 4   Diagnostic Criteria for Panic Disorder and Generalized Anxiety Disorder

Panic disorder (with or without agoraphobia)—DSM-III-R

A.   Panic attacks which on at least one occasion have been unexpected and not triggered by situations in which the person was the focus of others' attention.

B.   Four attacks within 4 weeks or one or more attacks followed by at least a month of persistent fear of having another attack.

C.   At least four of the following symptoms developed during at least one of the attacks:
       Shortness of breath (dyspnea) or smothering sensations
       Dizziness, unsteady feelings, or faintness
       Palpitations or accelerated heart rate (tachycardia)
       Trembling or shaking
       Sweating
       Choking
       Nausea or abdominal distress
       Depersonalization or derealization
       Numbness or tingling sensations (paresthesias)
       Flushes (hot flashes) or chills
       Chest pain or discomfort
       Fear of dying
       Fear of going crazy or of doing something uncontrolled

D.   During at least some of the attacks, at least four of the C symptoms developed suddenly and increased in intensity within 10 min of the beginning of the first C symptom noticed in the attack.

E.   It cannot be established that an organic factor initiated and maintained the disturbance (e.g., amphetamine or caffeine intoxication, hyperthyroidism).

Generalized anxiety disorder—DSM-III-R

A.   Unrealistic or excessive anxiety and worry (apprehensive expectation) about two or more life circumstances for a period of 6 months or longer.

B.   If another axis I disorder is present, the focus of the anxiety and worry in A is unrelated to it, (e.g., the anxiety or worry is not about having a panic attack; as in panic disorder).

C.   Does not occur only during the course of a mood disorder or a psychotic disorder and if there is another disorder present, the anxiety or worry is not related (e.g., fear of being embarrassed in public with social phobia, being contaminated with obsessive–compulsive disorder, gaining weight with anorexia nervosa).

D.   At least 6 of the following 18 symptoms:

Autonomic Hyperactivity	*Motor Tension*
Shortness of breath	Trembling, twitching
Palpitations, tachycardia	Muscle tension, aches
Sweating, cold clammy hands	Restlessness
Dry mouth	Easy fatigability
Dizziness or lightheadedness	
Nausea, diarrhea, abdominal distress	*Vigilance and Scanning*
Flushes (hot flashes) or chills	Feeling keyed up/on edge
Frequent urination	Exaggerated startle

Trouble swallowing/lump in throat	Difficulty concentrating
	Trouble falling/staying asleep
	Irritability

E.   It cannot be established that an organic factor initiated and maintained the disturbance (e.g., hyperthyroidism, caffeine intoxication).

Source: Adapted from Ref. 4. Diagnostic and Statistical Manual of Mental Disorders, Third Edition, Revised. Washington, DC: American Psychiatric Association, 1987 (with permission).

(e.g., dizziness, lightheadedness, palpitations, muscle tremors, weakness, palpitations) to signs of fluctuating viral activity. As with depression, there has also been a growing appreciation of the significant psychosocial morbidity of untreated anxiety disorders [23], including increased mortality due to suicide [97].

The Neurobiology of Anxiety Disorders

Katon has succinctly reviewed the major developments in the understanding of the neurobiology of panic disorder [55]. This literature continues to develop and focuses on the increasing evidence of biological abnormalities in patients with panic disorder, including a specific response to provocative testing, a positive response to pharmacological treatment, and accumulating evidence related to the genetics of the disorder [55]. Abnormalities in cerebral metabolism have been documented [81]. Specifically, there is evidence of alterations in the noradrenergic, serotonergic, and γ-aminobutyric acid (GABA) systems [55].

Pharmacotherapy of the Anxiety Disorders

There have been no published case reports or trials of anxiolytic therapy in CFS. Some patients are known to be taking a wide range of anxiolytic medications for a variety of reasons, some of which are unclear. The importance of distinguishing patients whose anxiety is of syndromal level arises from the advances in our understanding of the differential treatment response of the various anxiety disorders [55]. The treatment of anxiety has changed over the past decade, and there is now awareness of the roles for both pharmacotherapy and nonpharmacological management tailored specifically for each of the anxiety diagnoses [55].

Transient anxiety may be problematic for CFS patients. At times, this anxiety will be tied to specific stressors (e.g., performance anxiety, contact with relatives or friends who are critical of the patient or disparaging of the diagnosis). Alternatively, the anxiety may not appear to be associated with any external or intrapsychic stimulus that is observable by the patient or inferrable by the

Table 5 Studies of Anxiety Disorders in Chronic Fatigue Syndrome

Author [Ref.]	Year	Structured psychiatric interview and diagnostic criteria	Number of fatigue patients	CDC criteria	% With anxiety diagnoses		
					Before CFS	Current	Lifetime
Taerk et al. [92]	1987	DIS *DSM-III*	24	NR	NR	NR	PD = 13%; SPh = 25%; SocPh = 4% (not different from control group)
Wessely and Powell [98]	1989	SADS *RDC*	47	NR	NR	PhD = 4.3%; GAD = 2.1%	NR
Kruesi et al. [59]	1989	DIS *DSM-III*	28	100%	32%	NR	PD = 17.9%; SP = 28.6%
Gold et al. [32]	1990	DIS *DSM-III*	26	23% retrospective asst of sample	NR	NR	NR
Hickie et al. [47]	1990	SCID *DSM-III-R*	48	NR	PD = 2%	PD = 6.3%	NR
Katon et al. [54]	1991	SCID *DSM-III-R*	98	19% of sample	NR	NR	NR
Wood et al. [104]	1991	PSE *CATEGO*	34	NR	5.8%	Phobic anxiety neurosis = 11.8%; Generalized anxiety neurosis = 5.9%	NR

Abbrev: PD, panic disorder; SPh, simple phobia; SocPh, social phobia; GAD, generalized anxiety disorder; DIS, Diagnostic Interview Schedule; *DSM-III* and *III-R*, Diagnostic and statistical manual, 3rd ed. and 3rd ed. revised; SADS, Schedule for Affective Disorders and Schizophrenia; SCID, Structured Clinical Interview for *DSM-III-R*; *RDC*, Research Diagnostic Criteria; *CATEGO*, Computerized diagnostic system for ICD-9 diagnoses; PSE, Present State Examination. NR, not reported.

observer. The treatment of situational anxiety should focus primarily on nonpharmacological treatments, such as education about anxiety disorders; relaxation training; behavioral therapies, including graded desensitization or flooding with the anxiogenic stimulus [68]; or cognitive–behavioral techniques for anxiety control [22]. Often a partner, close friend, or family member can function as a "cotherapist" in assisting the patient to learn and practice these techniques and to identify situations for which their use could prevent or ameliorate anxiety. The use of medication with situational anxiety is more controversial, with medical opinion ranging from the view that it is contraindicated, through to finding medication acceptable in limited circumstances over discrete and relatively brief periods.

SLEEP DISTURBANCE AND CHRONIC FATIGUE SYNDROME

Sleep disturbance is a very common symptom in patients with CFS, and sleep disturbance either in the form of insomnia or hypersomnia constitutes one of the minor criteria in the current CFS case definition [48]. Formal studies of sleep disturbance in patients with CFS are beginning [60,73–75,103].

Moldofsky and colleagues [73–75] were the first to describe a sleep abnormality in CFS with the finding of the alpha-delta sleep pattern [45,72] that had been originally described in fibromyalgia [72]. The alpha-delta sleep pattern is a disturbance of non-REM sleep, in which the deep delta waves of stage III and IV sleep are interrupted by bursts of high-amplitude alphalike rhythms. It is now thought that this disruption in sleep is associated with a variety of posttraumatic and other pain disorders, rheumatoid arthritis, and fibrositis. The alpha-delta sleep pattern is a suitable target for pharmacological treatment.

As the relation between sleep and CFS has come under greater scrutiny, a variety of other sleep disorders have been demonstrated, including nocturnal myoclonus, sleep apnea of both central and peripheral origin, and others [13,60,76,103]. Further research awaits more detailed documentation of these abnormalities and emphasizes the importance of evaluating patients for sleep complaints, as there are a number of effective treatments for many of the primary sleep disorders.

The Neurobiology of Sleep Disturbance in Chronic Fatigue Syndrome

Moldofsky conducted pioneering work investigating the relation of the sleep–wake system and cytokine and cellular immune functioning [75]. He concluded that there is a reciprocal relation between the two systems and that interference with either the immune or sleep–wake systems has effects on the other system and will be accompanied by the symptoms of CFS. He suggests that disordered regulation of cytokines, such as interferon-α, interleukin-1 (IL-1), and interleukin-2 (IL-2), as are postulated to occur in CFS, results in alterations in both the immune and sleep–wake systems.

Pharmacotherapy of Sleep Disorders in Chronic Fatigue Syndrome

A variety of agents have been used to treat the alpha-delta sleep disturbance in patients with fibromyalgia, including chlorpromazine [72], low-dose tricyclic antidepressants [35], L-tryptophan [20] and, more recently, the cyclopyrrolone derivative zopiclone (Imovane), which is a short-acting hypnotic agent belonging to a novel chemical class structurally unrelated to existing hypnotics [26].

Although benzodiazepines and chloral derivatives may be helpful in the short-term, they distort sleep architecture and typically lose their efficacy over several weeks. Regular use of benzodiazepines is also problematic because their withdrawal produces rebound insomnia. Patients with initial insomnia may be helped by a sedating tricyclic antidepressant (e.g., amitriptyline, trazodone, doxepine). It has also been suggested that zopiclone, a novel cyclopyrrolone derivative, may be useful in both inducing and maintaining sleep in this group.

Approaches to the treatment of the alpha-delta sleep disturbance has involved the use of either a tricyclic antidepressant, zopiclone, or L-typtophan. A double-blind, controlled study of the use of zopiclone in the treatment of sleep abnormalities in fibromyalgia discerned a significant reduction in daytime tiredness and subjective sleep complaints, although there was no change in the polysomnographic record [26]. Further studies with zopiclone in fibromyalgia and CFS are presently underway. Zopiclone is reported to produce only slight changes in sleep architecture, with some delay in REM sleep, but no change in total duration of REM sleep, and a minimal decrease in stage 1 sleep, with an increase in stage 2 sleep [26]. L-Tryptophan is said to decrease REM latency and total REM sleep, but increase non-REM sleep and total sleep duration, and has improved sleep in fibromyalgia [20].

PRACTICAL GUIDE TO PSYCHOPHARMACOLOGY IN CHRONIC FATIGUE SYNDROME

General Strategies in Psychopharmacology

With the foregoing background, we can now turn to a discussion of how and when to use psychotropic drugs in CFS patients. The use of psychotropic medications in CFS requires an appreciation of the general principles of psychotropic drug use as outlined in Table 6. The ability to take a collaborative stance with the patient forms the cornerstone of effective pharmacotherapy. This

Table 6   General Principles of Psychopharmacological Treatment

---

 1. Psychotropic medication use requires a collaborative patient–physician relationship.
 2. Determine if an axis I diagnosis (e.g., major depression, panic disorder, generalized anxiety disorder) exists based on a comprehensive clinical assessment.
 3. If there is no axis I diagnosis, and pharmacotherapy is to be directed toward target symptoms, then define the frequency, intensity, of the target symptoms to assess drug effect (e.g., muscle aches, sleep disturbance, sleep disturbance, decreased mood, impaired concentration, pain, appetite disturbance, panic attacks).
 4. Review and document pretreatment symptoms that may be confused with medication side effects (e.g., headache, dry mouth, lightheadedness)
 5. Discuss with the patient the various alternative drugs that might be effective:
    Side effects that need to be avoided or side effects that may be advantageous (e.g., sedation)
    Possibility of drug interactions
    Relative or absolute contraindications to using a particular drug (e.g., benzodiazepines in substance abusers, tricyclic antidepressant in a patient with a cardiac conduction defect)
 6. Involve the patient in choosing the drug with the best risk/benefit ratio and cost-effectiveness.
 7. Educate the patient about the drug, how to initiate treatment, increase drug dose, common side effects (time duration and what can be done to decrease them), when to call for advice. Elicit patient's agreement to call and speak with the physician before discontinuing.
 8. Initiate therapy at the lowest possible dose and increase slowly as tolerated.
 9. When possible introduce one drug at a time to allow monitoring of effect.
10. Avoid polypharmacy unless clearly indicated.
11. Be aware of the various psychological meanings that patients attach to drugs (e.g., a sign of weakness, "crutch," magical cure).
12. Complete drug trial and document results. Endpoints for a completed trial include (1) positive outcome; (2) trial must be discontinued because of intolerable side effects; (3) ineffective after adequate length of time at adequate dose.

---

notion of a therapeutic alliance is based on the premise that both the physician and the patient share a determination to work together to ensure an adequate therapeutic drug trial. Although a therapeutic alliance is desirable for any drug trial, it is critical for a trial of psychotropic medication, as these medications are typically associated with a delayed onset of action, have a range of nuisance side effects that may be difficult to tolerate, particularly early in the course of treatment when it is still too early for perceivable benefit. As indicated earlier, these medications and their use are associated with social stigma. Psychotropic medication use is particularly problematic for patients who interpret it as a sign that their physician does not "believe them." Psychotropic medication use is also more problematic in patients with heightened sensitivity to medication side effects that may occur because of increased preoccupation with or sensitivity to bodily symptoms, which may be a long-standing characteristic of the patient's personality style or may be a response limited to periods of illness. In CFS, there seems to be a heightened sensitivity to side effects of medications, the basis of which is poorly understood. Many patients will describe themselves as never having had difficulties taking medications premorbidly, but following the onset of the illness find that they are exquisitely sensitive to the side effects of all medications. Some also report that they became intolerant of alcohol following the development of the illness.

As was discussed earlier in the chapter, the strongest indication for using psychotropic medication(s) is the finding of a psychiatric disorder, such as major depression, panic disorder, or generalized anxiety disorder. To reach such a diagnosis involves gathering data from the patient, including a review of the symptoms for these disorders (see Tables 2 and 4), and questioning the patient about past personal and family history of psychiatric disorder. A mental status examination is also needed, at which time observations are made of general behavior, an assessment of mood including both the physician's observations and the patient's subjective experience of their mood, a review of the neurovegetative changes of depression and somatic symptoms of anxiety, an evaluation of thought content (including lowered self-esteem, hopelessness, and helplessness), and a specific assessment concerning suicidality.

At times, a psychiatric consultation may be useful to clarify diagnostic questions or to obtain recommendations about psychotropic medication. Unfortunately, many patients resist such a consultation because of fears that the consultation labels them as "crazy" or have concerns about rejection by family and friends. Burszatjn and Barsky described techniques for facilitating patient acceptance of a referral for psychiatric consultation [14]. A psychiatric consultation is more likely to be accepted when phrased in terms of coping with the understandable stresses associated with medical illness and parallels are drawn with the use of psychiatric consultation for patients with cancer, heart disease, and other physical disorders. It is also helpful for the referring physician to provide reassurance that they will continue to care for the patient and that the consultation is not an attempt to "dump" them. Finally, many otherwise reluctant patients are willing to accept a consultation when they understand that it will help or reassure their physician in dealing better with their illness (i.e., "the consultation will be of use to me in caring for you"). Consultation is most likely to yield useful recommendations when a psychiatrist is chosen who has experience in the assessment and treatment of patients with comorbid medical and psychiatric disorders or has experience in working with chronic pain.

If suicidal ideation is present, the potential lethality of any drug must be considered and, when there is a choice, a drug with lower lethality in overdose should be chosen. For example, a selective serotonin reuptake inhibitor would be preferable to a tricyclic antidepressant. For drugs with lethal potential, consideration must be given to the quantity to be dispensed at any one time (e.g., for a tricyclic, the lethal dose may as low as 1.0 g of imipramine, which is equivalent to a 1-week supply at full therapeutic doses). Patients with suicidal ideation who are being managed on an outpatient basis should be impressed with the necessity to seek care (e.g., contact the physician or attend at the nearest emergency department) if the suicidal ideation increases in intensity to the point at which they are unsure of their ability to contain their impulses to inflict harm on themselves.

The medication should be initiated at the lowest possible dose and increased slowly. Patients need to understand that the trade-off is between a slow increase and decreased side effects, but also a delayed onset of action versus a more rapid escalation of dose, with a quicker onset of action, but potentially greater side effects. Patients should be encouraged to increase the dose at their own pace with this trade-off in mind. For many patients, it may be preferable to have a very slow increase that can be tolerated, even though this will mean a significant delay in the onset of efficacy. For example, a depressed patient in a psychiatric outpatient clinic treated with an antidepressant will typically be within the therapeutic dose range immediately if fluoxetine is used and within 7–10 days if a tricyclic antidepressant is used. For some depressed CFS patients it may take 4–8 weeks to get into a tolerable therapeutic dose range with either drug, resulting in a delay in the onset of clinical effect, but with the advantage that it may allow the patient to have a full drug trial, which they would have been unable to achieve had it been escalated more quickly.

PSYCHOPHARMACOLOGY OF SPECIFIC PSYCHIATRIC DIAGNOSES

Depression

The antidepressants used in the treatment of CFS are shown in Table 7. There is some debate among practitioners about which drug should be the first line of treatment. At this time, there is a general consensus that the drug of first choice is either a selective serotonin reuptake inhibitor or a second-generation tricyclic antidepressant. Some clinicians advocate the use of doxepine or amitriptyline if problems with insomnia are profound, although when used in full therapeutic dose for the mood disorder, they are likely to be too sedating to be easily tolerated by the CFS patient, and it is often better to use a hypnotic agent during the time that the patient is being established on the antidepressant therapy.

All of the antidepressant agents share the property of delayed onset of symptomatic improvement. Typically, there is improvement in biological functions (e.g., sleep, appetite, libido, diurnal variation) before an improvement in

Table 7 Pharmacotherapy of Major Depression in Chronic Fatigue Syndrome

Class	Example	Starting dose	Usual therapeutic dose	Frequency (%) of adverse effects at therapeutic doses [10,70]	
				>10%	>30%
Tricyclic antidepressants	Nortriptyline	10 mg qhs	40–200 mg qhs	Dry mouth, constipation, fatigue/weakness	
	Desipramine	10 mg qhs	75–300 mg qhs	Dry mouth, tachycardia	
Selective serotonin-reuptake inhibitors	Fluoxetine	2.5–5 mg qam	20 mg qam (max. 80 mg qam)	Insomnia, excitement/agitation, headache, anorexia, GI distress, fine tremor	
	Sertraline	50 mg[a]	50–200 mg[a]	Dry mouth, headache, dizziness, fine tremor, insomnia	GI distress
	Paroxetine	10 mg qam	10–50 mg qam	Dry mouth, headache, constipation, sweating, drowsiness/sedation, fine tremor, GI distress	
Monocyclic antidepressants	Bupropion	75 mg	225–450 mg[b]	Dry mouth, blurred vision, constipation, sweating, insomnia, excitement/agitation, headache, orthostatic hypotension, tachycardia	
Monoamine oxidase inhibitors	Phenelzine	15 mg qam	45–90 mg[c]	Blurred vision, excitement/agitation, insomnia, drowsiness/sedation, orthostatic hypotension, tachycardia, constipation, GI disturbance, weight gain, sexual disturbance	Dry mouth

[a]With evening meal.
[b]Divided into tid doses.
[c]Divided doses: last dose by 6 pm and by noon if insomnia is a side effect.

more cognitive and affective aspects of depression (e.g., anhedonia, hopelessness, guilt, suicidal thoughts, low motivation). Initial improvement in sleep and appetite may be seen in some patients within the first 7–10 days of treatment, whereas a full 6 weeks at a therapeutic dose may be required before there is significant improvement of the symptoms of major depression.

It is possible to monitor the plasma level of tricyclic antidepressant medications; however, knowledge remains somewhat limited about the correlation between plasma levels and the clinical actions of antidepressants [30]. The association between plasma level and clinical effect is best documented for nortriptyline, which has a curvilinear response curve with a "therapeutic window" of 50–150 ng/ml. Routine monitoring is not recommended, but it still may be of value in specific situations, such as to assess nonresponders after a presumably adequate dose, in patients with comorbid medical conditions for whom it may be advantageous to use the lowest possible therapeutic dose, in patients for whom excessive side effects are problematic, or in patients for whom there are questions about compliance.

"Augmentation" techniques may be useful when there has been no response to standard doses of an antidepressant over an adequate duration of treatment. Drugs that enhance the activity of antidepressants include: triiodothyronine (T_3) [51], lithium [24], and other antidepressants (e.g., adding desipramine or trazodone to fluoxetine) [77]. Beneficial effects of adding lithium to a regimen of tricyclic antidepressants in three patients with fibromyalgia has been described [94].

Anxiety Disorders

In the treatment of anxiety disorders, it is important to distinguish among those patients who have recurrent and disruptive panic attacks requiring pharmacological blockade of the attacks, those with infrequent panic attacks for whom medication is used to symptomatically treat individual panic attacks, and those with a diagnosis of generalized anxiety disorder. Table 8 outlines the treatments for panic disorder.

Sleep Disorders

Treatment of the sleep disorders accompanying CFS is aimed at offering the patient a better quality of life and may actually bring about a decrease in symptoms, as has been documented in FM. Before embarking on pharmacotherapy for sleep difficulties, it is important to assess and advise CFS patients about basic sleep hygiene (e.g., limited caffeine-containing compounds, establishing a regular sleep–wake cycle, abolishing daytime napping, getting out of bed if not able to sleep). Medications used to treat sleep disorders in CFS are shown in Table 9.

Table 8 Pharmacotherapy of Panic Disorder in Chronic Fatigue Syndrome

Class	Example	Starting dose	Usual therapeutic dose	Frequency (%) of adverse effects at therapeutic doses [10,70]		Comments
				>10%	>30%	
Tricyclic anti-depressants	Desipramine	10 mg qhs	70–300 mg qhs	Dry mouth, tachycardia		
	Imipramine	10 mg qhs	75–300 mg qhs	Blurred vision, constipation, sweating, delayed micturition, drowsiness/sedation, insomnia, excitement/agitation, headache, fine tremor, tachycardia, GI distress, weight gain	Dry mouth, orthostatic hypotension	
Selective serotonin reuptake inhibitors	Fluoxetine	2.5 mg qam	2.5–20 mg qam	Insomnia, excitement/agitation, headache, anorexia, GI distress, fine tremor		

				Adverse effects	
Monoamine oxidase inhibitors	Phenelzine	15 mg qam	45–90 mg[a]	Dry mouth	
				Blurred vision excitement/agitation, insomnia, drowsiness/sedation, orthostatic hypotension, tachycardia, constipation, GI disturbance, weight gain, sexual disturbance	
Antipanic benzodiazepines	Alprazolam Clonazepam	0.25 mg tid 0.25 mg bid	1.5–6 mg[b] 0.75–3 mg[a]	*Adverse effects* Rare, often disappear with dosage adjustment CNS depression, drowsiness, ataxia, confusion, disorientation Abrupt discontinuation contraindicated Discontinuation can produce withdrawal, rebound, or relapse	Use in patients with personal or family history of alcohol or drug abuse is relatively contraindicated. Use in patients who have trouble containing anger should be avoided. Discontinuation should be by no more than 0.25–05 mg alprazolam equivalents/wk.

[a]Divided into bid or tid dosing.
[b]Divided into tid or qid dosing.

Table 9 Pharmacotherapy of Insomnia in Chronic Fatigue Syndrome

Class	Example	Starting dose	Usual therapeutic dose	Side effects [10,70]	Comments
L-Tryptophan		1 g qhs	1–5 g qhs	GI distress (nausea and vomiting)	Potential for hyperserotonergic syndrome (i.e., diaphoresis, hyperreflexia, myoclonus, nausea, diarrhea, restlessness) when used with other serotonergic drugs (e.g., SSRIs, MAOI)
Cyclopyrrolone	Zopiclone	3.75 mg qhs	7.5–15 mg qhs	Bitter taste, dry mouth, GI distress, "hangover"	
Antidepressants	Amitriptyline	10 mg qhs	10–50 mg hs	Dry mouth, blurred vision, constipation, orthostatic hypotension, "hangover"	If insomnia associated with significant mood disturbance, use medications and doses as in Table 7.
	Doxepine	10 mg qhs	10–50 mg hs	Dry mouth, blurred vision, constipation, drowsiness/sedation, orthostatic hypotension, weight gain, "hangover"	
	Trazondone	50 mg qhs	50–100 mg hs	GI distress (nausea), orthostatic hypotension, "hangover"	

CONCLUSIONS

Pharmacotherapy is an important component in the comprehensive rehabilitation of patients with CFS. The integration of pharmacotherapy with other treatment modalities including cognitive–behavioral therapy and psychotherapy has been described by Sharpe [87] and Wessely and colleagues [101].

Controlled trials of the use of psychotropic medication in CFS are eagerly awaited. In the interim, clinicians must be guided by the available literature and clinical wisdom as they collaborate with the patient in the goal of improving function and reducing distress.

As part of a comprehensive treatment program, pharmacotherapy can bring about a significant improvement in the quality of life for patients who struggle with an illness such as CFS that remains so incompletely understood.

REFERENCES

1. Abbey SE, Garfinkel PE. Chronic fatigue syndrome and the psychiatrist. Can J Psychiatry 1990, 35:625–33.
2. Abbey SE, Garfinkel PE. Chronic fatigue syndrome and depression: cause, effect or covariate. Rev Infect Dis 1991; 13(suppl 1):S73–83.
3. Adams F, Quesada JR, Gutterman JU. Neuropsychiatric manifestations of human leukocyte interferon therapy in patients with cancer. JAMA 1984; 252:938–41.
4. American Psychiatric Association. Diagnostic and statistical manual of mental disorders. 3rd ed, revised. Washington, DC: American Psychiatric Association, 1987.
5. American Psychiatric Association. DSM-IV draft criteria, 3/1/93. Washington, DC: American Psychiatric Association, 1993.
6. Barsky AJ, Goodson, JD, Lane RS, Cleary PD. The amplification of somatic symptoms. Psychosom Med 1988; 50:510–19.
7. Behan PO, Behan WMH, Bell EJ. The postviral fatigue syndrome—an analysis of the findings in 50 cases. J Infect 1985; 10:211–22.
8. Bennett RM, Gatter RA, Campbell SM, et al. A comparison of cyclobenzaprine and placebo in the management of fibrositis. Arthritis Rheum 1988; 31:1535–42.
9. Berlin RM, King SL, Blythe DG. Symptomatic improvement of chronic fatigue with fluoxetine in ciguatera fish poisoning. Med J Aust 1992; 157:567.
10. Bezchlibnyk-Butler KZ, Jeffries JJ. Clinical handbook of psychotropic drugs, 4th revised ed. Toronto: Hogrefe & Huber Publishers, 1994.
11. Buchwald D, Sullivan JL, Komaroff AL. Frequency of chronic active Epstein–Barr virus infection in a general medical practice. JAMA 1987; 257:2303–7.
12. Buchwald D, Goldenberg DL, Sullivan JL, Komaroff AL. The "chronic, active Epstein–Barr virus infection" syndrome and primary fibromyalgia. Arthritis Rheum 1987; 30:1132–6.
13. Buchwald D. Discussion of fibromyalgia, sleep disorder and CFS. In: Brock GR, Whelan J, eds. Chronic fatigue syndrome. Ciba Foundation Symposium 173. Toronto: John Wiley & Sons, 1993; 277–278.

14. Burszatjn H, Barsky AJ. Facilitating patient acceptance of a psychiatric referral. Arch Intern Med 1985; 145:73–5.

15. Butler S, Chalder T, Ron M, Wessely S. Cognitive behaviour therapy in chronic fatigue syndrome. J Neurol Neurosurg Psychiatry 1991; 54:153–8.

16. Cadet JL, Lohr JB. Neuropsychiatric aspects of infectious and inflammatory diseases of the central nervous system. In: Hales RE, Yudofsky SC, eds. The American Psychiatric Press textbook of neuropsychiatry. Washington, DC: American Psychiatric Press, 1987:339–50.

17. Cadie M, Nye FJ, Storey P. Anxiety and depression after infectious mononucleosis. Br J Psychiatry 1976; 128:559–61.

18. Carette S, McCain GA, Bell DA, et al. Evaluation of amitriptyline in primary fibrositis. Arthritis Rheum 1986; 29:655–9.

19. Caruso I, Sarzi Puttini PC, Boccassini L. Double-blind study of dothiepin versus placebo in the treatment of primary fibromyalgia syndrome. Int Med Res 1987; 15:154–9.

20. Caruso I, Sarzi Puttini P, Cazzola M, Azzolini V. Double-blind study of 5-hydroxytryptophan versus placebo in the treatment of primary fibromyalgia syndrome. J Int Med Res 1990; 18:201–9.

21. Cassem N. Depression. In: Cassem N, ed. Massachusetts General Hospital handbook of general hospital psychiatry. St. Louis: Mosby Year Book, 1991.

22. Clark DM. Anxiety states: panic and generalized anxiety. In: Hawton K, Salkovskis PM, Kirk J, Clark DM, eds. Cognitive behaviour therapy for psychiatric problems. Oxford: Oxford University Press, 1989:52–96.

23. Cowley DS, Roy-Byrne PP. Panic disorder: psychosocial aspects. Psychol Ann 1988; 18:464–7.

24. de Montigny D, Grunberg F, Mayer A. Lithium indices rapid relief of depression in tricyclic antidepressant drug non-responders. Br J Psychiatry 1981; 138:252–6.

25. Denicoff KD, Rubinow DR, Papa MZ, Simpson C, Seipp CA, Lotze MT, Change AE, Rosenstein D, Rosenberg SA. The neuropsychiatric effects of treatment with interleukin-2 and lymphokine-activated killer cells. Ann Intern Med 1987; 107:293–300.

26. Drewes AM, Andreasen A, Jennum P, Nielsen KD. Zopiclone in the treatment of sleep abnormalities in fibromyalgia. Scand J Rheumatol 1991; 20:288–93.

27. Dubois RE, Seeley JK, Brus, I, Sakamoto K, Ballow M, Harada S, Behtold TA, Pearson G, Purtilo DT. Chronic mononucleosis syndrome. South Med J 1984; 77:1376–82.

28. Finestone DH, Ober SK. Fluoxetine and fibromyalgia. JAMA 1990; 264:2869–70.

29. Folstein MFL, McHugh PR. The neuropsychiatry of some specific brain disorders. In: Lade M, ed. Mental disorders and somatic illness. vol 2. Handbook of psychiatry. Cambridge: Cambridge University Press, 1983: 107–18.

30. Gelenberg AJ, Bassuk EL, Schoonover SC. The practitioner's guide to psychoactive drugs. 3rd ed. New York: Plenum Medical, 1991.

31. Geller SA. Treatment of fibrositis with fluoxetine hydrochloride. Am J Med 1989; 87:594–5.

32. Gold D, Bowden R, Sixbey J, et al. Chronic fatigue: a prospective clinical and virologic study. JAMA 1990; 264:48–53.

33. Goldenberg DL, Felson DT, Dinerman H. A randomized controlled trial of amitriptyline and naproxen in the treatment of patients with fibromyalgia. Arthritis Rheum 1986; 29:1371–7.

34. Goldenberg DL. Fibromyalgia and its relation to chronic fatigue syndrome, viral illness and immune abnormalities. J Rheumatol 1989; 16(suppl 19):91–3.

35. Goldenberg DL. A review of the role of tricyclic medications in the treatment of fibromyalgia syndrome. J Rheumatol 1989; 16(suppl 19):137–9.

36. Goldenberg DL, Simms RW, Geiger A, Komaroff AL. High frequency of fibromyalgia in patients with chronic fatigue seen in a primary care practice. Arthritis Rheum 1990; 33:381–7.

37. Goodnick PJ, Extein I. Bupropion and fluoxetine in depressive subtypes. Ann Clin Psychiatry 1989; 1:119–22.

38. Goodnick PJ. Bupropion in chronic fatigue syndrome [letter]. Am J Psychiatry 1990; 147:1091.

39. Goodnick PJ, Sandoval R, Brickman AL, Klimas NG. Bupropion treatment of fluoxetine-resistant chronic fatigue syndrome. Biol Psychiatry 1992; 32:834–8.

40. Goodnick PJ, Sandoval R. Psychotropic treatment of chronic fatigue syndrome and related disorders. J Clin Psychiatry 1993; 54:13–20.

41. Gracious B, Wisner KL. Nortriptyline in chronic fatigue syndrome: a double blind, placebo-controlled single case study. Biol Psychiatry 1991; 30:405–8.

42. Greenwood R. Residual mental disorders after herpesvirus infections. In: Kurstak E, Lipowski ZJ, Morozov PV, eds. Viruses, immunity and mental disorders. New York: Plenum, 1987:65–80.

43. Guyatt GH, Heyting A, Jaeschke R, Keller J, Adachi JD, Roberts RS. N of 1 randomized trials for investigating new drugs. Contr Clin Trials 1990; 11:88–100.

44. Hamaty D, Valentine JL, Howard R, et al. The plasma endorphin, prostaglandin and catecholamine profile of patients with fibrositis treated with cyclobenzaprine and placebo: a 5-month study. J Rheumatol 1989; 16(suppl 19):164–8.

45. Hauri P, Hawkins DR. Alpha-delta sleep. Electroenceph Clin Neurophysiol 1973; 34:233–7.

46. Hendler N, Leahy W. Psychiatric and neurologic sequelae of infectious mononucleosis. Am J Psychiatry 1978; 135:842–4.

47. Hickie I, Lloyd A, Wakefield D, et al. The psychiatric status of patients with the chronic fatigue syndrome. Br J Psychiatry 1990; 156:534–40.

48. Holmes GP, Kaplan JE, Gantz NM, et al. Chronic fatigue syndrome: a working case definition. Ann Intern Med 1988; 108:387–9.

49. Hyman SE, Nestler EJ. The molecular foundations of psychiatry. Washington, DC: American Psychiatric Press, 1993.

50. Jaeschke R, Adachi J, Guyatt G, Keller J, Wong B. Clinical usefulness of amitriptyline in fibromyalgia: the results of 23 N-of-1 randomized controlled trials. J Rheumatol 1991; 18:447–51.

51. Joffe RT, Singer W. A comparison of triiodothyronine and thyroxine in the potentiation of tricyclic antidepressants. Psychiatry Res 1990; 32:241–51.

52. Jones JF, Ray CG, Minnich LL, Hicks MJ, Kibler R, Lucas DO. Evidence for active Epstein–Barr virus infection in patients with persistent, unexplained illnesses: elevated anti-early antigen antibodies. Ann Intern Med 1985; 102:1–7.

53. Jones JF, Straus SE. Chronic Epstein–Barr virus infection. Annu Rev Med 1987; 38:195–209.

54. Katon WJ, Buchwald DS, Simon GE, Russo JE, Mease PJ. Psychiatric illness in patients with chronic fatigue and those with rheumatoid arthritis. J Gen Intern Med 1991; 6:277–85.

55. Katon W. Panic disorder in the medical setting. Washington, DC: American Psychiatric Press, 1991.

56. Katon WJ, Walker EA. The relationship of chronic fatigue to psychiatric illness in community, primary care and tertiary care samples. In: Bock GR, Whelan J, eds. Chronic fatigue syndrome. Ciba Foundation Symposium 173. Toronto: John Wiley & Sons, 1993:193–211.

57. Katon W, Russo J. Chronic fatigue syndrome criteria: a critique of the requirement for multiple physical complaints. Arch Intern Med 1992; 152:1604–9.

58. Klimas NG, Morgan R, van Riel F, Fletcher MA. Observations regarding use of an antidepressant, fluoxetine, in chronic fatigue syndrome. In: Goodnick PJ, Klimas, NG, eds. Chronic fatigue and related immune deficiency syndromes. Washington, DC: American Psychiatric Press, 1993:95–108.

59. Kruesi MJP, Dale J, Straus SE. Psychiatric diagnoses in patients who have chronic fatigue syndrome. J Clin Psychiatry 1989; 50:53–6.

60. Krupp LB, Mendelson WB. Sleep disorders in chronic fatigue syndrome. In: Horn J, ed. Sleep '90. Bochum Pontenagel Press, 1990:261–3.

61. Lishman WA. Organic psychiatry: the psychological consequences of cerebral disorder. 2nd ed. Boston: Blackwell Scientific, 1987.

62. Lloyd A, Hickie I, Wakefield D, Boughton C, Dwyer J. A double-blind, placebo-controlled trial of intravenous immunoglobulin therapy in patients with chronic fatigue syndrome. Am J Med 1990; 89:561–8.

63. Lloyd AR, Hickie I, Brockman A, Hickie C, Wilson A, Dwyer J, Wakefield D. Immunologic and psychologic therapy for patients with chronic fatigue syndrome: a double-blind, placebo-controlled trial. Am J Med 1993; 94:197–203.

64. Lustman PJ, Harper GW, Griffith LS, Clouse RE. Use of the diagnostic interview schedule in patients with diabetes mellitus. J Nerv Ment Dis 1986; 174:743–6.

65. Lynch S, Seth R, Montgomery S. Antidepressant therapy in the chronic fatigue syndrome. Br J Gen Pract 1991; 41:339–42.

66. Manu P, Matthews DA, Lane TJ. Panic disorder among patients with chronic fatigue. South Med J 1991; 84:451–6.

67. Manu P, Lane TJ, Matthews DA. Chronic fatigue syndromes in clinical practice. Psychother Psychosom 1992; 58:60–8.

68. Marks IM. Fears, phobias and rituals: panic, anxiety and their disorders. New York: Oxford University Press, 1987.

69. Mattson K, Niiranen A, Iivanainen M, Farkkila M, Bergstron L, Holsti LR, Kauppinen J-L, Cantell K. Neurotoxicity of interferon. Cancer Treat Rep 1983; 67:958–61.

70. Maxmen JS. Psychotropic drugs: fast facts. New York: WW Norton & Co, 1991.

71. McBride SJ, McCluskey DR. Treatment of chronic fatigue syndrome. Br Med Bull 1991; 47:895–907.

72. Moldofsky H, Scarisbrick P, England R, Smythe H. Musculoskeletal symptoms and non-REM sleep disturbance in patients with "fibrositis syndrome" and healthy subjects. Psychosom Med 1975; 37:341–51.

73. Moldofsky H, Saskin P, Lue FA. Sleep and symptoms in fibrositis syndrome after febrile illness. J Rheumatol 1988; 15:1701–4.

74. Moldofsky H. Nonrestorative sleep and symptoms after a febrile illness in patients with fibrositis and chronic fatigue syndrome. J Rheumatol 1989; 16(suppl 19):150–3.

75. Moldofsky H. Fibromyalgia, sleep disorder and chronic fatigue syndrome. In: Brock GR, Whelan J, eds. Chronic fatigue syndrome. Ciba Foundation Symposium 173. Toronto: John Wiley & Sons, 1993; 262–79.

76. Morriss R, Sharpe M, Sharpley AL, Cowen PJ, Hawton K, Morris J. Abnormalities of sleep in patients with the chronic fatigue syndrome. Br Med J 1993; 306:1161–6.

77. Nelson JC, Mazure CM, Bowers MB, Jatlow PI. A preliminary open study of the combination of fluoxetine and desipramine for rapid treatment of major depression. Arch Gen Psychiatry 1991; 48:303–7.

78. Peterson PK, Shepard J, Macres M, Schenck C, Crosson J, Reichtman D, Lurie N. A controlled trial of intravenous immunoglobulin G in chronic fatigue syndrome. Am J Med 1990; 89:554–60.

79. Quimby LG, Gratwick GM, Whitney CD, Block SR. A randomized trial of cyclobenzaprine for the treatment of fibromyalgia. J Rheumatol 1989; 16(suppl 19):140–3.

80. Ray C. Chronic fatigue syndrome and depression: conceptual and methodological ambiguities. Psychol Med 1991; 21:1–9.

81. Reiman EM. The study of panic disorder using positron emission tomography. Psychiatry Dev 1987; 5:63–78.

82. Robins E, Guze SB. Suicide and primary affective disorder. Am J Psychiatry 1970; 126:107–11.

83. Rodin G, Craven J, Littlefield C. Depression in the medically ill: an integrated approach. New York: Brunner/Mazel, Publishers, 1991.

84. Salit IE. Sporadic postinfectious neuromyasthenia. Can Med Assoc J 1985; 133:659–63.

85. Saskin P, Moldofsky H, Lue FA. Sleep and posttraumatic rheumatic pain modulation disorder (fibrositis syndrome). Psychosom Med 1986; 43:319–23.

86. Scudds RA, McCain G. Rollman GB, Harth M. Improvements in pain responsiveness in patients with fibrositis after successful treatment with amitriptyline. J Rheumatol 1989; 16(suppl 19):98–103.

87. Sharpe M. Psychiatric management of PVFS. Br Med Bull 1991; 47:989–1005.

88. Smedley H, Katrak M, Sikora K, Wheeler T. Neurological effects of recombinant human interferon. Br Med J 1983; 286:262–4.

89. Stewart D. Emotional disorders misdiagnosed as physical illness: environmental hypersensitivity, candidiasis hypersensitivity, and chronic fatigue syndrome. Int J Ment Health 1990; 19:56–68.

90. Straus SE, Tosato G, Armstrong G, Lawley T, Preble OT, Henle W, Davey R, Pearson G, Epstein J, Brus I, Blaese RM. Persisting illness and fatigue in adults with evidence of Epstein–Barr virus infection. Ann Intern Med 1985; 102:7–16.

91. Straus SE, Dale JK, Tobi M, Lawley T, Preble O, Blaese RM, Hallahan C, Henle W. Acyclovir treatment of the chronic fatigue syndrome: lack of efficacy in a placebo-controlled trial. N Engl J Med 1988; 319:1692–8.

92. Taerk GS, Toner BB, Salit IE, Garfinkel PE, Ozersky S. Depression in patients

with neuromyasthenia (benign myalgic encephalomyelitis). Int J Psychiatry Med 1987; 17:49–56.

93. Tavoni A, Vitali C, Bombardier D, et al. Evaluation of *S*-adenosylmethionine in primary fibromyalgia. Am J Med 1987; 83(suppl A):107–10.

94. Tyber M. Lithium carbonate augmentation therapy in fibromyalgia. Can Med Assoc J 1990; 143:902–4.

95. Webb HE, Parsons LM. Treatment of the post-viral fatigue syndrome—rationale for the use of antidepressants. In: Jenkins R, Mowbray J, eds. Post-viral fatigue syndrome. Chichester: John Wiley & Sons, 1991:297–304.

96. Wells KB, Stewart A, Hays RD, Burnham A, Rogers W, Daniels M, Berry S, Greenfield S, Ware J. The functioning and well-being of depressed patients: results from the medical outcome study. JAMA 1989; 262:914–9.

97. Weissman MM, Klerman GL, Markowitz JS, Ouellette R. Suicidal ideation and suicide attempts in panic disorders and attacks. N Engl J Med 1989; 321:1209–14.

98. Wessely S, Powell R. Fatigue syndromes: a comparison of chronic "postviral" fatigue with neuromuscular and affective disorders. J Neurol Neurosurg Psychiatry 1989; 52:940–8.

99. Wessely S, David A, Butler S, Chalder T. Management of chronic (post-viral) fatigue syndrome. J R Coll Gen Pract 1989; 39:26–9.

100. Wessely S. Old wine in new bottles: neurasthenia and "ME." Psychol Med 1990; 20:35–53.

101. Wessely S, Butler S, Chalder T, David A. The cognitive behavioural management of the post-viral fatigue syndrome. In: Jenkins R, Mowbray J, eds. Post-viral fatigue syndrome. Chichester: John Wiley & Sons, 1991:305–34.

102. Wessely S. The neuropsychiatry of CFS. In: Brock GR, Whelan J, eds. Chronic fatigue syndrome. Ciba Foundation Symposium 173. Toronto: John Wiley & Sons, 1993:212–37.

103. Whelton C, Salit I, Moldofsky H. Sleep, Epstein–Barr virus infection, musculoskeletal pain, and depressive symptoms in chronic fatigue syndrome. J Rheumatol 1992; 19:939–43.

104. Wood GC, Bentall RP, Gopfert M, Edwards RHT. A comparative psychiatric assessment of patients with chronic fatigue syndrome and muscle disease. Psychol Med 1991; 21:619–28.

105. Wysenbeek AJ, Mor F, Lurie Y, Weinberger A. Imipramine for the treatment of fibrositis: a therapeutic trial. Ann Rheum Dis 1985; 44:752–3.

106. Demitrack MA, Gold PW, Dale JK, Krahn DD, Kling MA, Straus SE. Plasma and cerebrospinal fluid monoamine metabolism in patients with chronic fatigue syndrome: preliminary findings. Biol Psychiatry 1992; 32:1065–77.

107. Moldofsky H, Warsh JJ. Plasma tryptophan and musculoskeletal pain in nonarticular rheumatism (fibrositis syndrome). Pain 1978; 5:65–71.

108. Morgane PJ. Monoamine theories of sleep: the role of serotonin—a review. Psychopharm Bull 1981; 17:13–17.

17

Cognitive–Behavioral Therapy and the Treatment of Chronic Fatigue Syndrome

Michael Sharpe
University of Oxford and Warneford Hospital,
Oxford, England

Frequently the patient remarks, "Yes doctor, I have done as you said, but I feel so tired." "That may be true" is the reply, "but you were just as tired last week, and then you were accomplishing nothing. The difference is that today you are so much nearer the goal."

G. A. Waterman 1909 [1]

In this chapter I will discuss the place of cognitive–behavioral therapy (CBT) in the management of patients who present with chronic fatigue syndrome (CFS). The chapter is organized as follows:

What is CBT?
Why treat CFS with CBT?
A cognitive–behavioral theory of CFS
Evidence for the efficacy of CBT in CFS
Practical guidelines for treatment

WHAT IS COGNITIVE–BEHAVIORAL THERAPY?

In addition to administering physical treatments, the good physician teaches patients about the nature of their illness and advises them about what they must do to enhance their recovery. Cognitive–behavioral therapy can be seen as a

435

specialized development of this traditional aspect of medical practice. Hence, the aim of CBT is to facilitate recovery by helping the patients reevaluate how they think about and manage their illness [2].

The Importance of Cognitions

The term *cognition* refers to a person's thoughts and beliefs. Cognative–behavioral therapy is based on the assumption that cognitions play an important role in determining a persons emotional state and behavior. Consequently, if those cognitions are inaccurate, unduly alarming, or excessively pessimistic, there will be important negative consequences for the patient. For example, if a man recovering from a myocardial infarction believes that even gentle exertion is very likely to trigger a life-threatening recurrence, he will feel understandably anxious when encouraged to increase his level of exercise, and he is likely to avoid doing so. Similarly, a patient who mistakenly believes that there is nothing he or she can do about their illness, is likely to feel helpless and depressed, and to make little active effort toward recovery.

By their influence on behavior and emotional state, cognitions can also influence physiological function (Fig. 1). Cognitions that lead to complete avoidance of exercise will have profound and predictable consequences, including loss of muscular and cardiovascular fitness, and a progressive reduction in the capacity for exercise [3]. Cognitions that arouse anxiety will increase activity in the sympathetic nervous system, resulting in tachycardia, breathlessness, and sweating [4], and those that tend to depress mood lead to sleep disturbance and loss of energy [5].

The Practice of Cognitive–Behavioral Therapy

If cognitions play an important role in a patient's distress, disability and pathophysiology, it should be possible to improve his or her condition by changing them; CBT is a form of psychotherapy that aims to do just this.

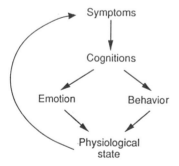

Figure 1 The central place of cognition in mediating behavioral, emotional, and physiological consequences of symptoms.

The initial task of CBT is to determine the presence and nature of illness-perpetuating cognitions. This is achieved by interview, and by the patient recording illness-related thoughts in a diary. Those thoughts and beliefs that may be considered to be either inaccurate or unhelpful can then be reevaluated. Reevaluation is achieved by examining with the patients the evidence on which their belief is based. This evidence comes both from medical research, and from the patient's own experience. Hence, once it has been determined that a cardiac patient who remained disproportionately disabled after myocardial infarction is unnecessarily fearful of activity, his or her belief in the likelihood of an exercise-induced recurrence can be examined. For some patients a review of the medical evidence may be sufficient to convince them that they have overestimated the risk, but for others the personal experience of being active without mishap is necessary. Therefore, CBT uses both discussion and planned "behavioral experiments" in which the patient tries out previously avoided activities to determine whether his or her beliefs are accurate and whether the feared negative consequences actually occur.

Applications of Cognitive-Behavioral Therapy

Cognitive therapy was initially developed as a treatment for anxiety and depression. This form of therapy is now the treatment of choice for phobias, and is of proved effectiveness in panic, eating disorders, and depression [6]. A second application of CBT is as an adjunct to pharmacological therapy in the treatment of physical disease, where CBT has been shown to improve patients' well-being, functioning, and quality of life [7]. A third application is in the treatment of patients with physical symptoms unexplained by organic disease. Cognitive therapy has been shown in clinical trials to be effective in reducing distress, symptoms, and disability in patients with atypical chest pain, back pain, headache, irritable bowel syndrome, and hypochondriasis [reviewed in 8].

WHY TREAT CHRONIC FATIGUE SYNDROME WITH COGNITIVE—BEHAVIORAL THERAPY?
Chronic Fatigue Syndrome Is a Syndrome Not a Disease

Fatigue is among the most common of patients' complaints [9]. A small proportion of such patients will have well-recognized and treatable organic disease. Usually, however, no pathological process can be identified [10]. The illness may then be regarded as "idiopathic." A patient whose fatigue is idiopathic, persistent, and causing impairment of physical and mental functioning may be diagnosed as suffering from CFS [11,12], a condition associated with considerable distress, disability, and occupational morbidity [13]. Attempts have been made to delineate specific fatigue syndromes from the large heterogeneous category [14] of "idiopathic chronic fatigue." These include more restrictively defined chronic fatigue syndromes [15,16], "postviral fatigue syndrome" [17], and "myalgic encephalomyelitis" (ME) [18]. Although each has its advocates, none of these specific syndromes have yet been validated by the identification of a particular etiology, prognosis, or response to treatment [19]; therefore, a broad definition of CFS is preferred [20].

However, patients who meet criteria for this broadly defined CFS may also fulfil criteria for other syndromes of uncertain cause in which fatigue and pain are prominent symptoms [19]. These include chronic pain syndromes [21], fibromyalgia [22], and anxiety and depressive disorders [23]. Chronic fatigue syndrome is also clinically similar to neurasthenia [24,25] and effort syndrome [26], conditions prevalent in the earlier years of this century.

There Are No Specific Treatments for Chronic Fatigue Syndrome

There is, as yet, no accepted therapy for patients with CFS. The etiology is controversial. Treatments aimed at modifying hypothetical pathological processes, such as persistent virus infection or impaired immune function, have not been effective and are expensive and invasive to administer [27,28].

A Pragmatic Approach Is Appropriate

There is a case, therefore, for taking a pragmatic approach to therapy. This approach does not seek to identify occult causes of CFS, but rather, concentrates on the modification of identifiable factors that may be inhibiting recovery in the particular patient being treated. An individual assessment is required to identify those factors that (1) are likely to be playing a role in perpetuating that particular patient's symptoms, distress, and disability, and (2) are amenable to modification. The factors likely to be identified by this approach are listed in Table 1.

Inactivity and Lack of Physical Fitness
Marked reductions in activity are typical of many patients with CFS, some resorting to prolonged periods of bed rest. Many patients are physically unfit

Table 1 Factors That May Perpetuate CFS

Lack of physical fitness
Depression and anxiety
Sleep disturbance
Chronic life stresses
Inaccurate or unhelpful illness beliefs

[29]. Inactivity causes a range of physical and mental symptoms, similar to those reported by patients with CFS. These include muscle wasting, changes in the cardiovascular response to exertion, depressed mood, postural hypotension, and impaired thermoregulation [30]. In the inactive person, these effects can be reversed by a program of gradual increases in activity [31], although this may result in transient exacerbations of certain symptoms, particularly muscle pain [32]. Such graded increases in overall activity level are a central component of general rehabilitation programs [33]. There also is evidence that graded increases in activity are of benefit to patients with the syndromes of fibromyalgia [34], and anxiety and depression of mild to moderate severity [35].

Depression and Anxiety

Depression and anxiety are highly prevalent in almost all systematic descriptions of patients diagnosed as suffering from CFS [36,37]. Fatigue, impaired concentration, muscular pains, and other symptoms of CFS are common features of the syndromes of depression and anxiety [4,5]. Indeed, patients with CFS may be symptomatically indistinguishable from those with uncomplicated depression [23]. Anxiety and depression may be effectively treated with antidepressant drugs. However, patients with CFS are often intolerant of such medication [13]. Cognitive–behavioral therapy is an alternative approach to treatment of these conditions, which has been found, at least in some studies, to be of similar efficacy to drug therapy [38,39].

Sleep Disturbance

Both subjectively reported and objectively measurable disturbance of sleep patterns are common in patients with CFS [13,40]. The observed abnormalities include excessive sleep, and interrupted or inadequate sleep, both of which can cause daytime fatigue [41]. These sleep disturbances can be treated using cognitive and behavioral techniques [42].

Life Stresses

Careful inquiry into the life circumstances of patients with CFS frequently reveals major ongoing social stresses and difficulties, particularly in the areas of employment and relationships [37]. Such difficulties are known to exacerbate anxiety and depression, and may inhibit functional recovery from illness. Patients with CFS can be helped to tackle and resolve such difficulties during treatment with CBT using practical problem-solving techniques [43].

Illness-Related Cognitions

Patients with CFS commonly believe that they have a serious physical disease, despite the absence of abnormal physical findings [23]. Consequently, they are fearful of doing anything that causes an exacerbation of their symptoms, in the belief that this will lead to prolonged disability and deterioration of the disease

[13]. Such beliefs are likely to perpetuate distress and disability, and to discourage rehabilitation. Cognitive–behavioral therapy is well suited to helping patients reevaluate such beliefs [2].

Therefore, it can be argued, on purely pragmatic grounds, that CBT has a place in the management of patients with CFS. This form of treatment could plausibly help patients cope more effectively with the illness, whatever its original cause, and whether or not persistent viral infection and immune dysfunction are playing a role.

A COGNITIVE–BEHAVIORAL THEORY OF CHRONIC FATIGUE SYNDROME

A more radical case has been made for the application of CBT to CFS. Exponents of this view argue that the illness-related cognitions and associated behavior observed in patients with CFS do not merely determine adjustment to a mystery illness, but are actually play a central role in perpetuating the illness [44,45].

Such a cognitive–behavioral theory of CFS aims to describe how certain cognitions and behaviors could account for the symptoms, distress, and disability that constitute CFS [44,46]. Interestingly, this idea is not new. The theory is similar to those proposed many years ago for neurasthenia [47], and effort syndrome [48], and more recently chronic pain [49], fibromyalgia [50], and other medically unexplained syndromes [8].

A cognitive–behavioral theory of CFS was first proposed by Wessely et al. in London [44]. This model focused on the avoidance of activity. The cognitive–behavioral theory developed in Oxford pays more attention to the patients' cognitions. It is based on two principal assumptions:

Cognitions Play a Central Role in Perpetuating the Symptoms, Distress, and Disability

Clinical experience of patients with CFS suggests that three main types of cognitions are likely to lead to perpetuation of the illness. These concern the nature of the illness, the significance of the symptoms, and the patient's ability to perform his or her normal activities.

Beliefs About Illness

Patients commonly believe that they have a mysterious, untreatable, physical disease, best managed by prolonged rest [23]. A detailed history often reveals how the mystery and uncertainty surrounding CFS led to the adoption of this belief. In the early stages, their own doctor may have failed to provide them with a convincing explanation of, or effective therapy for, their illness [51]. At the same time, magazine articles, patient self-help literature, and alternative medical therapists confidently offered a simple explanation in terms of a physical disease, such as postviral fatigue syndrome or Myalgic Encephalomyelitis. Accounts of these "mystery illnesses" are often accompanied by strong advice to rest [13]. Although the patient may also have been offered explanations of his or her symptoms in terms of emotional disorder (anxiety and depression), patients frequently prefer an explanation that does not carry the social stigma of inadequacy, blame, and personal weakness, associated with mental illness [52].

The cognitive—behavioral theory assumes that belief in a primarily physical disease as a cause for the symptoms is both inaccurate and unhelpful to the patient. It is inaccurate because, although various biological abnormalities have been identified in patients with CFS, no disease process has yet been established [12]. On the contrary, in many patients, the symptoms can be more easily explained as resulting from known and modifiable psychological and physiological processes [30]. A belief in physical disease may also be considered unhelpful to patients if it focuses their attention on the somatic symptoms [53], leads them to pursue ineffective and potentially damaging rest [13], encourages them to seek ineffective and often expensive "cures," and fosters neglect of relevant psychological and interpersonal problems.

Beliefs About Symptoms

Patients frequently believe that the exacerbation of symptoms by activity indicates that the activity is worsening the disease process [13]. The evidence that gives rise to this belief may originate from two sources. The first is the patient's own observation that repeated attempts to increase his or her level of activity cause increased fatigue, muscular pains, and other symptoms. The second is the advice that the patient may have received from some self-help groups, nonmedical therapists, and doctors to stay within the "limits of the illness" [18].

The cognitive—behavioral theory assumes that these cognitions are both inaccurate and unhelpful. Although sudden or large increases in activity are likely to cause a temporary increase in symptoms, these exacerbations are understandable in terms of physical deconditioning, unaccustomed muscle use [32], and anxiety [54], and do not imply disease. These beliefs about the meaning of symptoms are also unhelpful to the patient if they lead to excessive limitation of activities, anxiety about somatic symptoms, and to the adoption of a lifestyle whereby symptoms dictate activity.

Beliefs About Performance and Responsibility

The third type of cognition of potential relevance to the perpetuation of CFS includes beliefs about performance and responsibility that make the resumption of normal activity after illness difficult. Our own experience of treating patients with CFS indicates that an extreme need to perform to a high standard [55], to meet all the expectations of others [56], and to always be emotionally strong, is common in patients referred to hospital with CFS. These beliefs are likely to be long-standing and may have contributed to the high level of achievement and stoicism reputed to characterize the personalities of persons who develop CFS [29,56].

The cognitive–behavioral theory assumes that the extreme form of these beliefs makes them both unrealistic and unhelpful to the patient. They are unrealistic because their rigidity does not take into account the inevitable fluctuations in the person's health or priorities. They lead the person holding them to overestimate what he or she can realistically expect of him or herself. They are unhelpful because the continual comparison of current performance with high premorbid standards leads to perceived failure, self-criticism, anxiety, and ultimately depression.

Cognitions, Behavior, Emotion, and Physiology Interact

It is hypothesized that the cognitions described perpetuate illness by leading to certain coping behaviors, emotional responses, and physiological states. The cognitions, behavior, emotion, and physiology then interact in self-perpetuating vicious circles.

Illness Onset

The cognitive–behavioral model proposes that the illness may be precipitated by stress, by infection, or by a combination of these factors. In the face of adversity, the patient who holds the aforementioned personal beliefs about performance and weakness tends to push on without complaining, until he or she eventually collapses with exhaustion. An explanation in terms of postviral fatigue offers a plausible explanation, and also avoids the stigma of blame, weakness, and failure associated with a psychological explanation. Once the illness has become viewed as a physical disease, medical, rather than psychological, help is sought. Difficulties in work or relationships may remain unresolved, while rest and sleep are pursued in an attempt to regain energy.

The pursuit of rest may alleviate symptoms in the short term. In the longer term, chronic inactivity, disturbed sleep, and emotional distress tend to have the opposite effect. Increasing psychological and physiological intolerance of physical and mental activity results. However, unmet responsibilities will tend to lead the typically conscientious CFS sufferers to make anxious attempts to regain their previous levels of activity. Their physiological and psychological state dooms these attempts to failure and gives rise to activity-associated increases in symptoms. Anxiety and depression are reinforced and further attempts at tackling problems and meeting responsibilities avoided.

Thus, it is possible to see how the patient with CFS could become locked into a self-perpetuating cycle of symptoms, unhelpful thoughts and beliefs, causing avoidance of activity, emotional distress, and physiological changes, which themselves, lead to further symptoms and so on (Fig. 2).

HOW EFFECTIVE IS COGNITIVE–BEHAVIORAL THERAPY IN THE TREATMENT OF CHRONIC FATIGUE SYNDROME?

Several centers are already treating patients with CFS using a cognitive–behavioral approach. To date, however, there have been only two published studies that have formally evaluated CBT in samples of patients specifically diagnosed as having CFS. Other studies are currently in progress, including a controlled trial in Oxford.

The National Hospital Study

The first study was a carefully evaluated case series of outpatients and inpatients at the National Hospital For Nervous Diseases in London [57] (Table 2). The form of CBT employed in this study focused on overcoming avoidance of activity. Treatment was by a skilled nurse–therapist for a mean of 7.5 hr over a

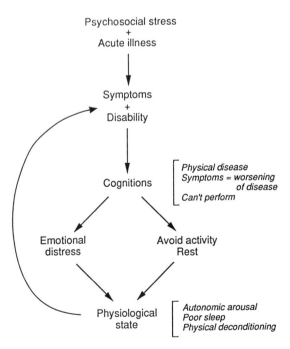

Figure 2 An outline of the cognitive–behavioral model of CFS.

Table 2 National Hospital Study

Parameter	Definition
Setting	Tertiary referral neurological hospital in UK
Patients	50 patients with CFS (Oxford criteria)
Design	Uncontrolled case series
Treatment	Behavioral therapy (mean 7.5 hr) and antidepressant medication (20 patients)
Results	32 patients agreed to treatment
	22 improved at end of therapy
Conclusion	Patients can improve
	Behavioral therapy may be useful

number of months. Patients who met criteria for depressive disorders were also treated with an antidepressant drug.

Fifty severely disabled patients who met the criteria for CFS [11] were offered treatment. Eighteen patients refused. Of the 32 patients treated, there was a clinically significant improvement in symptoms and functioning for 22/32 (69%), which was maintained at 3 months follow-up. The improvements in many cases were marked, and resulted in return to work. However five patients dropped out before treatment was completed, and four were judged to be unchanged at completion of treatment. One patient deteriorated, an outcome that the authors ascribe to a worsening depressive disorder

Although these results were encouraging, the study suffered from methodological limitations. First, it did not include a control group or independent assessment of outcome. Second, the refusal and dropout rate was too high to adequately evaluate its effectiveness. Finally, the use of combined pharmacological and nonpharmacological treatment makes it difficult to determine which was the most important. Nonetheless, this study indicated that something could be done for patients with CFS, and highlighted the potential application of CBT as a treatment.

The Prince Henry Hospital Study

The second published study was from Sydney, Australia [58] (Table 3). This was a controlled trial of CBT, compared with medical management, in combination with a trial of immunotherapy and placebo in a four-cell design. The patients all met the Australian criteria for CFS [15]. The form of CBT was similar to that employed in the National Hospital Study, with an emphasis on graded increases in activity. There was also an explanatory booklet and involvement of family members. The therapy was administered by a psychiatrist and was relatively brief (six biweekly sessions of less than 1 hr).

Table 3 Prince Henry Hospital Study

Parameter	Definition		
Setting	Tertiary referral fatigue clinic in Australia		
Patients	68 patients meeting Australian criteria for CFS		
Design	Randomized controlled trial (4 cells)		
		Immunotherapy	Placebo
	CBT	1	2
	Standard medical care	3	4
Treatment	Behavioral (less than 6 hr)		
Results	All patients improved in mood and fatigue		
	No specific effect of CBT		
Conclusion	This type of therapy no better than supportive medical care		

Sixty-eight patients were recruited, and none either refused CBT or dropped out from this treatment. The results indicated that this form of CBT offered little benefit over standard medical management in terms of reduction of fatigue, distress, or disability. Both groups experienced a reduction in fatigue and depression over the 7-month follow-up period, but no reduction in disability.

One might conclude from this study that CBT is no more effective than careful medical follow-up in patients with CFS. However, we first need to ask whether the design of the study was capable of answering this question and, in particular, whether the form of CBT given was appropriate. The CBT used focused on the benefits of increased activity, but had three major limitations. First it was too brief. The patients had been ill for a mean of 5.5 years and as long as 28 years, and it is unrealistic to expect that such brief treatment could make much impact in such chronic cases. Indeed, the results suggest that the therapy did not even produce an increase in the patients' overall level of activity. Second, the therapy does not appear to have questioned the patients' attribution of symptoms to organic disease. Indeed, the patients' belief that they had a primarily physical disease, requiring medical treatment, may have been unwittingly reinforced by the design of the study, which required that patients also receive injections. The authors' observation that patient improvement was correlated with their *belief* that they had received active immunotherapy supports this contention. Third, although it is reported that many of the patients were suffering from depressive disorder, neither the content nor the duration of the therapy was adequate to address this component of the illness.

Given the shortcomings of the form of CBT employed and in the design of this study, it is not surprising that little benefit was observed. Better-designed trials of more potent forms of CBT are required.

The Oxford Study

We are currently conducting a randomized, controlled trial of outpatient CBT. Patients who meet criteria for CFS [46] are recruited from an infectious disease outpatient clinic. A total of 60 patients will be randomized either to "treatment as usual" or to CBT. Treatment as usual comprises (usually conservative) management by the general practitioner, and "alternative" therapies sought by the patient. The CBT consist of 16, 1-hr sessions of individual CBT from a psychiatrist or psychologist, given over 4 months. The therapy is based on the cognitive theory of CFS, as described in the foregoing, and is tailored to the individual. As well as graded increases in activity, the therapy addresses the patients' attribution of symptoms to physical disease, unrealistic expectations of themselves, and the negative thinking of depression. Outcome is measured in terms of global ratings, symptom severity, and functional impairment.

The intervention employed in this study may not be optimal. For some patients even 16 sessions is likely to be too brief. Furthermore, combining CBT with more closely supervized activity programs or with antidepressant drug treatment may confer additional benefits. However, our preliminary results indicate that it is possible to engage almost all patients in this form of therapy, and that most are able to increase their level of activity. We have found that therapy is often difficult to complete in even 16 sessions. This is because, although patients are initially reluctant to consider the relevance of psychological factors, once this block is overcome, major sources of dissatisfaction (such as choice of career, relationships with family) often emerge. The reduction of depression and anxiety may depend on the resolution of these problems.

Although almost all the patients we have treated have improved, final judgment about the effectiveness of this form of CBT, as compared with standard medical care, will have to await completion of the trial. A brief outline of the treatment follows.

PRACTICAL GUIDELINES

For the reader interested in learning more about cognitive therapy there are several useful texts [e.g., 2,59]. There are also specialist accounts of the application of CBT to medically unexplained somatic symptoms [8]. Finally, there are several descriptions of the application of CBT specifically to patients with CFS [44–46,57]. The main components of CBT for CFS are shown in Table 4.

Assessment

Individual assessment is essential, as the importance of the various etiological factors may vary among individuals. The assessing physician should first ensure that the patient is not suffering from a medical or psychiatric illness that requires

Table 4 CBT in the Treatment of CFS

Assessment
   Exclude physical disease
   Assess cognitions and behaviors
Engagement in treatment
   Agree formulation of illness
   Agree realistic and valued goals
Cognitive components
   Education about CFS
   Reduce concern about symptoms
   Challenge excessive perfectionism
   Problem-solving
Behavioral components
   Graded increase in activity
   Relaxation

specific treatment. This can be achieved by a careful medical and psychiatric history and examination. The use of extensive laboratory investigation is unrewarding [60] and may be psychologically harmful to the patient by increasing their concern about missed organic disease. The assessment should also determine the presence of depression, anxiety, sleep disturbance, and inquire into the patient's beliefs and concerns about the nature, cause, and effects of his or her illness.

Engagement in Treatment

Patients are more likely to agree to treatment if they feel the therapist accepts their illness as real and not "all in the mind." The therapist should describe how it can be understood by using the theory outlined, together with the information gathered during the assessment, to produce an individualized account.

Many patients will have spent a considerable amount of time looking for a specific physical cause for their fatigue, in the hope that this will lead to a simple cure. The failure of this search to produce a solution should be discussed. The patient is then invited to try the alternative approach of CBT for a set period (say 4 months) so that the possible benefits of this "new" approach can be assessed.

Goals for treatment should be explicitly negotiated and agreed with the patient. Goals should be clearly defined and based on what the patient would realistically like to be able to do in the future. It is important to also explicitly discuss continuing medical investigation and parallel treatments. The continuation of these is likely to be a distraction from the CBT.

Specific Techniques

For clarity cognitive and behavioral components of treatment are described separately, although they are usually employed in parallel.

Cognitive Components

There are four main components: The first is to provide education about the nature of CFS and the relevance of cognitions to its perpetuation. Patients have often read a great deal about the condition, not all of which is either accurate or helpful. The therapist should be honest, direct, and as consistent as is possible within the limitations of our current understanding.

The second component is concerned with reducing excessive concern about activity-induced symptoms. When increases in activity level result in a short-term exacerbation of fatigue and other symptoms, the patient is likely to have thoughts such as: "If I do more I'll be unwell for days." Patients are asked to keep a record of these thoughts and, in discussion with the therapist, to generate less catastrophic alternatives, such as "I'm bound to feel more fatigued initially because I am not used to exercise, but with practice I will be able to do more." The evidence for and against these alternative propositions should be reviewed. If evidence is lacking "behavioral experiments" can be performed. For example, by recording symptoms carefully while gradually increasing activity, it is possible to test the hypothesis that increases in activity will lead to a persistent increase in symptoms.

The third cognitive component is the challenging of the patient's belief that they must always perform at premorbid levels. "All-or-nothing" perfectionistic beliefs about standards and responsibilities may be maintaining depressed mood, and must be questioned if graded increases in behavior are to be achieved. Such cognitions may also be perpetuating emotional distress. Repeated challenging of negative thoughts about failure may be necessary to alleviate anxiety and depression.

The final cognitive component is helping the patient to deal with life problems. Occupational and interpersonal difficulties may become serious obstacles to recovery unless the patient has a strategy for dealing with them. Problem-solving techniques can help the patient break down problems into manageable components, and to generate more effective solutions.

Behavioral Components

The adoption of increases in activity is planned as a behavioral experiment. The aim is to provide the patient with evidence that activity may be performed without harm. The emphasis, therefore, is on practicing activities at regular intervals, regardless of the occurrence of symptoms. These activities should be consistent with the patient's short-term goals. They may include walking, swimming, domestic tasks, and socializing. Tasks are graded in terms of how difficult they are, and introduced gradually in stages. During the early stages of treatment, the patient will experience an increase in symptoms, and it is imperative that the therapist predicts this. The symptoms usually decrease over time, and when they are associated with anxiety, may be reduced by relaxation techniques. In addition to carrying out the planned activity, the patient should also have planned rest. Only when symptom reduction or increased tolerance to activity has occurred are new targets set.

Treatment Sessions

Outpatients are usually seen for approximately 1 hr at a time. Typically between 5 and 20 sessions are required. Each session should begin with setting an agenda. There are usually several issues to work on, and it is important to cover the essential ones in the time allowed. Once treatment is under way, the general approach remains the same. Homework tasks are reviewed and problems discussed. The emphasis is on self-help.

Treatment Issues

Several important issues must be considered in planning treatment:

Treatment of Depression

Depressive disorder merits treatment, whether it is considered to be a primary or a secondary problem. Both CBT and increasing activity will tend to reduce depression. If depression is severe, treatment with antidepressant medication is indicated.

Inpatient Versus Outpatient

Most patients can be treated as outpatients. However, if the patient is bed-bound, inpatient treatment may be required. There are difficulties in using medical wards for this purpose unless nurses are trained in behavioral therapy. The principles of treatment are the same as for outpatients, but the goals for activity may have to be initially very modest (e.g., getting out of bed for meals).

Insurance Benefits

Problems may also arise if the patient requests a diagnosis the doctor feels is inappropriate, or wants certification of permanent invalidity. Although many patients are severely disabled, this should not be considered a *permanent* state until an adequate trial of treatment has been undertaken. The loss of existing benefits without guarantee of alternative income is a potential obstacle to recovery.

Treatment Problems

Problems commonly arise in treatment and can be predicted from the theory outlined in the foregoing.

Failure to Achieve an Increase in the Patient's Activity

The most likely reasons for the patient failing to increase his or her activity level are (1) too large an increase in activity was planned, (2) the patient has doubts about the safety or value of the treatment, (3) there is some other block to increasing activity, such as fear of failure. The problem is best managed by reviewing and revising the targets and eliciting and challenging any inaccurate or exaggerated concerns about the significance of symptoms and implications of failure.

Unwillingness by the Patient to Accept That Psychological Factors Are Relevant to Treatment

Patients may express a marked unwillingness to accept any treatment that is seen to imply that they have psychological problems or psychiatric illness. Clinical experience suggests that the objection to psychological approaches commonly results from a concern that, if the illness is labeled as psychological or psychiatric, it implies fault or weakness on the part of the patient. This erroneous belief should be specifically addressed.

Lack of Patient Enthusiasm About Treatment Goals

Initial progress may stall as the patient approaches an initially agreed goal (e.g., return to premorbid career). It is important to ensure that the target is desired by, and of real value to, the patient. A review of goals may be required.

CONCLUSIONS

There are strong arguments for considering the use of CBT in the treatment of patients with CFS. It is possible to engage almost all patients in cognitive–behavioral treatment. There is some evidence that this approach can improve disability and symptoms in at least a proportion. The overall efficacy of, and indications for, CBT in CFS require further clarification. Questions about the effectiveness of CBT in CFS are more complicated than they first seem. Cognitive therapy is not a unitary treatment, but rather, a therapeutic approach. The cognitive–behavioral theory of CFS is still being developed, and the optimum type and duration of CBT required remains uncertain. Furthermore, CFS as a diagnosis is unlikely to represent a unitary condition. A more realistic question is, therefore, which form of CBT (if any) is effective in which patients with CFS. Despite these uncertainties CBT already offers a logical alternative to therapeutic nihilism.

ACKNOWLEDGMENTS

I wish to acknowledge the contribution of Dr. Simon Wessely, Ms Trudie Chalder, Ms Ann Hackman, Dr. Christina Surawy, Ms Ivana Klimes, and Dr. Keith Hawton to the development of a cognitive–behavioral approach to chronic fatigue syndrome. The Oxford study is supported by the Wellcome Trust.

REFERENCES

1. Waterman GA. The treatment of fatigue states. J Abnorm Psychol 1909; 4:128–39.
2. Cognitive behaviour therapy for psychiatric problems: a practical guide. Oxford: Oxford Medical Publications, 1989.
3. Kottke FJ. The effect of limitation of activity upon the human body. JAMA 1966; 196:825–30.
4. Tyrer P. Institute of Psychiatry Maudsley monograph 23: the role of bodily feelings in anxiety. Oxford: Oxford University Press, 1976.
5. Mathew RJ, Weinman ML, Mirabi M. Physical symptoms of depression. Br J Psychiatry 1981; 139:293–6.
6. Beck AT. Cognitive therapy. A 30-year retrospective. Am Psychol 1991; 46:368–75.
7. Sensky T. Cognitive therapy with patients with chronic physical illness. Psychother Psychosom 1989; 52:26–32.
8. Sharpe MC, Peveler R, Mayou R. The psychological treatment of patients with functional somatic symptoms: a practical guide. J Psychosom Res 1992; 36:515–29.
9. Kroenke K, Arrington ME, Manglesdorff D. The prevalence of symptoms in medical outpatients and the adequacy of therapy. Arch Intern Med 1990; 150:1685–9.
10. Valdini AF, Steinhardt S, Feldman E. Usefulness of a standard battery of laboratory tests in investigating chronic fatigue in adults. Fam Pract 1989; 6:286–91.
11. Sharpe MC, Archard LC, Banatvala JE, et al. A report—chronic fatigue syndrome: guidelines for research. J R Soc Med 1991; 84:118–21.
12. Schluederberg A, Straus SE, Peterson PK, et al. Chronic fatigue syndrome research: definition and medical outcome. Ann Intern Med 1992; 117:325–31.
13. Sharpe MC, Hawton KE, Seagraott V, Pasvol G. Patients who present with fatigue: a follow up of referrals to an infectious diseases clinic. Br Med J 1992; 305:147–52.
14. Schwartz MN. The chronic fatigue syndrome—one entity or many? N Engl J Med 1988; 319:1726–8.
15. Lloyd AR, Wakefield D, Boughton CR, Dwyer J. What is myalgic encephalomyelitis? Lancet 1988; 1:1286–7.
16. Holmes GP, Kaplan JE, Gantz NM, et al. Chronic fatigue syndrome: a working case definition. Ann Intern Med 1988; 108:387–9.
17. Behan PO, Behan MH. Postviral fatigue syndrome. Crit Rev Neurobiol 1988; 4:157–79.
18. Dowsett EG, Ramsay AM, McCartney RA, Bell EJ. Myalgic encephalomyelitis—a persistent enteroviral infection? Postgrad Med J 1990; 66:526–30.

19. Sharpe MC, Fatigue and chronic fatigue syndrome. Curr Opin Psychiatry 1992; 5:207–12.

20. Straus SE. Defining the chronic fatigue syndrome [editorial; comment]. Arch Intern Med 1992; 152:1569–70.

21. Blakely AA, Howard RC, Sosich RM, Murdoch JC, Menkes DB, Spears GF. Psychiatric symptoms, personality and ways of coping in chronic fatigue syndrome. Psychol Med 1991; 21:347–62.

22. Goldenberg DL, Simms RW, Geiger A, Komaroff AL. High frequency of fibromyalgia in patients with chronic fatigue seen in a primary care practice. Arthritis Rheum 1990; 33:381–7.

23. Wessely S, Powell R. Fatigue syndromes: a comparison of chronic "postviral" fatigue with neuromuscular and affective disorder. J Neurol Neurosurg Psychiatry 1989; 52:940–8.

24. Greenberg D. Neurasthenia in the 1980s: chronic mononucleosis, chronic fatigue syndrome, and anxiety and depressive disorders. Psychosomatics 1990; 31:129–37.

25. Wessely S. Old wine in new bottles: neurasthenia and "ME." Psychol Med 1990; 20:35–53.

26. Wood P. Da Costa's syndrome (or effort syndrome). Br Med J 1941; 1:767–72.

27. Straus SE, Dale JK, Tobi M, et al. Acyclovir treatment of the chronic fatigue syndrome; lack of efficacy in a placebo controlled trial. N Engl J Med 1988; 319:1692–8.

28. Straus SE. Intravenous immunoglobulin treatment for the chronic fatigue syndrome. Am J Med 1991; 89:551–2.

29. Riley MS, O'Brien CJ, McClusky DR, Bell NP, Nicholls DP. Aerobic work capacity in patients with chronic fatigue syndrome. Br Med J 1990; 301:953–6.

30. Sharpe MC, Bass C. Pathophysiological mechanisms in somatization. Int Rev Psychiatry 1992; 4:81–97.

31. Salit B, Blomqvist G, Mitchell JH. Response to exercise after bedrest and after training. Circulation 1986; 38:

32. Edwards RHT. Muscle fatigue and pain. Acta Med Scand 1986; 711(supp):179–88.

33. Vignos PJ. Physical models of rehabilitation in neuromuscular disease. Muscle Nerve 1983; 5:323–38.

34. McCain GA, Bell DA, Mai FM, Holliday PD. A controlled study of the effects of a supervised cardiovascular fitness training programme on the manifestations of primary fibromyalgia. Arthritis Rheum 1988; 31:1135–41.

35. Sexton H, Maere A, Dahl NH. Exercise intensity and reduction in neurotic symptoms. Acta Psychiatr Scand 1989; 80:231–5.

36. Manu P, Dale A, Matthews MD, Lane TJ. The mental health of patients with a chief complaint of chronic fatigue; a prospective evaluation and follow-up. Arch Intern Med 1988; 148:2213–7.

37. Wood GC, Bentall RP, Gopfert M, Edwards RHT. A comparative psychiatric assessment of patients with chronic fatigue syndrome and muscle disease. Psychol Med 1991; 21:619–28.

38. Beck AT, Rush AJ, Shaw BF, Emery G. Cognitive therapy of depression. New York: Guilford Press, 1979.

39. Clark DM. A cognitive approach to panic. Behav Res Ther 1986; 24:461–70.

40. Morriss R, Sharpe MC, Sharpley A, Morris J, Cowen P, Hawton KE. Chronic fatigue syndrome: a disorder of sleep? Br Med J 1993; 306:1161–4.

41. Horne JA, Dimensions to sleepiness. In: Monk TH, ed. Sleep, sleepiness and performance. London: John Wiley & Sons, 1991:169–95.

42. Sloan EP, Hauri P, Bootzin R, Morin C, Stevenson M, Shapiro C. The nuts and bolts of behavioural therapy for insomnia. J Psychosom Res 1993; 37(suppl 1):19–37.

43. Hawton KE, Kirk J. Problem-solving. In: Hawton K, Salkovskis PM, Kirk J, Clark DM, eds. Cognitive behaviour therapy for psychiatric problems. Oxford: Oxford Medical Publications, 1989:406–27.

44. Wessely S, David AS, Butler S, Chalder T. Management of chronic (post-viral) fatigue syndrome. J R Coll Gen Pract 1989; 39:26–9.

45. Sharpe MC. Psychiatric management of PVFS. Br Med Bull 1991; 47:989–1006.

46. Sharpe MC, Non-pharmacological approaches to treatment. In: Chronic fatigue syndrome. Ciba Found Symp 1993; 173:298–317.

47. Hurry JB. The vicious circles of neurasthenia and their treatment. London: Churchill, 1915.

48. Wood P. Aetiology of Da Costa's syndrome. Br Med J 1941; 1:845–50.

49. Philips HC. The psychological management of chronic pain: a manual. New York: Springer-Verlag, 1988.

50. Nielson WR, Walker C, McCain G. Cognitive behavioural treatment of fibromyalgia syndrome: preliminary findings. J Rheumatol 1992; 19:98–103.

51. Ware NC. Suffering and the social construction of illness: the delegitimation of illness experience in chronic fatigue syndrome. Med Anthropol Q 1992; 6:347–61.

52. Abbey SE. Somatization, illness attribution and the sociocultural psychiatry of chronic fatigue syndrome. In: Chronic fatigue syndrome. Ciba Found Symp 1993; 173:238–61.

53. Pennebaker JW. The psychology of physical symptoms. New York: Springer-Verlag, 1982.

54. Salkovskis PM, Clark DM. Affective responses to hyperventilation: a test of the cognitive model of panic. Behav Res Ther 1990; 28:51–61.

55. Komaroff AL. Chronic fatigue syndromes: relationship to chronic viral infections. J Virol Methods 1988; 21:3–10.

56. Ware NC, Kleinman A. Culture and somatic experience: the social course of illness in neurasthenia and chronic fatigue syndrome. Psychosom Med 1992; 54:546–60.

57. Butler S, Chalder T, Ron M, Wessely S. Cognitive behaviour therapy in chronic fatigue syndrome. J Neurol Neurosurg Psychiatry 1991; 54:153–8.

58. Lloyd AR, Hickie I, Brockman A, et al. Immunologic and psychologic therapy for patients with chronic fatigue syndrome: a double blind placebo controlled trial. Am J Med 1993; 94:197–203.

59. Persons JB. Cognitive therapy in practice: a case formulation approach. New York: WW Norton & Co, 1989.

60. Lane TJ, Matthews DA, Manu P. The low yield of physical examinations and laboratory investigations of patients with chronic fatigue. Am J Med Sci 1990; 299:313–8.

Index

About the Editor

Stephen E. Straus is Chief of the Laboratory of Clinical Investigation and Senior Investigator and Head, Medical Virology Section, Laboratory of Clinical Investigation, National Institute of Allergy and Infectious Diseases, National Institutes of Health, Bethesda, Maryland. The author or coauthor of over 300 professional papers and abstracts that reflect his research interests in molecular biology, pathophysiology, and the treatment and prevention of herpesvirus infections, he is a Fellow of the Infectious Diseases Society of America and a member of the Association of American Physicians, the American Society for Microbiology, the American Federation for Clinical Research, and the American Society for Clinical Investigation. Dr. Straus received the B.S. degree (1968) in life sciences from the Massachusetts Institute of Technology, Cambridge, and the M.D. degree (1972) from the Columbia University College of Physicians and Surgeons, New York, New York.

DATE DUE

NOV 2 0 2007			
DEC 2 8 2007			

DEMCO 38-296